LIVER TUMORS

Edited by **Alexander Julianov**

Liver Tumors
Edited by Alexander Julianov

Published by InTech

Janeza Trdine 9, 51000 Rijeka, Croatia

Publishing Process Manager Anja Filipovic

Technical Editor Teodora Smiljanic

Cover Designer InTech Design Team

Additional hard copies can be obtained from orders@intechopen.com

Liver Tumors, Edited by Alexander Julianov
p. cm.
ISBN 978-953-51-0036-2

For EU product safety concerns:
IN TECH d.o.o., Prolaz Marije Krucifikse Kozulić 3, 51000 Rijeka, Croatia,
info@intechopen.com or visit our website at intechopen.com.

Meet the editor

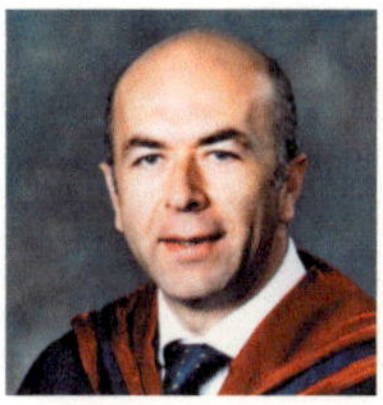

Dr Alexander Julianov, MD, PhD, FACS is a well-recognized expert in HPB-surgery and abdominal surgical oncology. Board certified in Surgery and Oncology, he is the author of more than 120 scientific publications, including pioneer works in the fields of treatment of liver tumors and laparoscopic surgery. Dr Julianov also serves as the Editor and Reviewer in various journals, and has been rewarded with local and international honors (American College of Surgeons International Guest Award, ISS/SIC Foundation Grant, Korea University Medical Center Appreciation Plaque etc.). He is the Clinical Director and Chief of Department of Surgery at Thracian University Hospital, Stara Zagora, Bulgaria.

Contents

Preface

"It is a most gratifying sign of the rapid progress of our time that our best textbooks become antiquated so quickly."

Theodor Billroth (1829-1894)

In the last few years the knowledge about liver tumors has progressed rapidly involving many fields of science such as molecular biology and genetics, pharmacology, imaging techniques, invasive radiology and surgery, etc. That is why the above Billroth's sentence is becoming more actual than ever.

The overriding goal in development of this book has been the mobilization of information related to the very selected key topics in the biology, diagnosis and management of liver tumors. Experts from clinics and laboratories from around the world, including Europe, North America and Asia shared their knowledge and experience gained in the understanding and management of primary and metastatic liver cancer. Conflicting opinions in some chapters will be noted, but they allow the reader to assess the points of view of experts with different approaches to a particular problem.

This book is oriented towards clinicians and scientists in the field of the management of patients with liver tumors. As many unresolved problems regarding primary and metastatic liver cancer still await investigation, I hope this book can serve as a tiny step on a long way that we need to run on the battlefield of liver tumors.

Alexander Julianov, MD, PhD, FACS
Clinical Director and Chief, Department of Surgery
Thracian University Hospital
Associate Professor of Surgery
Thracian University
Stara Zagora, Bulgaria

1

Molecular Genetics and Genomics of Hepatocellular Carcinoma

Dilek Colak[1] and Namik Kaya[2]
[1]*Department of Biostatistics, Epidemiology and Scientific Computing, King Faisal Specialist Hospital and Research Centre, Riyadh,*
[2]*Department of Genetics, King Faisal Specialist Hospital and Research Centre, Riyadh, Saudi Arabia*

1. Introduction

Hepatocellular carcinoma (HCC) is a major type of liver cancer and third leading cause of cancer-related deaths worldwide. It is often diagnosed at an advanced stage, and hence typically has a poor prognosis. The advances in high-throughput "omics" technologies (genomics, transcriptomics, proteomics) parallel to the availability of high-density microarrays and next-generation sequencing technologies feature important advances in understanding of the complex biological processes underlying tumorigenesis and metastasis of HCC, and uncovering promising biomarkers with clinical potential. Ultimately, the trend will be toward a personalized medicine that will improve diagnosis, treatment and prevention of primary liver cancer. In this chapter, we present an overview of most up-to-date developments regarding these approaches toward an understanding of molecular mechanisms of HCC and for the development of novel biomarkers and cancer therapeutics targets.

2. Background

Hepatocellular carcinoma (HCC) is the most common primary cancer originating in the liver, the fifth most common cancer type, and is the third leading cause of cancer mortality worldwide [1-2]. It is often diagnosed at an advanced stage, leading to poor prognosis. Recent reports show that HCC is becoming more widespread and has dramatically increased in North America, Western Europe and Japan [2-4]. Early detection of HCC, especially detection of early/small HCC, followed by the appropriate treatment would significantly alter the prognosis and reduce the number of tumor-related deaths. Though inspiring progress has been made in understanding the molecular mechanisms of HCC, there is still lack of complete understanding of the disease perhaps due to complexities associated with the HCC such as intricacy of liver transcriptome, viral infection, liver regeneration, and other confounding factors, that have been major limitations for developing useful biomarkers for the detection and early diagnosis as well as identification of novel therapeutic targets for HCC.

The advances in high-throughput "omics" technologies such as genomics, transcriptomics, proteomics, and metabolomics combined with the availability of high-density microarrays and low-cost high-throughput parallel sequencing technologies and their analyses using different bioinformatics tools and algorithms are providing unprecedented biological insights related to HCC. Global molecular profiling studies of HCC are providing a comprehensive view of genomic aberrations and expression changes that occur during the carcinogenic process. Hence, the knowledge gained from continuing research efforts on HCC undoubtedly facilitates the understanding of molecular mechanism of HCC pathogenesis, and to provide the best therapy for each cancer patient and to improve patient management. This approach will create a foundation for personalized therapeutics and treatments and expectantly will be available in the near future alongside the unprecedented advancement of next-generation sequencing technologies. These technologies already began to identify novel genes that may have a driver force for HCC pathobiology [5]. Identification of such driver genes within each tumor will highly likely be a source for the development of novel therapeutic targets for the malignancies for each HCC-affected individual.

Our aim in this chapter is to focus on the current advances in the genomics field of HCC as well as recent progress using next-generation deep sequencing technologies, and the current shift towards integrative approaches using data from these advanced technologies that will help better understanding of HCC and for the development of novel biomarkers and cancer therapeutics targets.

3. Genomic alterations in liver cancer

Current advances in microarray technologies has resulted in high-dimensional genomic data sets and profoundly improved our understanding of genomic imbalances in the context of its role in carcinogenesis; first, with the introduction of copy number variation (CNV) concept in addition to single nucleotide polymorphisms (SNP), and second, with the improved mapping of such CNVs throughout the whole genome of patients versus normal individuals. While very early observations have identified CNVs as "chromosomal polymorphisms" that are several megabases in size, the lower end of the size range of CNVs continues to drop that is consistent with the pace of technological advancement [6]. With their inclusion of coding genes, it is hardly surprising that CNVs play a role in human health and disease, although their role is only recently being recognized, first in the context of Mendelian disorders and more recently in complex diseases [7-8]. The presence of these polymorphisms, either at small (SNPs or mutations) or large (CNVs and CNAs) scale as well as regions comprising loss of heterozygosity (LOH) blocks are, therefore, likely to contribute to cancer formation [9-11]. The genomic modifications in a tumor represents a structural fingerprint that may include the transcriptional control mechanisms and locally impact gene expression levels [10, 12].

Initial array platforms utilizing either spotted clones inserted in bacterial artificial chromosomes (BACs) or in situ synthesized oligos on chip surfaces have been applied to HCC samples to better understand the role of genomic aberrations at the DNA level. These microarray-based assays are called array comparative genomic hybridization (aCGH) technique since they are a modified version of the comparative genomic hybridization (CGH) approach applied to microarrays. Numerous studies have investigated chromosomal alterations associated with HCC using both CGH and aCGH techniques (as reviewed by Moinzadeh *et al.* [9]). Moreover, two leading microarray companies have developed similar assays containing only SNP probes. This approach was initiated by Affymetrix Inc. then later applied by Illumina Inc. Both companies have come up with different SNP assays comprising different numbers of unique SNP probe sets. While the aCGH approach provides much higher resolution over standard microscope-based banding techniques in terms of cytogenetics analysis, SNP arrays bring two main advantages over the other techniques including aCGH: LOH and uniparental disomy detection, and more diverse applications, such as utilization in association studies based on both SNP as well as CNV calls.

Later, higher density arrays having hundreds of thousands or even currently more than a million unique probe sets targeting CNVs and SNPs have been employed in HCC research and identified critical regions of the genome likely to be involved in molecular carcinogenesis of HCC. Such critical regions commonly exhibit either deletion or increased gene dosage, leading to changes in DNA copy number variations/polymorphisms (CNVs/CNPs), aberrations/abnormalities (CNAs) or contain LOH blocks in various cancers, including HCC [9, 13-15].

It is plausible that such HCC-specific CNVs and LOH blocks spanning from several kilobases to megabases comprise critical driver genes that may play a leading role in hepatocarcinogenesis and contain the genetic factors involved in HCC [14, 16-17]. In one of those early studies, Luo *et al.* utilized an integrated approach of DNA and RNA level analyses for HCC, and investigated overlapping genome-wide transcriptomic and genomic alterations among hepatocellular carcinomas (HCC), hepatoblastomas (HPBL), tissue adjacent to HCC and normal liver tissue derived from normal livers and hepatic resections [14]. In their study, genomic imbalances between 27 HCC samples and matching normal controls were determined using low density oligonucleotide arrays. The results indicated that several regions on chromosome 7, 8, 10 and 12 harbor numerous genomic aberrations. Further investigations revealed that many of these changes do not cause remarkable gene expression alterations. However, among other genes, two genes, GPC3 and TIEG, were found to have significant correlation between their copy numbers and expression changes. Further investigations of these two genes in a larger cohort (484 hepatic tissue and normal samples) confirmed the expression differences in HCC samples. Additional studies investigating the role of GPC3 expression in poorer clinical outcome revealed this gene may have a possible role on HCC aggressiveness and therefore may predict the HCC outcome [14].

In a more recent study, Chen *et al.* employed Affymetrix's 500K SNP arrays with an average of 6 kb distance between its unique SNP probes to examine 13 different HCC cell lines in addition to some other cancer cell lines as well as 45 archived primary HCCs [18]. Numerous common and novel aberrations were observed in multiple cancer lines confirming previously known HCC-related cytogenetic regions detected by low-resolution methods and refining their breakpoints and boundaries, and also introducing previously unknown critical genomic regions associated with HCC. Among 653 amplicons and 57 homozygous deletions (HDs) detected by the arrays using different cell lines, 126 amplicons and 6 HDs were selected and tested to identify novel HCC-related genes. Further analysis of such aberrant regions yielded two genes, FNDC3BB and SLC29A2, consistently up-regulated in multiple HCC data sets. Knock-down studies using short hairpin RNAs targeting both genes showed decreased cell proliferation, tumor formation, and anchorage-independent growth in xenograft models in nude mice confirmed a possible pivotal role of these genes in growth and tumor formation in subsets of HCC samples. Up-regulation of either gene is proposed to be activated through STAT3 signaling pathway which is a well-known phenomenon in HCC progression usually triggered by cytokines such as interleukin-6 [19-22].

In another study, Clifford *et al.* used Affymetrix SNP 6.0 assay comprising probes for detection of CNVs and SNPs, each has more than 900,000 unique oligos, totaling nearly 1.9 million probe sets [23]. In their study, a large number of samples exceeding 1100 cases including histopathologically confirmed HCC and liver cirrhosis (LC) samples as well as normal controls with Korean and Chinese ethnicity were analyzed in two stages; each having different subsets of patients and controls. Based on their analysis, two SNPs were found to diverge significantly between HCC versus LC group and therefore considered a likely factor influencing transitional events from cirrhosis to hepatocellular carcinogenesis. Interestingly, the first SNP, rs2551677, is not within close proximity of any known gene, the closest gene DDX18 being 175 kb upstream of the SNP. The second SNP, rs2880301, is positioned on intron 1 of TPTE2 encoding a homolog of PTEN tumor suppressor gene and is the first time reported to be associated with carcinogenesis [23]. Additionally, three SNPs (rs9267673, rs2647073, and rs3997872) were found to be strongly associated with HCC only and were not presenting any additive/multiplicative effect. The first SNP, rs9267673, is in close proximity of C2 gene unlike the other two SNPs, rs2647073 and rs3997872, associated with SNPs falling into linkage disequilibrium of two different HLA group genes: The rs2647073 with HLA-DRB1, HLA-DRB6, HLA-DRB5, and HLA-DRA whereas the rs3997872 with HLA-DQA1, HLA-DQB1, HLA-DQA2, and HLA-DQB2 loci. The associations were independently confirmed using TAGMAN assays indicating the validity of the SNP study. When they analyzed probes targeting copy number polymorphisms, eight CNV loci including six germline CNVs were identified to be significantly associated with liver carcinogenesis. One of the germline CNVs showing a high level of association with HCC is located on a small region on p arm of chromosome 1 where no gene is known. Five other CNVs found to be linked to HCC involving *KNG1, C4orf29, LARP2, ALDH7A1, PHAX, C5orf48, LMNB1, SRPK2, PUS7,* and *TMPO* genes. Among these CNVs, two involving TRG@ and TRA@ had the strongest association to HCC. Moreover, a functional pathway and network analyses carried out using 1000 most significant SNPs associated with HCC. Among the critical pathways "antigen processing and presentation" is found the most significantly overrepresented pathway with *p*-value of $1x10^{-11}$ indicating the strongest association to HCC. Overall, these observations indicate involvement of immune system in constitutional susceptibility to HCC and HCC carcinogenesis which was suggested by clinical observations and animals models previously.

In a recent study, Jia *et al.* searched for critical somatic CNVs in 58 HCC tumor samples with adjacent non-tumor samples using Affymetrix 6.0 assay and identified 1241 regions [24].

These regions were then interrogated in search of dysregulated genes and 362 differentially expressed genes were identified. Among these, 20 genes were further evaluated functionally and *TRIM35, HEY1,* and *SNRPE* were confirmed to be involved in HCC by various functional experiments. Involvement of these genes, *TRIM35* as tumor suppressor, and *HEY1* and *SNRPE* as potential oncogenes, in HCC is novel.

4. Global gene expression profiling of liver cancer

During the past two decades, discoveries on the global gene expression profiling technologies emerged one after the other. Subtractive hybridization, differential display, SAGE, microarrays and more recently next generation sequencing techniques appeared as cutting-edge tools to study genome-wide transcriptional profiling differences in nearly all different types of tissues. With the rapid advances in these technologies, the medicine, particularly cancer genomics, is evolving into numerous dimensions.

The microarrays had a great impact from the way we look at the transcriptome and the way we understand the biology and complexity of it. Microarray expression technologies have allowed the simultaneous analysis of thousands of transcripts that cover nearly the entire genome [25]. Hence, gene expression microarrays, that are providing a comprehensive view of the transcriptional changes that occur during the carcinogenic process, have been applied with great success to the molecular profiling of HCC which has resulted in a much more detailed molecular classification scheme as well as in the identification of potential gene signature sets, molecular biomarkers, prediction of early recurrence and patient survival [26-29].

Over the last decade, numerous studies have applied this technology, and identified a number of candidate genes useful as biomarkers in cancer staging, prediction of recurrence and prognosis, and treatment selection. Considering the complexity of the HCC carcinogenesis many genes may be involved in the initiation and progression of the cancer, and therefore a comprehensive expression analysis using microarray technology has great potential to discover new genes involved in carcinogenesis, as well as may highlight the functional modules and pathways altered in HCC. Indeed, some of the new target molecules that were identified using this technology have been used to develop new serum diagnostic markers and therapeutic targets against HCC to benefit patients.

The first report of cDNA microarray analysis of hepatocellular carcinoma (HCC) by Lau *et al.* [30] studied the gene expression using about 4000 known human genes in 10 pairs of HCC and non-tumorous tissues. Since then numerous studies have been published to date in the context of genome-wide expression profiling of HCC liver. The microarray analyses of HCC highlighted activation of important pathways in liver carcinogenesis, such as wingless-type (WNT), p53, transforming growth factor (TGF)-β, MAPK signalling pathways [31-34] as well as novel genes with altered expression, such as *MARKL1, VANGL1, PEG10, BMAL2, HLA-DR, GPC3,* and *ROBO1.*

Over the past 10 years, the microarray-based gene expression profiling has been used to identify gene signatures associated with etiological factors, histological phenotypes, and clinical phenotypes, as well as unveiling novel subtypes of HCC previously unrecognized by conventional methods [26, 35-36] . Most cases of HCC originate from chronic liver disease caused by hepatitis viral infection, including hepatitis B virus (HBV) and hepatitis C virus (HCV), exposure to aflatoxin B1 in mold, and alcohol abuse. In this context, gene signatures associated with different etiologies have also been reported [37-39]. Microarray studies indicated that HBV and HCV viral infections lead to the development of liver cancer by different molecular mechanisms [32, 38-39]. Okabe *et al.* analyzed expression profiles of 20 primary HCCs by using cDNA microarrays consisting of 23,040 genes, and compared HBV- with HCV-related HCC [32]. The authors identified a gene signature that is correlated with the infection status, and found that genes that are involved in drug metabolism and carcinogen detoxification were differentially regulated between HCV-based and HBV-based HCC. In another study, Iizuka *et al.* [38] performed genome-wide expression profiling 45 HCC (14 HBV- and 31-HCV-associated) and identified 83 genes whose expression significantly differed between the two types of HCCs. The HBV-associated HCC showed significantly up-regulation of imprinted genes (H19 and IGF2) and genes related to signal transduction, transcription, and metastasis. On the other hand, HCV-associated HCC displayed up-regulation of genes related to detoxification and immune response. Delpuech *et al.* showed that HBV-associated HCC altered different cellular pathways, those controlling apoptosis, p53 signalling and G1/S transition, whereas the HCV-related HCC resulted in an over-expression of the TGF-beta induced gene [31].

Microarray gene expression profiling together with prediction models have been used in numerous studies to identify gene signatures in tumor or surrounding non-tumorus tissues that can predict vascular invasion, metastasis, post-surgical recurrence, survival, and response to therapy. These signatures may aid in identifying patients most likely to benefit from surgery and chemotherapeutic treatment.

Vascular invasion (VI) is an unfavorable prognostic factor for early HCC recurrence. There have been several microarray studies which identified gene signatures that correlated with VI. Ho *et al.* [40] identified 14 genes correlated with VI, which can classify patients with high or low risk of VI development and recurrence after curative hepatectomy. In another study, Budhu *et al.* reported a 17-gene signature expressed in noncancerous hepatic tissues with venous metastasis, capable of predicting recurrence after surgical hepatectomy, with 79% accuracy [41]. Similarly, Wang *et al.* identified a 57-gene signature to predict disease recurrence at diagnosis (84% sensitivity) [42].

Using supervised machine learning methods on the gene expression data, Nam *et al.* identified 240 genes that classified samples into different histological grades, from low-grade DNs to primary HCC [43]. Kim *et al.* reported 44 genes that can discriminate HBV-positive HCC from non-tumor liver tissues [44]. Iizuka *et al.* [26] reported a gene signature of 12 genes that can predict HCC patients at high risk of early intra-hepatic recurrence (IHR) after curative surgery (93% sensitivity). Similarly, Kurokawa *et al.* [45] identified a 20-gene signature which could predict early IHR after curative resection. In another study, a 3-gene signature (HLA-DRA, DDX17, and LAPTM5) found to be predictor of recurrence after curative hepatectomy, which predicted early IHR with 81% accuracy in the validation group [46].

Researchers also used microarrays to identify gene signatures as predictors of survival after surgical resection. Lee *et al.* analyzed the gene expression profile of 91 HCC samples using unsupervised classification approach which divided the patients into two subclasses with significant differences in survival [29]. The authors also identified genes that accurately predicted the length of survival. Functional analyses indicated that genes related to cell proliferation, anti-apoptosis, and cell cycle regulators were found to be predictor of poor prognosis. Other microarray studies reported c-Met- and TGF-beta regulated genes that are highly associated with the length of survival [47-48].

HCC is a challenging malignancy; most cases of HCC are diagnosed in an advanced stage, and, therefore, treatment options are limited. Hence, it is important to diagnose it at early stage. DNA microarray studies attempted to identify markers for early HCC [27, 49]. Recently considerable attention has been placed on global gene expression studies as well as genomic aberrations in order to understand the pathogenesis of HCC, and to look for possible early markers of detection [14, 16-17, 28, 34, 49-51]. Furthermore, combining cross-species comparative and/or functional genomics approaches from human and animal models of HCC along with genomic DNA copy number alterations enhances the ability to identify robust predictive markers for HCC [13, 36, 52-54]. Thus, characterization of diverse HCC subgroups using the array technologies together with improved analytical approaches are crucial for better management of the disease, especially in the era of personalized medicine approach in HCC treatment.

5. Global miRNA expression profiling of HCC

One of the most important findings of the analysis on the human genome is identification of a significant number of sequences encoding non-coding RNA molecules such as small nucleolar RNAs and microRNAs also known as miRNAs [55-56]. MicroRNAs, single-stranded RNAs typically 21-23 nucleotide long, are untranslated molecules that have capability to bind complementary sequences resulting in their silence, therefore, regulating the expression of their target genes. Some of these molecules have currently been intensely studied and their biogenesis, structure and function are now known and some other small regulatory RNAs are yet to be discovered. Among these different RNAs species, miRNAs holds special attention due to its properties and potential use as therapeutic targets for cancer. Currently around 6000 miRNAs from multiple species have been annotated in different databases. These miRNAs target and regulate around 30% of all protein coding genes in mammals. It has been shown that the miRNAs regulate processes essential to differentiation, apoptosis, cell growth, adhesion, and cell death [57-58]. Recently, due to its oncogenic and tumor suppression activities, these molecules exploited for various cancers, including HCC [59-63].

The genomic instability, transcriptional regulation, and epigenetic alteration have been identified to contribute to the abnormal expression of miRNAs in HCC. Furthermore, the aberrant expression of certain miRNAs is correlated with clinical features of HCC, indicating their potential to serve as diagnostic and prognostic biomarkers of HCC [64-65]. Some aberrantly expressed miRNAs may have a direct role in liver tumorigenesis, and could promote differentiation, cell cycle progression, angiogenesis and invasion, such as mir-221 and mir-21 [59]. Murakami *et al.* identified eight miRNAs with altered expression in HCC, which discriminated HCC samples from non-tumor with 97.8% accuracy [66]. Similarly, Huang *et al.* identified 24 abberrantly expressed miRNAs [67]. Toffanin *et al.* studied miRNA profiling of HCC samples that was previously profiled for mRNA and copy number (CN) changes [65]. The authors identified three subclasses of HCC based on miRNA profiles. The other studies identified miRNA signatures that predicted metastasis potential, recurrence and survival [64, 68-69]. Since the miRNAs are stable in blood, more recently, the circulating miRNAs have been reported as diagnostic markers for various cancers, including the HCC [70-72].Therefore, identification of miRNAs and their protein-coding target genes is important to understand the mechanisms of hepatocarcinogenesis, and reveals new biomarkers for diagnosis, prognosis and therapeutic targets.

6. Deep sequencing of HCC using next-generation sequencing technologies

Current advances in genomics technologies have been first seen as revolution of microarrays and then recently appeared as high-throughput parallel sequencing techniques. The resolute advance of fluorescence-based standard Sanger technique seemingly stretched to its limits for technical enhancements. At the same time soaring demand for low-cost and high-output sequencing has driven the development of superior technologies that allow massively parallel sequencing processes, producing millions and billions of sequences at once [73-74]. Therefore, it was inevitable to see the replacement of standard sequencing methods to newly emerging advanced sequencing technologies called next generation sequencing technologies. These technologies initially appeared as relatively high-cost difficult techniques for practical use and believed to be useful for only whole genome sequencing of different species. But soon these perceptions were evaded radically. Today, the state of DNA sequencing technologies is in a greater flux than ever before. With this foreseeable evolution, comes new possibilities not only in the field of large-scale genomic sciences from medicine to agriculture and plant sciences coupled with new challenges in data storage and analysis, but also for practical use such as clinical utilization for routine diagnostics[74-78]. Currently, several methods are already established, made significant impact on the field of genomics by having reputable track record for many different published applications and some are in the process of building confidence, some are yet to be tested and perfected[78-84].

The first study of HCC using the next-generation sequencing technology for deep sequencing appeared most recently [5]. Using Illumina's Genome Analyzer IIx system, also called GAIIx, Totoki *et al.* sequenced genomic libraries from a normal Japanese male and hepatitis C-positive HCC sample. Both samples' sequence reads had an almost complete match to a human reference sequence covering 99.79% and 99.69% for lymphocyte (normal male) and HCC sample genomes, respectively. Nearly ~3 million nucleotide variations were recorded from each genome, yielding 84,555 bases more variations in lymphocyte genome perhaps due to presence of chromosomal alterations in tumor genome and 11,731 of these changes in HCC were somatically acquired. There were several interesting results related to nucleotide changes in the study. First, it was found that occurrence of somatic substitutions was varied between genic and intergenic regions, significantly lower in the genic regions (consisting of coding and noncoding exons, and introns) in comparison to its counterpart intergenic regions. This was explained either by negative selection of lethal mutations in the genic regions or by the existence of specific molecules responsible for the repair of transcribed region. Second, presence of germline variations was significantly lesser in the coding regions relative to the non-coding regions. Third, the ratio of nonsynonymous to synonymous variations (N/NS) either somatic or germline origins differed in HCC and was significantly lower than that of somatically originated substitutions. To explain this, authors highlighted the influence of positive selections happening in exons causing survival of tumor cells or favored negative selection of somatic variations over germline substitutions on the coding exons. Fourth, the preferred somatic substitutions included T>C/A>G and C>T/G>A transitions. Fifth, in addition to 81 confirmed somatic substitutions common to both genomes (all in protein coding regions), 670 small deletions and insertions were identified and seven of which were validated. Among these variations, some of the changes seemed more critical since they were located on the previously annotated tumor suppressor genes for HCC and other cancer types. Moreover, authors decided to resequence exons potentially harboring malignant changes in 96 HCC and control samples as well as 21 HCC cell lines. These efforts yielded two critical somatic mutations p.Phe190Leu and p.Gln212X in *LRRC30.*

Besides the nucleotide changes, small deletions and insertions, 22 verified chromosomal rearrangements were identified. These rearrangements were mostly intra-chromosomal and in close proximity with some known copy number regions. These chromosomal rearrangements led four different fusion transcripts that involve transcriptional regulation of BCORL1-ELF4 [5]. Then using the deep whole exome sequencing approach (76X or more coverage) a nonsense mutation in TSC1 gene was also identified in a subset of tumor cells.

As demonstrated in this study, further next-generation sequencing studies have the potential to reveal novel genes/mutations and likely critical pathways that can be utilized for the biomarker discovery and identification of novel therapeutic targets for HCC. Besides, the next-generation technologies have already been proven to be useful for genomic studies on some cancers [85-94]. Moreover, once affordable prices are reached, such next generation sequencing techniques will create an amazing opportunity to look for genome-wide DNA and/or RNA level differences and methylation patterns in many cancer types at an affordable cost and will open doors for daily diagnostics and personalized medicine [86] [95-96].

7. Animal models and comparative genomics of HCC

Developing animal models of HCC provide an experimental ground for dissecting the genetic and biological complexities of human cancer and contribute to our ability to identify and characterize pathogenic modifications relevant to various stages of cancer development and progression. [97-98]. Several models of constitutive, conditional and inducible models of HCC were developed inducing genetic manipulations and investigating the genetic changes. The results usually are comparable to that found in humans [99]. Each model appears to have its own advantages and disadvantages [100]. Recent studies, including our own, demonstrated the usefulness of modeling human cancer in diethylnitrosamine (DEN)-induced in rats [54] as well as in genetically engineered mice [97, 101].

The recent studies have used cross-species comparative genomics approach, that identifies genes that are conserved in animal models of cancer and in human cancer, that would facilitate the identification of critical regulatory modules conserved across species in the expression profiles and to understand the molecular pathogenesis of various cancers, including HCC [36, 54, 101-103]. The cross-species comparative analysis of animal models and human HCCs would provide new therapeutic strategies to maximize the efficiency of treatments.

8. Integrative and comparative analyses of HCC for identification of novel therapeutic targets and biomarker discovery

It has been shown that CNAs have clear impact on expression levels in a variety of tumors [9, 13, 15]. The presence of such CNAs and LOH may contribute to cancer formation [9-11]. Integrating the gene expression with the CNA data reveals the chromosomal regions with concordantly altered genomic and transcriptional status in tumors [12, 52, 104]. The pattern of genomic modifications in a tumor represents a structural fingerprint that may include the transcriptional control mechanisms and locally impact gene expression levels [10, 12]. Therefore, focusing on differentially-expressed genes with concomitant altered DNA copy number may identify novel early HCC markers of malignant transformation, progression and survival [17].

The studies using integrative analysis of genomic aberrations with the expression profiling demonstrated the usefulness of this approach to identify the likely drivers of cancer [105] and helped better understand the processes affected by the drivers/passenger factors and led to obtain novel insights into pathobiology of HCC [17, 54, 105].

In this context, we performed cross-species and integrative genomic analysis to identify potential biomarker genes for early HCC [54]. In this study, we first developed a rat model of early HCC as well as liver regeneration post-hepatectomy and compared them to normal liver using a microarray approach. We then performed a cross-species comparative analysis coupled with CNAs of early human HCCs to identify the critical regulatory modules conserved across species. We identified 35 gene signature conserved across species, with more than 50% mapping to human CNA regions associated with HCC [54]. Combining cross-species comparative and/or functional genomics approaches from human and animal models of HCC along with genomic DNA copy number alterations enhances the ability to identify robust predictive markers for HCC [13, 36, 52-54].

9. Future directions

Elucidating the molecular pathogenesis of HCC on human samples has been an onerous task due to certain limitations such as varying etiologies among studied patients, changes likely to arise during the different stages of the disease or progression of HCC, and heterogeneity of the disease. Moreover, the success of studies is hampered by the fact that hepatic transcriptome is among the most complex of any organ, and the study of tumor formation in liver can be thorny and complicated by the continuous change of the transcriptome during liver regeneration after hepatectomy. Besides, cancer progresses through a series of histopathological stages during which genetic alterations accumulate and, in consequence, the pattern of genetic expression changes complicates the interpretation of the genetic changes in human HCC. These limitations have hampered development of proper therapeutics that was further complicated by recurrences even after aggressive local therapies.

The advances in high-throughput "omics" and next-generation sequencing technologies have been providing unprecedented biological insights related to pathogenesis of HCC. Undoubtedly, comparative and integrative genomics approaches are promising to lead to novel and robust biomarkers for improved diagnosis, prognosis, and treatment of HCC. The systems approach via the integration of data reflecting alterations at genomic, transcriptomic, proteomic, and epigenomics levels will ultimately converge toward a personalized medicine that will improve diagnosis, treatment and prevention of liver cancer.

10. References

[1] El-Serag HB, Rudolph KL: Hepatocellular carcinoma: epidemiology and molecular carcinogenesis. *Gastroenterology* 2007, 132:2557-2576.

[2] Altekruse SF, McGlynn KA, Reichman ME: Hepatocellular carcinoma incidence, mortality, and survival trends in the United States from 1975 to 2005. *J Clin Oncol* 2009, 27:1485-1491.

[3] Nguyen MH, Whittemore AS, Garcia RT, Tawfeek SA, Ning J, Lam S, Wright TL, Keeffe EB: Role of ethnicity in risk for hepatocellular carcinoma in patients with chronic hepatitis C and cirrhosis. *Clin Gastroenterol Hepatol* 2004, 2:820-824.

[4] Farazi PA, DePinho RA: Hepatocellular carcinoma pathogenesis: from genes to environment. *Nat Rev Cancer* 2006, 6:674-687.

[5] Totoki Y, Tatsuno K, Yamamoto S, Arai Y, Hosoda F, Ishikawa S, Tsutsumi S, Sonoda K, Totsuka H, Shirakihara T, et al: High-resolution characterization of a hepatocellular carcinoma genome. *Nat Genet* 2011, 43:464-469.

[6] Geschwind DH: DNA microarrays: translation of the genome from laboratory to clinic. *Lancet Neurol* 2003, 2:275-282.

[7] Lupski JR: Genomic rearrangements and sporadic disease. *Nat Genet* 2007, 39:S43-47.

[8] Lupski JR: Genome structural variation and sporadic disease traits. *Nat Genet* 2006, 38:974-976.

[9] Moinzadeh P, Breuhahn K, Stutzer H, Schirmacher P: Chromosome alterations in human hepatocellular carcinomas correlate with aetiology and histological grade--results of an explorative CGH meta-analysis. *Br J Cancer* 2005, 92:935-941.

[10] Albertson DG, Collins C, McCormick F, Gray JW: Chromosome aberrations in solid tumors. *Nat Genet* 2003, 34:369-376.

[11] Zhao X, Weir BA, LaFramboise T, Lin M, Beroukhim R, Garraway L, Beheshti J, Lee JC, Naoki K, Richards WG, et al: Homozygous deletions and chromosome amplifications in human lung carcinomas revealed by single nucleotide polymorphism array analysis. *Cancer Res* 2005, 65:5561-5570.

[12] Pollack JR, Sorlie T, Perou CM, Rees CA, Jeffrey SS, Lonning PE, Tibshirani R, Botstein D, Borresen-Dale AL, Brown PO: Microarray analysis reveals a major direct role of

DNA copy number alteration in the transcriptional program of human breast tumors. *Proc Natl Acad Sci U S A* 2002, 99:12963-12968.

[13] Cifola I, Spinelli R, Beltrame L, Peano C, Fasoli E, Ferrero S, Bosari S, Signorini S, Rocco F, Perego R, et al: Genome-wide screening of copy number alterations and LOH events in renal cell carcinomas and integration with gene expression profile. *Mol Cancer* 2008, 7:6.

[14] Luo JH, Ren B, Keryanov S, Tseng GC, Rao UN, Monga SP, Strom S, Demetris AJ, Nalesnik M, Yu YP, et al: Transcriptomic and genomic analysis of human hepatocellular carcinomas and hepatoblastomas. *Hepatology* 2006, 44:1012-1024.

[15] Tsafrir D, Bacolod M, Selvanayagam Z, Tsafrir I, Shia J, Zeng Z, Liu H, Krier C, Stengel RF, Barany F, et al: Relationship of gene expression and chromosomal abnormalities in colorectal cancer. *Cancer Res* 2006, 66:2129-2137.

[16] Su WH, Chao CC, Yeh SH, Chen DS, Chen PJ, Jou YS: OncoDB.HCC: an integrated oncogenomic database of hepatocellular carcinoma revealed aberrant cancer target genes and loci. *Nucleic Acids Res* 2007, 35:D727-731.

[17] Woo HG, Park ES, Lee JS, Lee YH, Ishikawa T, Kim YJ, Thorgeirsson SS: Identification of potential driver genes in human liver carcinoma by genomewide screening. *Cancer Res* 2009, 69:4059-4066.

[18] Chen CF, Hsu EC, Lin KT, Tu PH, Chang HW, Lin CH, Chen YJ, Gu DL, Lin CH, Wu JY, et al: Overlapping high-resolution copy number alterations in cancer genomes identified putative cancer genes in hepatocellular carcinoma. *Hepatology* 2010, 52:1690-1701.

[19] Moran DM, Mattocks MA, Cahill PA, Koniaris LG, McKillop IH: Interleukin-6 mediates G(0)/G(1) growth arrest in hepatocellular carcinoma through a STAT 3-dependent pathway. *J Surg Res* 2008, 147:23-33.

[20] Moran DM, Mayes N, Koniaris LG, Cahill PA, McKillop IH: Interleukin-6 inhibits cell proliferation in a rat model of hepatocellular carcinoma. *Liver Int* 2005, 25:445-457.

[21] Basu A, Meyer K, Lai KK, Saito K, Di Bisceglie AM, Grosso LE, Ray RB, Ray R: Microarray analyses and molecular profiling of Stat3 signaling pathway induced by hepatitis C virus core protein in human hepatocytes. *Virology* 2006, 349:347-358.

[22] Moran DM, Koniaris LG, Jablonski EM, Cahill PA, Halberstadt CR, McKillop IH: Microencapsulation of engineered cells to deliver sustained high circulating levels of interleukin-6 to study hepatocellular carcinoma progression. *Cell Transplant* 2006, 15:785-798.

[23] Clifford RJ, Zhang J, Meerzaman DM, Lyu MS, Hu Y, Cultraro CM, Finney RP, Kelley JM, Efroni S, Greenblum SI, et al: Genetic variations at loci involved in the immune response are risk factors for hepatocellular carcinoma. *Hepatology* 2010, 52:2034-2043.

[24] Jia D, Wei L, Guo W, Zha R, Bao M, Chen Z, Zhao Y, Ge C, Zhao F, Chen T, et al: Genome-wide copy number analyses identified novel cancer genes in hepatocellular carcinoma. *Hepatology* 2011.

[25] Asyali MH, Colak D, Demirkaya O, and Inan MS: Gene Expression Profile Classification: A Review. Current Bioinf. 2006, 1:55-73.

[26] Iizuka N, Oka M, Yamada-Okabe H, Nishida M, Maeda Y, Mori N, Takao T, Tamesa T, Tangoku A, Tabuchi H, et al: Oligonucleotide microarray for prediction of early

intrahepatic recurrence of hepatocellular carcinoma after curative resection. *Lancet* 2003, 361:923-929.

[27] Jia HL, Ye QH, Qin LX, Budhu A, Forgues M, Chen Y, Liu YK, Sun HC, Wang L, Lu HZ, et al: Gene expression profiling reveals potential biomarkers of human hepatocellular carcinoma. *Clin Cancer Res* 2007, 13:1133-1139.

[28] Ye QH, Qin LX, Forgues M, He P, Kim JW, Peng AC, Simon R, Li Y, Robles AI, Chen Y, et al: Predicting hepatitis B virus-positive metastatic hepatocellular carcinomas using gene expression profiling and supervised machine learning. *Nat Med* 2003, 9:416-423.

[29] Lee JS, Chu IS, Heo J, Calvisi DF, Sun Z, Roskams T, Durnez A, Demetris AJ, Thorgeirsson SS: Classification and prediction of survival in hepatocellular carcinoma by gene expression profiling. *Hepatology* 2004, 40:667-676.

[30] Lau WY, Lai PB, Leung MF, Leung BC, Wong N, Chen G, Leung TW, Liew CT: Differential gene expression of hepatocellular carcinoma using cDNA microarray analysis. *Oncol Res* 2000, 12:59-69.

[31] Delpuech O, Trabut JB, Carnot F, Feuillard J, Brechot C, Kremsdorf D: Identification, using cDNA macroarray analysis, of distinct gene expression profiles associated with pathological and virological features of hepatocellular carcinoma. *Oncogene* 2002, 21:2926-2937.

[32] Okabe H, Satoh S, Kato T, Kitahara O, Yanagawa R, Yamaoka Y, Tsunoda T, Furukawa Y, Nakamura Y: Genome-wide analysis of gene expression in human hepatocellular carcinomas using cDNA microarray: identification of genes involved in viral carcinogenesis and tumor progression. *Cancer Res* 2001, 61:2129-2137.

[33] Boyault S, Rickman DS, de Reynies A, Balabaud C, Rebouissou S, Jeannot E, Herault A, Saric J, Belghiti J, Franco D, et al: Transcriptome classification of HCC is related to gene alterations and to new therapeutic targets. *Hepatology* 2007, 45:42-52.

[34] Wurmbach E, Chen YB, Khitrov G, Zhang W, Roayaie S, Schwartz M, Fiel I, Thung S, Mazzaferro V, Bruix J, et al: Genome-wide molecular profiles of HCV-induced dysplasia and hepatocellular carcinoma. *Hepatology* 2007, 45:938-947.

[35] Yu GR, Kim SH, Park SH, Cui XD, Xu DY, Yu HC, Cho BH, Yeom YI, Kim SS, Kim SB, et al: Identification of molecular markers for the oncogenic differentiation of hepatocellular carcinoma. *Exp Mol Med* 2007, 39:641-652.

[36] Lee JS, Thorgeirsson SS: Comparative and integrative functional genomics of HCC. *Oncogene* 2006, 25:3801-3809.

[37] Iizuka N, Oka M, Yamada-Okabe H, Hamada K, Nakayama H, Mori N, Tamesa T, Okada T, Takemoto N, Matoba K, et al: Molecular signature in three types of hepatocellular carcinoma with different viral origin by oligonucleotide microarray. *Int J Oncol* 2004, 24:565-574.

[38] Iizuka N, Oka M, Yamada-Okabe H, Mori N, Tamesa T, Okada T, Takemoto N, Tangoku A, Hamada K, Nakayama H, et al: Comparison of gene expression profiles between hepatitis B virus- and hepatitis C virus-infected hepatocellular carcinoma by oligonucleotide microarray data on the basis of a supervised learning method. *Cancer Res* 2002, 62:3939-3944.

[39] Honda M, Kaneko S, Kawai H, Shirota Y, Kobayashi K: Differential gene expression between chronic hepatitis B and C hepatic lesion. *Gastroenterology* 2001, 120:955-966.

[40] Ho MC, Lin JJ, Chen CN, Chen CC, Lee H, Yang CY, Ni YH, Chang KJ, Hsu HC, Hsieh FJ, Lee PH: A gene expression profile for vascular invasion can predict the recurrence after resection of hepatocellular carcinoma: a microarray approach. *Ann Surg Oncol* 2006, 13:1474-1484.
[41] Budhu A, Forgues M, Ye QH, Jia HL, He P, Zanetti KA, Kammula US, Chen Y, Qin LX, Tang ZY, Wang XW: Prediction of venous metastases, recurrence, and prognosis in hepatocellular carcinoma based on a unique immune response signature of the liver microenvironment. *Cancer Cell* 2006, 10:99-111.
[42] Wang SM, Ooi LL, Hui KM: Identification and validation of a novel gene signature associated with the recurrence of human hepatocellular carcinoma. *Clin Cancer Res* 2007, 13:6275-6283.
[43] Nam SW, Park JY, Ramasamy A, Shevade S, Islam A, Long PM, Park CK, Park SE, Kim SY, Lee SH, et al: Molecular changes from dysplastic nodule to hepatocellular carcinoma through gene expression profiling. *Hepatology* 2005, 42:809-818.
[44] Kim BY, Lee JG, Park S, Ahn JY, Ju YJ, Chung JH, Han CJ, Jeong SH, Yeom YI, Kim S, et al: Feature genes of hepatitis B virus-positive hepatocellular carcinoma, established by its molecular discrimination approach using prediction analysis of microarray. *Biochim Biophys Acta* 2004, 1739:50-61.
[45] Kurokawa Y, Matoba R, Takemasa I, Nagano H, Dono K, Nakamori S, Umeshita K, Sakon M, Ueno N, Oba S, et al: Molecular-based prediction of early recurrence in hepatocellular carcinoma. *J Hepatol* 2004, 41:284-291.
[46] Somura H, Iizuka N, Tamesa T, Sakamoto K, Hamaguchi T, Tsunedomi R, Yamada-Okabe H, Sawamura M, Eramoto M, Miyamoto T, et al: A three-gene predictor for early intrahepatic recurrence of hepatocellular carcinoma after curative hepatectomy. *Oncol Rep* 2008, 19:489-495.
[47] Kaposi-Novak P, Lee JS, Gomez-Quiroz L, Coulouarn C, Factor VM, Thorgeirsson SS: Met-regulated expression signature defines a subset of human hepatocellular carcinomas with poor prognosis and aggressive phenotype. *J Clin Invest* 2006, 116:1582-1595.
[48] Coulouarn C, Factor VM, Thorgeirsson SS: Transforming growth factor-beta gene expression signature in mouse hepatocytes predicts clinical outcome in human cancer. *Hepatology* 2008, 47:2059-2067.
[49] Kaposi-Novak P, Libbrecht L, Woo HG, Lee YH, Sears NC, Coulouarn C, Conner EA, Factor VM, Roskams T, Thorgeirsson SS: Central role of c-Myc during malignant conversion in human hepatocarcinogenesis. *Cancer Res* 2009, 69:2775-2782.
[50] Shackel NA, Seth D, Haber PS, Gorrell MD, McCaughan GW: The hepatic transcriptome in human liver disease. *Comp Hepatol* 2006, 5:6.
[51] Smith MW, Yue ZN, Geiss GK, Sadovnikova NY, Carter VS, Boix L, Lazaro CA, Rosenberg GB, Bumgarner RE, Fausto N, et al: Identification of novel tumor markers in hepatitis C virus-associated hepatocellular carcinoma. *Cancer Res* 2003, 63:859-864.
[52] Garraway LA, Widlund HR, Rubin MA, Getz G, Berger AJ, Ramaswamy S, Beroukhim R, Milner DA, Granter SR, Du J, et al: Integrative genomic analyses identify MITF as a lineage survival oncogene amplified in malignant melanoma. *Nature* 2005, 436:117-122.

[53] Thorgeirsson SS, Lee JS, Grisham JW: Molecular prognostication of liver cancer: end of the beginning. *J Hepatol* 2006, 44:798-805.

[54] Colak D, Chishti MA, Al-Bakheet AB, Al-Qahtani A, Shoukri MM, Goyns MH, Ozand PT, Quackenbush J, Park BH, Kaya N: Integrative and comparative genomics analysis of early hepatocellular carcinoma differentiated from liver regeneration in young and old. *Mol Cancer* 2010, 9:146.

[55] Ross JS, Carlson JA, Brock G: miRNA: the new gene silencer. *Am J Clin Pathol* 2007, 128:830-836.

[56] Zhang B, Farwell MA: microRNAs: a new emerging class of players for disease diagnostics and gene therapy. *J Cell Mol Med* 2008, 12:3-21.

[57] Kloosterman WP, Plasterk RH: The diverse functions of microRNAs in animal development and disease. *Dev Cell* 2006, 11:441-450.

[58] Zamore PD, Haley B: Ribo-gnome: the big world of small RNAs. *Science* 2005, 309:1519-1524.

[59] Gramantieri L, Fornari F, Callegari E, Sabbioni S, Lanza G, Croce CM, Bolondi L, Negrini M: MicroRNA involvement in hepatocellular carcinoma. *J Cell Mol Med* 2008, 12:2189-2204.

[60] Negrini M, Gramantieri L, Sabbioni S, Croce CM: microRNA involvement in hepatocellular carcinoma. *Anticancer Agents Med Chem* 2011, 11:500-521.

[61] Law PT, Wong N: Emerging roles of microRNA in the intracellular signaling networks of hepatocellular carcinoma. *J Gastroenterol Hepatol* 2011, 26:437-449.

[62] Ji J, Wang XW: New kids on the block: diagnostic and prognostic microRNAs in hepatocellular carcinoma. *Cancer Biol Ther* 2009, 8:1686-1693.

[63] Huang S, He X: The role of microRNAs in liver cancer progression. *Br J Cancer* 2011, 104:235-240.

[64] Sato F, Hatano E, Kitamura K, Myomoto A, Fujiwara T, Takizawa S, Tsuchiya S, Tsujimoto G, Uemoto S, Shimizu K: MicroRNA profile predicts recurrence after resection in patients with hepatocellular carcinoma within the Milan Criteria. *PLoS One* 2011, 6:e16435.

[65] Toffanin S, Hoshida Y, Lachenmayer A, Villanueva A, Cabellos L, Minguez B, Savic R, Ward SC, Thung S, Chiang DY, et al: MicroRNA-based classification of hepatocellular carcinoma and oncogenic role of miR-517a. *Gastroenterology* 2011, 140:1618-1628 e1616.

[66] Murakami Y, Yasuda T, Saigo K, Urashima T, Toyoda H, Okanoue T, Shimotohno K: Comprehensive analysis of microRNA expression patterns in hepatocellular carcinoma and non-tumorous tissues. *Oncogene* 2006, 25:2537-2545.

[67] Huang YS, Dai Y, Yu XF, Bao SY, Yin YB, Tang M, Hu CX: Microarray analysis of microRNA expression in hepatocellular carcinoma and non-tumorous tissues without viral hepatitis. *J Gastroenterol Hepatol* 2008, 23:87-94.

[68] Ji J, Shi J, Budhu A, Yu Z, Forgues M, Roessler S, Ambs S, Chen Y, Meltzer PS, Croce CM, et al: MicroRNA expression, survival, and response to interferon in liver cancer. *N Engl J Med* 2009, 361:1437-1447.

[69] Budhu A, Jia HL, Forgues M, Liu CG, Goldstein D, Lam A, Zanetti KA, Ye QH, Qin LX, Croce CM, et al: Identification of metastasis-related microRNAs in hepatocellular carcinoma. *Hepatology* 2008, 47:897-907.

[70] Mitchell PS, Parkin RK, Kroh EM, Fritz BR, Wyman SK, Pogosova-Agadjanyan EL, Peterson A, Noteboom J, O'Briant KC, Allen A, et al: Circulating microRNAs as stable blood-based markers for cancer detection. *Proc Natl Acad Sci U S A* 2008, 105:10513-10518.

[71] Huang Z, Huang D, Ni S, Peng Z, Sheng W, Du X: Plasma microRNAs are promising novel biomarkers for early detection of colorectal cancer. *Int J Cancer* 2010, 127:118-126.

[72] Qu KZ, Zhang K, Li H, Afdhal NH, Albitar M: Circulating microRNAs as biomarkers for hepatocellular carcinoma. *J Clin Gastroenterol* 2011, 45:355-360.

[73] Mardis ER: A decade's perspective on DNA sequencing technology. *Nature* 2011, 470:198-203.

[74] Mardis ER: New strategies and emerging technologies for massively parallel sequencing: applications in medical research. *Genome Med* 2009, 1:40.

[75] Mardis ER: The impact of next-generation sequencing technology on genetics. *Trends Genet* 2008, 24:133-141.

[76] Varshney RK, Nayak SN, May GD, Jackson SA: Next-generation sequencing technologies and their implications for crop genetics and breeding. *Trends Biotechnol* 2009, 27:522-530.

[77] Imelfort M, Duran C, Batley J, Edwards D: Discovering genetic polymorphisms in next-generation sequencing data. *Plant Biotechnol J* 2009, 7:312-317.

[78] Zhou X, Ren L, Meng Q, Li Y, Yu Y, Yu J: The next-generation sequencing technology and application. *Protein Cell* 2010, 1:520-536.

[79] Zhang J, Chiodini R, Badr A, Zhang G: The impact of next-generation sequencing on genomics. *J Genet Genomics* 2011, 38:95-109.

[80] Mardis ER: Next-generation DNA sequencing methods. *Annu Rev Genomics Hum Genet* 2008, 9:387-402.

[81] Morozova O, Marra MA: Applications of next-generation sequencing technologies in functional genomics. *Genomics* 2008, 92:255-264.

[82] Zhou X, Ren L, Li Y, Zhang M, Yu Y, Yu J: The next-generation sequencing technology: a technology review and future perspective. *Sci China Life Sci* 2010, 53:44-57.

[83] Simon SA, Meyers BC: Small RNA-mediated epigenetic modifications in plants. *Curr Opin Plant Biol* 2011, 14:148-155.

[84] Simon SA, Zhai J, Nandety RS, McCormick KP, Zeng J, Mejia D, Meyers BC: Short-read sequencing technologies for transcriptional analyses. *Annu Rev Plant Biol* 2009, 60:305-333.

[85] Ramsingh G, Koboldt DC, Trissal M, Chiappinelli KB, Wylie T, Koul S, Chang LW, Nagarajan R, Fehniger TA, Goodfellow P, et al: Complete characterization of the microRNAome in a patient with acute myeloid leukemia. *Blood* 2010, 116:5316-5326.

[86] Mardis ER: Cancer genomics identifies determinants of tumor biology. *Genome Biol* 2010, 11:211.

[87] Ding L, Wendl MC, Koboldt DC, Mardis ER: Analysis of next-generation genomic data in cancer: accomplishments and challenges. *Hum Mol Genet* 2010, 19:R188-196.

[88] Mardis ER, Wilson RK: Cancer genome sequencing: a review. *Hum Mol Genet* 2009, 18:R163-168.

[89] Link DC, Schuettpelz LG, Shen D, Wang J, Walter MJ, Kulkarni S, Payton JE, Ivanovich J, Goodfellow PJ, Le Beau M, et al: Identification of a novel TP53 cancer susceptibility mutation through whole-genome sequencing of a patient with therapy-related AML. *JAMA* 2011, 305:1568-1576.
[90] Ley TJ, Ding L, Walter MJ, McLellan MD, Lamprecht T, Larson DE, Kandoth C, Payton JE, Baty J, Welch J, et al: DNMT3A mutations in acute myeloid leukemia. *N Engl J Med* 2010, 363:2424-2433.
[91] Mardis ER, Ding L, Dooling DJ, Larson DE, McLellan MD, Chen K, Koboldt DC, Fulton RS, Delehaunty KD, McGrath SD, et al: Recurring mutations found by sequencing an acute myeloid leukemia genome. *N Engl J Med* 2009, 361:1058-1066.
[92] Ding L, Ellis MJ, Li S, Larson DE, Chen K, Wallis JW, Harris CC, McLellan MD, Fulton RS, Fulton LL, et al: Genome remodelling in a basal-like breast cancer metastasis and xenograft. *Nature* 2010, 464:999-1005.
[93] Ding L, Getz G, Wheeler DA, Mardis ER, McLellan MD, Cibulskis K, Sougnez C, Greulich H, Muzny DM, Morgan MB, et al: Somatic mutations affect key pathways in lung adenocarcinoma. *Nature* 2008, 455:1069-1075.
[94] Ley TJ, Mardis ER, Ding L, Fulton B, McLellan MD, Chen K, Dooling D, Dunford-Shore BH, McGrath S, Hickenbotham M, et al: DNA sequencing of a cytogenetically normal acute myeloid leukaemia genome. *Nature* 2008, 456:66-72.
[95] Walter MJ, Graubert TA, Dipersio JF, Mardis ER, Wilson RK, Ley TJ: Next-generation sequencing of cancer genomes: back to the future. *Per Med* 2009, 6:653.
[96] Mardis ER: The $1,000 genome, the $100,000 analysis? *Genome Med* 2010, 2:84.
[97] Lee JS, Chu IS, Mikaelyan A, Calvisi DF, Heo J, Reddy JK, Thorgeirsson SS: Application of comparative functional genomics to identify best-fit mouse models to study human cancer. *Nat Genet* 2004, 36:1306-1311.
[98] Perez-Carreon JI, Lopez-Garcia C, Fattel-Fazenda S, Arce-Popoca E, Aleman-Lazarini L, Hernandez-Garcia S, Le Berre V, Sokol S, Francois JM, Villa-Trevino S: Gene expression profile related to the progression of preneoplastic nodules toward hepatocellular carcinoma in rats. *Neoplasia* 2006, 8:373-383.
[99] Fausto N, Campbell JS: Mouse models of hepatocellular carcinoma. *Semin Liver Dis* 2010, 30:87-98.
[100] Wu L, Tang ZY, Li Y: Experimental models of hepatocellular carcinoma: developments and evolution. *J Cancer Res Clin Oncol* 2009, 135:969-981.
[101] Sweet-Cordero A, Mukherjee S, Subramanian A, You H, Roix JJ, Ladd-Acosta C, Mesirov J, Golub TR, Jacks T: An oncogenic KRAS2 expression signature identified by cross-species gene-expression analysis. *Nat Genet* 2005, 37:48-55.
[102] Paoloni M, Davis S, Lana S, Withrow S, Sangiorgi L, Picci P, Hewitt S, Triche T, Meltzer P, Khanna C: Canine tumor cross-species genomics uncovers targets linked to osteosarcoma progression. *BMC Genomics* 2009, 10:625.
[103] Ellwood-Yen K, Graeber TG, Wongvipat J, Iruela-Arispe ML, Zhang J, Matusik R, Thomas GV, Sawyers CL: Myc-driven murine prostate cancer shares molecular features with human prostate tumors. *Cancer Cell* 2003, 4:223-238.
[104] Patil MA, Chua MS, Pan KH, Lin R, Lih CJ, Cheung ST, Ho C, Li R, Fan ST, Cohen SN, et al: An integrated data analysis approach to characterize genes highly expressed in hepatocellular carcinoma. *Oncogene* 2005, 24:3737-3747.

[105] Akavia UD, Litvin O, Kim J, Sanchez-Garcia F, Kotliar D, Causton HC, Pochanard P, Mozes E, Garraway LA, Pe'er D: An integrated approach to uncover drivers of cancer. *Cell* 2010, 143:1005-1017.

2

The *Hcs7* Mouse Liver Cancer Modifier Maps to a 3.3 Mb Region Carrying the Strong Candidate *Ifi202b*

Andrea Bilger, Elizabeth Poli, Andrew Schneider,
Rebecca Baus and Norman Drinkwater
McArdle Laboratory for Cancer Research,
University of Wisconsin School of Medicine and Public Health,
Madison, WI
USA

1. Introduction

Genes that affect a person's chance of developing hepatocellular carcinoma (HCC), as *BRCA1* and *BRCA2* affect a person's chance of developing breast or ovarian cancer, have been difficult to detect. The vast majority of liver cancers can be attributed to Hepatitis B or C virus infection, aflatoxin exposure, or alcoholic cirrhosis, alone or in combination (Montalto et al., 2002). This high background of predisposing environmental factors makes identifying less penetrant genetic contributors more difficult. Familial patterns of susceptibility to liver cancer independent of environmental factors have helped identify a few monogenic metabolic syndromes (*e.g.*, hemochromatosis; Dragani, 2010). However, the analysis of liver tumors points to a variety of other genes that affect liver tumor development. The patterns of chromosome gain and loss in liver cancers worldwide reveal several regions that are gained or lost in up to 86% of tumors, including gains of 1q, 6p, 8q, and 20q, and losses of 1p, 4q, 6q, 8p, 13q, 16q, and 17p (Lau and Guan, 2005; Chochi et al., 2009; Zhang et al., 2010). Chromosome analyses combined with genome-wide association studies have revealed candidate HCC modifier genes for some of these regions, such as *PAPSS1* on chromosome 4q and *HCAP1* on chromosome 17p (Wan et al., 2004; Shih et al., 2009).

Mice present an independent model of liver carcinogenesis for which external variables such as chemical exposure can be controlled and the genetics is manipulable. Different inbred strains of mice develop cancers at different frequencies. Because these differences are genetic, and the mice are homozygous due to inbreeding, causative genes can be identified through positional cloning.

Inbred mouse strains differ dramatically in their susceptibility to both spontaneous and carcinogen-induced HCC. Females of the C57BR/cdJ strain, for example, develop up to 50-fold more tumors after a single injection of N,N-diethylnitrosamine (DEN) than females of the related, relatively resistant C57BL/6J (B6) strain. We have recently mapped the predominant locus responsible for this difference to a 6 Mb region on Chromosome 17 (Peychal et al., 2009). This region corresponds to part of the chromosome 6p region amplified in the majority of late-stage HCC (Santos et al., 2007; Chochi et al., 2009).

The C3H/HeJ strain (C3H), highly susceptible to both spontaneous and carcinogen-induced HCC, develops up to 50-fold more liver tumors than the B6 strain after a single carcinogen treatment (Drinkwater and Ginsler, 1986). We previously reported mapping the predominant locus responsible for this susceptibility, *Hcs7*, to distal Chromosome 1 (Bilger et al., 2004). This chromosomal region corresponds in part to the 1q21-24 chromosomal region amplified in up to 86% of human liver cancers (Lau and Guan, 2005; Chochi et al., 2009; Zhang et al., 2010). C3H alleles on mouse Chromosome 1 confer a dominant 15-fold increased susceptibility to male mice and a semi-dominant 5-fold increased susceptibility to female mice carrying C3H alleles (Bilger et al., 2004).

Here we analyze the effect of C3H Chromosome 1 alleles on spontaneous hepato-carcinogenesis, on apoptosis and mitosis after DEN treatment, and on preneoplastic lesion growth. We have mapped the *Hcs7* modifier to a 3.3 Mb region and used expression and CGH arrays to identify the *Ifi202b* gene as a strong candidate for this locus.

2. Materials and methods

2.1 Mice

B6 and C3H mice were purchased from the Jackson Laboratory (Bar Harbor, Maine) and bred in our facilities. All mice were housed in plastic cages on corncob bedding (Bed O'Cobs, Anderson Cob Division, Maumee, OH), fed Purina 5020 diet (9% fat; St. Louis, MO), and given acidified tap water *ad libitum*. Mice were inspected daily and weighed monthly.

Lines derived from the B6.C3H-Ch1 recombinant strain (Bilger et al., 2004) were generated as follows. B6 females were mated with B6.C3H-Ch1 males heterozygous for the congenic region. Markers between *D1Mit285* and *D1MIT17* were used to identify recombinants, and breakpoints were mapped more finely with additional markers. Males and females from a given recombinant line were then intercrossed to generate homozygotes. Heterozygous or homozygous mice were mated with B6 to generate heterozygous experimental progeny (Figures 1 and 3, and Table 3) or homozygotes were intercrossed to generate homozygous experimental progeny (Tables 1 and 2). Tested parental B6.C3H-Ch1 were homozygous.

Lines derived from B6.BR-Ch1 were generated by mating B6 females with B6.BR-Ch1 males heterozygous for the congenic region. The markers *D1Mit143*, *D1Mit17*, and two additional microsatellite markers at 172.9 and 176.9 Mb were used to identify recombinants. (The lack of SNPs or SSLPs between B6 and BR in this region prevented refinement of these breakpoints.) Heterozygotes were intercrossed to generate homozygous lines. B6 females were then crossed with homozygous congenic males to generate experimental progeny.

The C3H.B6-Ch1 line carrying B6 alleles for distal Chromosome 1 on a C3H genetic background was generated by crossing C3B6F1 (N1) mice with C3H mice and selecting C3H.B6 N2 mice carrying B6 alleles at *D1Mit143*, *D1Mit15*, *D1Mit166*, and *D1Mit461*. Backcrossing to C3H and selection of these B6 alleles was continued for eight additional generations to generate C3.B6(*D1Mit143-D1Mit461*)N10, or "C3H.B6-Ch1" (Figure 3) mice.

2.2 Genotyping

DNA was prepared from spleen tissue by Proteinase K treatment/ammonium acetate/isopropyl alcohol precipitation as described (Bilger et al., 2004) or from spleen, tail, or toe tissue by alkaline lysis (modified from Truett et al., 2000). Approximately 2 mm^3 of spleen or 10 mm^3 of tail or toe tissue was incubated in 200 µl lysis solution (25 mM NaOH, 0.2 mM EDTA) at 95°C for 20-60 minutes and then neutralized by the addition of 200 µl 40 mM Tris (pH 8.0). After agitation for approximately 30 seconds and centrifugation for five minutes at 13.5 krpm, 0.25 to 2 µl of the supernatant was used directly for genotyping as described (Bilger et al., 2004).

2.3 Tumor and preneoplastic lesion induction and assessment

Tumors were induced by a single intraperitoneal injection of DEN (Eastman Kodak Co., Rochester NY; 0.1 µmol/g body weight) dissolved in tricaprylin (a.k.a. trioctanoin; Sigma, St. Louis, MO) 12 ± 1 days after birth. Mice, all male, were sacrificed by CO_2 asphyxiation. For prenoplastic lesion volume analysis, mice were sacrificed at 16 or 24 weeks of age (Table 2) and representative sections of the liver were frozen immediately on dry ice and stained for glucose-6-phosphatase activity as described (Bugni et al., 2001). Glucose-6-phosphatase deficiency is a hallmark of the majority of preneoplastic lesions in DEN-treated mice (Bugni et al., 2001). For tumor analysis, mice were sacrificed at 32 weeks of age (Figure 1, Figure 3). Livers were removed and weighed, and all tumors larger than 1 mm in diameter were counted. Liver tumors were sampled at random, fixed in RNAlater (Qiagen, Valencia, CA) at 4°C, then drained of RNAlater and transferred to -80°C. Spleens were collected as a source of DNA and frozen on dry ice. All tumors were scored by a single observer blind to genotype. To assess spontaneous tumors (Table 1), mice were allowed to age to 15 months without undergoing any procedures. Tumors larger than 1 mm in diameter were counted.

To assess apoptosis, mitosis, and RNA expression immediately following DEN injection, male mice were either left untreated or injected with DEN (0.1 µmol/g body weight), at 12 days of age between 11 a.m. and 3 p.m.. Mice were sacrificed one, two, or three days later between 3 and 6 p.m.. One half of each left lobe and half of each half of the medial lobe were placed in formalin at 4°C. Half of the remaining parts of the left and medial lobes were placed in RNAlater at 4°C. The remaining portions of the left and medial lobes were frozen in pre-chilled tubes on dry ice and transferred to -80°C.

Formalin-fixed tissue was sectioned and stained with hematoxylin and eosin (H&E). Hepatocytes, apoptoses, and mitoses were counted under 600× magnification.

2.4 Microarray analysis of gene expression

RNA was purified from 20-70 mg liver or liver tumor tissue fixed in RNAlater using an RNeasy MIDI kit (Qiagen, Valencia, CA) as directed, except 50% ethanol, rather than 70% ethanol, was added to the homogenized lysate. Fluorescently labeled cDNAs were generated using Agilent Quick-Amp Labeling kits and hybridized in competition with a mixed-sex, whole-tissue liver cDNA control to Agilent Whole Mouse Genome arrays (Item #G4122F, Agilent, Santa Clara, CA). Arrays were scanned using an Agilent DNA Microarray Scanner G2505C.

2.5 Comparative genomic hybridization

Genomic DNA from male spleens was prepared using a standard Proteinase K/ammonium acetate/isopropyl alcohol precipitation protocol as described (Bilger et al., 2004), except DNA was treated with RNase A, which was then precipitated with ammonium acetate before the final DNA precipitation. Genomic DNA of either line 1R5 or inbred C3H mice was then labeled and mixed with control genomic B6 DNA, for dual-color CGH, and hybridized to the MM 8_WG_CGH_1of8 chip. This array has 50-75 nucleotide probes spaced at an average of 650 bp, covering all of Chr 1 and Chr 2 through position 123959568. Results were analyzed by Nimblegen CGH Services, using the CGH-segMNT algorithm (Roche Nimblegen, Madison, WI).

2.6 Statistical analysis

The significance of differences between tumor multiplicity data sets was determined by the Wilcoxon rank-sum test, using Mstat software (version 5.4, McArdle Laboratory for Cancer Research; URL, http://www.mcardle.wisc.edu/mstat). All *P*-values were calculated on the basis of a two-sided test, except in the case of spontaneous tumorigenesis, for which we were testing the one-sided hypothesis that C3H alleles that increase DEN-induced tumor multiplicity also increase spontaneous tumor multiplicity. Differences between RNA expression data sets were evaluated with the limma software package (Smyth, 2004), using a moderated t-statistic followed by FDR correction.

3. Results

3.1 A dominant modifier on Chr 1, *Hcs7*, maps to a 3.3 Mb region between 175.35 and 178.64 Mb

To map the Chromosome 1 modifier to a smaller region, we crossed B6 mice with B6.C3H-Ch1 congenic mice carrying *Hcs7* susceptibility alleles on Chromosome 1. Mice that had undergone recombination in the susceptibility region were selected and then bred again with B6 mice to generate heterozygous progeny cohorts for phenotyping. Male progeny were injected with DEN at 12 days and sacrificed at 32 weeks of age. The median number of tumors developed by males of each recombinant line is shown in Figure 1, below.

Most of the susceptibility conferred by *Hcs7* can be mapped to the distal end of the chromosome. Lines carrying C3H alleles only distal of *D1Mit143* at 165 Mb developed 5- to 12-fold more tumors than B6 (line 1R28: $P < 10^{-7}$; line 1R33: $P < 10^{-6}$; line 1R42: $P < 10^{-5}$). For lines 1R28 and 1R33, the number of tumors developed was not significantly different from the number developed by the homozygous B6.C3H-Ch1 parental congenic line (1R28: $P > 0.30$; line 1R33: $P > 0.11$).

Six of the seven recombinant lines that carry C3H from *D1Mit15* at 170 Mb to *D1Mit17* at 191 Mb near the telomere were highly susceptible. These six lines developed an average of eight times as many tumors as B6. The exception, line 1R5, carries this susceptibility region but was resistant (1R5 vs B6: $P > 0.35$). Comparative genomic hybridization revealed a potential explanation. In the distal susceptibility region, line 1R5 differs from C3H at the 5' end of the *Ifi202b* gene (Figure 2). While line 1R5 and C3H both carry polymorphisms that suggest duplication of part of this region relative to B6, line 1R5 also carries polymorphisms that reduce hybridization to the CGH probes relative to B6 and C3H. This effect could be due to deletion, rearrangement, or novel sequences.

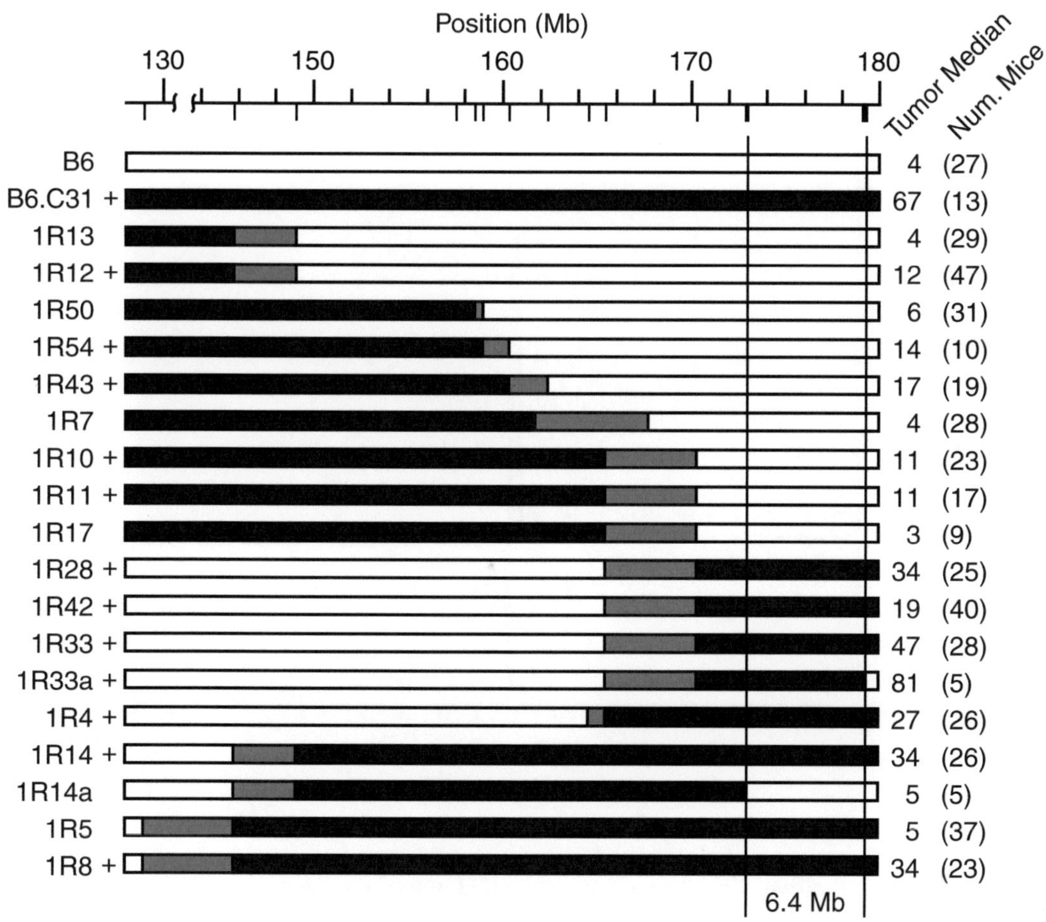

Fig. 1. C3H liver cancer susceptibility alleles map to distal Chromosome 1.

Male mice carrying C3H alleles on Chromosome 1 on a B6 genetic background were injected with DEN and liver tumors were counted at 32 weeks. The line designated B6.C31 refers to B6.C3H-Ch1. Regions inherited from B6 are shown in white; C3H regions are shown in black. Regions carrying a breakpoint between B6 and C3H alleles are shown in grey. The median tumor multiplicity and number of mice tested are shown to the right of each line. Lines that were significantly more susceptible than B6 are marked with a "+." The positions of markers along Chromosome 1 are shown as tics below the position axis at the top of the figure.

Two additional lines, derived from the susceptible 1R14 and 1R33 lines during the breeding of experimental progeny, suggested that *Hcs7* lies in a 6.4 Mb region carrying *Ifi202b*. Although few mice were phenotyped (five per line), the results for each line were significant. Line 33a, like its parent, was significantly more susceptible than B6 ($P < 10^{-3}$) and not significantly different from B6.C3H-Ch1 ($P > 0.55$). The distal breakpoint for line 1R33a is proximal of 179.3 Mb, suggesting that the minimal susceptibility region lies proximal of 179.3 Mb. Line 1R14a, unlike its parental line 1R14, was resistant to hepatocarcinogenesis. The difference between the lines is the distal breakpoint between 172.9 and 173.0 Mb in line

1R14a, suggesting that the minimal susceptibility region is distal of 172.9 Mb. Together, the two sublines suggest that *Hcs7* lies between 172.9 and 179.3 Mb.

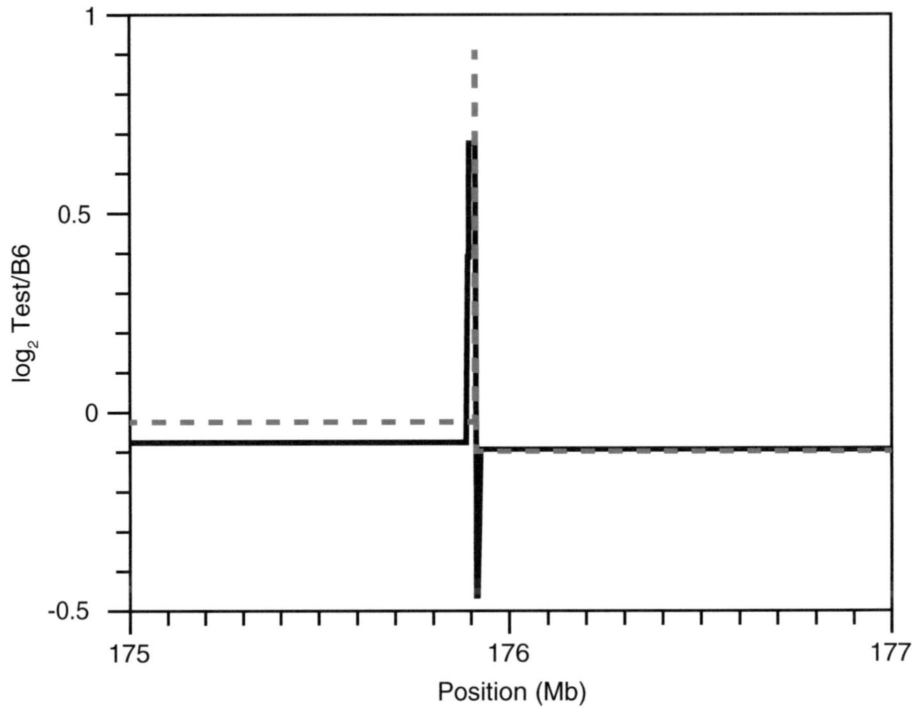

Fig. 2. The homozygous line 1R5 genome differs from C3H at *Ifi202b*.

Genomic DNA of either line 1R5 or inbred C3H was labeled and mixed with control genomic B6 DNA before hybridization to a chip carrying Chromosome 1 probes spaced 650 bp apart. The $\log_2$ ratio of the mean of the intensity of the 1R5 or C3H signal (Test) relative to B6 is plotted. C3H is shown as a dashed grey line; the 1R5 recombinant is shown as a solid black line.

Several other congenic lines that lacked the distal susceptibility region were significantly more susceptible than B6, developing three- to four-fold more tumors by 32 weeks (lines marked with plus signs, Figure 1; $P < 10^{-3}$ for all). These lines and the closely related congenic lines that are as resistant as B6 reveal a complex pattern of possibly interacting modifiers along proximal Chromosome 1. Resistant line 1R50, for example, carries more C3H than sensitive line 1R12, but it carries less C3H than sensitive line 1R54 (1R50 vs B6: $P > 0.06$; vs R12: $p < 10^{-2}$; vs 1R54: $p < 0.02$). Similarly, the C3H region carried by resistant line 1R7 extends farther distally than the C3H region carried by sensitive line 1R43. However, the resistance of line 1R7 might be explained by a unique B6 genotype at the proximal end of Chromosome 1 (proximal of 74 Mb).

To localize the distal Chromosome 1 liver cancer modifier further, we bred line 1R33 with B6 and selected males with breakpoints in or near the region between 172.9 and 179.3 Mb (Figure 3). These mice were bred with B6 females to generate experimental progeny that were injected with DEN at 12 days; tumors were counted at 32 weeks.

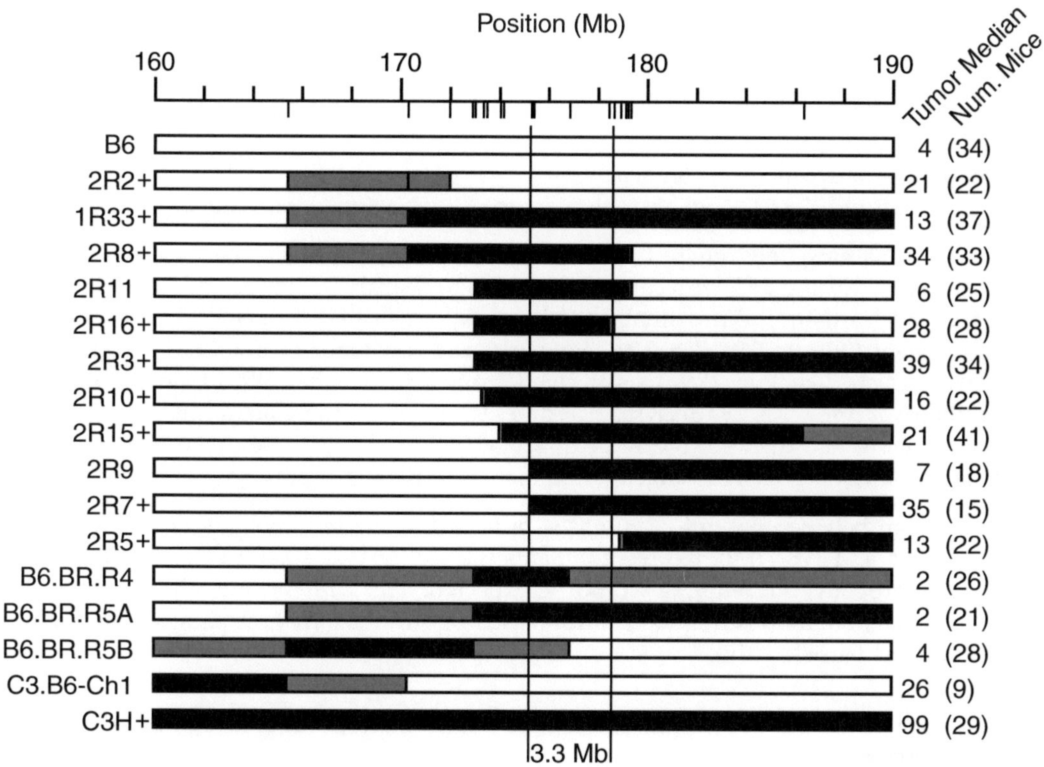

Fig. 3. C3H liver cancer susceptibility alleles map to a 3.3 Mb region between 175.35 and 178.64 Mb.

Male mice were injected with DEN and liver tumors were counted at 32 weeks. "B6" and "C3" mice were inbred; lines beginning with a "1" or "2" were B6.C3 congenic mice carrying C3H Chromosome 1 alleles on a B6 genetic background; "B6.BR." lines carry BR Chromosome 1 alleles on a B6 genetic background; and the C3H.B6-Ch1 (C3.B6-Ch1) line carries B6 Chromosome 1 alleles on a C3H background. Regions inherited from B6 are shown in white; C3H and BR regions are shown in black. Regions carrying a breakpoint between B6 and C3H alleles, or between B6 and BR alleles, are shown in grey. The median tumor multiplicity and number of mice tested are shown to the right of each line. Lines that were significantly more susceptible than B6 are marked with a "+." The positions of markers along Chromosome 1 are shown as tics below the position axis at the top of the figure.

Mice from line 2R16, which carries the smallest susceptibility region, developed 7-fold more tumors than B6 ($P < 10^{-5}$; Figure 3). This line carries C3H from 172.9 to 178.64 Mb, confirming and narrowing the location of the distal modifier. Line 2R16 was derived from line 2R3, which carries an additional ~14 Mb of C3H alleles distal of 178.64 Mb. Like 2R16, 2R3 was highly susceptible, developing 10-fold more tumors than B6 (line 2R3 vs. 2R16: $P > 0.12$; vs. B6: $P < 10^{-8}$). Line 2R8 has a larger congenic region than 2R16, extending up to 7.5 Mb farther proximally and ~ 700kb farther distally. This line was also highly susceptible, developing more than 8-fold more tumors than B6 ($P < 10^{-5}$). Together with the parental line 1R33 (again highly significantly different from B6), these lines establish that the *Hcs7* locus confers a 7- to 10-fold increase in tumor multiplicity and lies between 172.9 and 178.64 Mb. This region carries 132 genes (www.ensembl.org; 8/2011). Line 2R7, which extends distally from 175.35 Mb, was also highly susceptible relative to B6, developing almost 9-fold more tumors ($P < 10^{-5}$). In addition, line 2R7 is approximately 3-fold more susceptible than line 2R5, which carries C3H alleles distal of 178.9 Mb ($P < 0.02$). Together with the 2R16 results that place *Hcs7* between 172.9 and 178.64 Mb, these data suggest that *Hcs7* lies in the 3.3 Mb between 175.35 and 178.64 Mb. This region carries 44 genes (www.ensembl.org; 8/2011).

Again, the remaining lines suggest that the pattern of modifiers along the chromosome is complex. Lines 2R9 and 2R7 both carry C3H alleles to near the telomere and line 2R9 carries more C3H alleles than 2R7 proximally (their breakpoints differ by about 100 Kb), but line 2R9 is resistant (2R9 vs B6: $P > 0.24$). Similarly, the resistance of line 2R11 (2R11 vs. B6: $P > 0.09$), which, like line 2R9, was derived from sensitive line 2R3, together with the susceptibility of lines 2R2, 2R10, 2R15, 2R7, and 2R5, suggests there are additional modifiers both proximal to and distal of the 175.4 to 178.64 Mb minimal region. Alternatively, some lines may have undergone rearrangement in the susceptibility region.

Recombination between B6 and C3H was suppressed in the minimal susceptibility region, between 175.4 and 178.4 Mb. No recombinants were observed among approximately 1350 segregating progeny, although 24 would be expected. This difference is highly significant ($P < 10^{-6}$). Recombination is frequently suppressed by chromosomal rearrangements such as inversions (Kirkpatrick, 2010).

3.2 B6 alleles on distal Chr 1 are sufficient to suppress hepatocarcinogenesis on a C3H background

To determine whether B6 Chromosome 1 alleles can confer resistance to a sensitive C3H background (as C3H alleles confer sensitivity to a resistant B6 background), we generated C3H.B6-Ch1 congenics using ten generations of backcrossing B6 to C3H, selecting B6 alleles on distal Chromosome 1 at each generation. Heterozygous and homozygous congenic males and control inbred C3H males were injected with DEN at 12 days of age and their tumors were counted at 32 weeks (Figure 3). While heterozygosity for B6 alleles had no effect on tumorigenesis ($P>0.84$), homozygosity caused a 3.8-fold reduction in tumor multiplicity ($P<10^{-3}$).

3.3 C57BR/cdJ alleles between 175.35 and 178.64 Mb do not confer susceptibility

We have shown previously that distal Chromosome 1 carries a modifier that causes 5- to 6-fold increased susceptibility in male C57BR/cdJ (BR) mice relative to B6 mice (Poole and Drinkwater, 1996; Bilger et al., 2004). To determine whether this *Hcif2* (formerly *Hcf2*) modifier might involve the same locus that confers susceptibility to C3H, we used B6.BR-Ch1 congenic mice to derive mice carrying smaller congenic regions and counted their tumors at 32 weeks (Figure 3). The line carrying the largest BR region, B6.BR.R4, developed fewer tumors than B6 (though not significantly; $P > 0.37$). Similarly, lines B6.BR.R5A and B6.BR.R5B, which carry part of the minimal region and extend distally beyond 191 Mb (R5A) or proximally beyond 165 Mb (R5B), also developed the same number of tumors as B6 or fewer ($P > 0.86$ and $P > 0.68$, respectively). All three recombinant lines developed significantly fewer tumors than the parental B6.BR-Ch1 line (not shown; $P < 0.03$ for all). These results indicate that *Hcif2* is unlikely to lie in the 175.35 to 178.64 *Hcs7* region.

3.4 Haplotype analysis of sensitive and resistant strains

The CBA/J strain is a cousin to C3H. Like its relative, CBA/J is highly susceptible to liver tumorigenesis, and the dominant modifier mapped in crosses between CBA/J and B6 maps to distal Chromosome 1 (Bilger et al., 2004). Because these strains are likely to share a susceptibility allele, we generated a haplotype map of the minimal *Hcs7* region in CBA using SNPs obtained through the Imputed SNP Database (Szatkiewicz et al., 2008). Only SNPs that could be determined with greater than 80% confidence were included (Figure 4). This map suggests that CBA is highly related to the C3H strain through most of the *Hcs7* region, confirming the likelihood that these two sensitive strains share one or more susceptibility alleles.

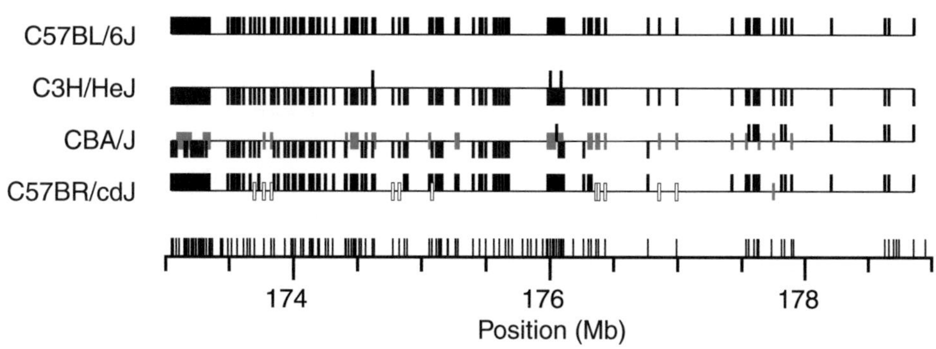

Fig. 4. Haplotype maps for the *Hcs7* interval.

Haplotypes were determined for each gene and intergenic region. B6 haplotypes are shown as tics above the bar. C3H haplotypes are shown as tics below the bar. Haplotypes unique to CBA are shown as grey tics centered on the bar, while haplotypes unique to BR are shown as outlined tics centered on the bar. The starting position of each gene is shown as a tic above the position axis.

3.5 C3H Chromosome 1 alleles increase spontaneous hepatocarcinogenesis

To determine whether *Hcs7* influences spontaneous as well as DEN-induced hepatocarcinogenesis, homozygous male mice were aged to 15 months and tumors were counted (Table 1). B6.C3H-Ch1 males developed significantly more liver tumors than B6 males (one-sided $P < 0.01$). The 4-fold higher multiplicity and the 2.5-fold higher incidence in this line closely resemble the higher multiplicity and incidence seen in inbred C3H males ($P > 0.85$). Similarly, line 1R33 males developed twice as many tumors and had 50% higher incidence than B6. The difference in tumor multiplicity was significant (one-sided $P < 0.04$). Males of the proximally congenic line 1R11, which developed approximately 3-fold more tumors than B6 when treated with DEN, had approximately 25% higher incidence and developed approximately 25% more spontaneous tumors than B6, but this difference was not significant (one-sided $P > 0.18$). This analysis of spontaneous tumor incidence indicates that the majority of the difference between C3H and B6 can be ascribed to alleles on Chromosome 1, including alleles in the *Hcs7* region.

Line	N	Incidence	Multiplicity
B6	46	0.21	0.28 ± 0.58
C3H	38	0.53	0.84 ± 1.10
B6.C3H-Ch1	17	0.47	1.35 ±2.21
1R33	31	0.35	0.65 ± 1.05
1R11	44	0.25	0.34 ± 0.71

Table 1. B6.C3H-Ch1 and 1R33 males are more susceptible to spontaneous liver tumors than B6.

Inbred and recombinant male mice were left untreated to 15 months of age and liver tumors were enumerated. N, the number of mice per group.

Many line 1R33 males developed severe skin disease. Twenty-eight males died or were euthanized prior to the 15-month time point (as compared to three B6, eight C3H, ten B6.C3H-Ch1, and eight line 1R11 males). These line 1R33 males developed skin problems with a frequency that differed from both B6 and the B6.C3H-Ch1 line, suggesting that multiple cooperating genes along Chromosome 1 must be derived from the same strain to prevent skin lesions. *Ifi202b* and neighboring genes have been implicated in autoimmune skin disease in distal Chromosome 1 congenic lines derived from B6 and the NZB (New Zealand Black) strain (Choubey et al., 2010; Panchanathan et al., 2011).

3.6 *Hcs7* affects early lesion growth

To determine when *Hcs7* influences tumorigenesis, we measured preneoplastic lesion size in B6, C3H, and congenic lines that had been treated with DEN at 12 days of age. Livers were collected at 16 and 24 weeks and frozen immediately on dry ice, followed by glucose-6-phosphatase staining to identify preneoplastic lesions. In the first experiment, lesions were measured in B6, line 1R11, and line 1R33 livers. By sixteen weeks, lesions in the moderately susceptible line 1R11 and the highly susceptible line 1R33 occupied 3.5 and 3.4 times, respectively, the volume occupied by B6 lesions ($P < 10^{-3}$ for both lines; Table 2). At 24 weeks, 1R11 lesions occupied 1.5-fold more volume than B6 lesions ($P > 0.15$), while 1R33 lesions occupied 2.0-fold more volume than B6 lesions ($P < 0.05$). This result indicates that the growth advantage of lesions in the congenic lines begins prior to 16 weeks.

A second experiment yielded results for line 2R8 that were very similar to those obtained for the larger 1R33 congenic. Line 2R8 lesions occupied 3.4-fold more volume than B6 lesions at 16 weeks; the ratio was 3.3-fold at 24 weeks. This result confirms that *Hcs7* modifies preneoplastic lesion growth. This second experiment included C3H males, which developed lesions that occupied significantly more volume than the congenic at both time points (16 wks: $P < 0.01$; 24 wks: $P < 10^{-4}$). C3H lesions occupied 17-fold more volume than B6 at 16 weeks, which increased to 33-fold more than B6 at 24 weeks. The magnitude of the growth effects in inbred C3H males suggests that *Hcs7* C3H alleles are not sufficient to recapitulate entirely the early lesion development seen in C3H inbred mice.

Experiment/age	N	Focus Volume Fraction (VF) ± SD	VF ratio
Experiment 1			
16 weeks			
B6	14	0.00098 ± 0.0011	-
1R33	19	0.0033 ± 0.0020	3.4
1R11	10	0.0034 ± 0.0022	3.5
24 weeks			
B6	18	0.022 ± 0.029	-
1R33	12	0.043 ± 0.040	2.0
1R11	9	0.033 ± 0.040	1.5
Experiment 2			
16 weeks			
B6	13	0.00071 ± 0.00062	-
2R8	12	0.0024 ± 0.0016	3.4
C3H	12	0.012 ± 0.011	17
24 weeks			
B6	12	0.0042 ± 0.0042	-
2R8	12	0.014 ± 0.012	3.3
C3H	11	0.14 ± 0.093	33

Table 2. Distal Chromosome 1 alleles influence net lesion growth before 16 weeks.

Male mice were treated at 12 days of age with DEN and sacrificed at 16 or 24 weeks of age. Frozen liver sections were evaluated for the presence and size distribution of glucose-6-phosphatase-deficient foci. N, number of animals per group; VF ratio, volume fraction ratio relative to B6.

3.7 *Hcs7* does not modify apoptosis or mitosis in the acute response to DEN injection

Other modifiers of DEN-induced hepatocarcinogenesis, such as IL-6 and IKKgamma, have been shown to affect apoptosis and/or mitosis within 72 hours of DEN administration (Maeda et al., 2005; Naugler et al., 2007). To determine whether the tumor susceptibility conferred by the *Hcs7* region affects mitosis or apoptosis rates during this acute response to DEN injection, we collected livers from line 2R8 males one, two, or three days after DEN injection at 12 days of age. Livers were fixed in formalin and stained with H&E. Mitoses and apoptoses were scored based on staining and morphology, under 600× magnification. Two microscopic fields centered on a portal vein and two fields centered on a central vein were scored. Hepatocytes were counted for 10-25 fields per strain and condition (*e.g.*, B6/DEN). Each field represented an equivalent number of hepatocytes per field (~330) in resistant and susceptible mice, independent of DEN treatment ($P > 0.07$ for all comparisons).

Rates of mitosis and apoptosis never differed significantly between B6 and line 2R8, whether or not mice were treated with DEN ($P > 0.10$ for all comparisons; Table 3). These results indicate that the tumorigenic effect of *Hcs7* does not involve acute changes in the rates of apoptosis or mitosis in response to DEN injection.

		Num. mice		Mitoses / field		Apoptoses / field	
Age	**Treatment**	**B6**	**2R8**	**B6**	**2R8**	**B6**	**2R8**
13 days	No DEN	7	11	1.50	1.25	0.50	0.50
14 days	No DEN	9	9	2.00	1.5	0.25	0.50
15 days	No DEN	7	8	1.40	1.00	0.30	0.25
13 days	DEN	7	7	0.5	0.5	0.30	0.25
14 days	DEN	9	11	2.25	2.50	0.25	0.50
15 days	DEN	7	12	2.00	1.85	0.50	0.55

Table 3. Mitosis and apoptosis do not differ significantly between line 2R8 and B6 during tumor initiation.

3.8 The *Hcs7*-interval genes most differentially expressed between C3H and B6 are immune genes

To identify potential candidate genes and pathways regulated by the *Hcs7* region, we collected livers from DEN-treated B6 and 2R8 mice at 13 days, 28 hours after DEN injection. RNA from these livers was reverse-transcribed and hybridized to Agilent whole-genome arrays, in competition with a B6 mixed-sex control, to identify differentially expressed genes. These arrays carry 43,379 probes representing most genes in the genome. Of the 44 genes in the 175.35 to 178.64 Mb region, 35 are represented by probes. The remaining nine include genes for three spliceosomal RNAs, two olfactory receptors, one protein of unknown function, and three pyrin-domain-containing genes. Genome-wide, *Ifi202b* is the only significantly differentially expressed transcript based on FDR correction ($q < 10^{-2}$). The expression of *Ifi202b* is 57-fold higher in line 2R8 than in B6.

To identify potential candidates that may not be expressed at 13 days, RNA from three B6 and three 2R8 tumors was reverse transcribed and hybridized individually in competition with the mixed-sex control DNA. Genome-wide, *Ifi202b* was again the only significantly differentially expressed transcript, with levels 48-fold higher in 2R8 tumors than in B6 tumors (genome-wide FDR $q < 0.05$). When limiting analysis of the expression array data set to only the 35 candidate genes in the 175.35 to 178.64 Mb minimal region, both *Ifi202b* and the closely related *Aim2* (*Absent in melanoma* 2) were expressed at significantly different levels ($q < 10^{-4}$ and $q < 10^{-2}$, respectively).

Recent resequencing of the C3H genome has revealed many SNPs in the *Hcs7* region. Data compiled by the Mouse Genome Database (MGD) at the Mouse Genome Informatics website (Blake et al., 2011; URL: http://www.informatics.jax.org; 8/2011) show that the C3H alleles of eight genes in the *Hcs7* region encode amino acids that differ from B6. *Ifi202b* carries a Thr/Ser polymorphism. The most dramatic changes lie in *Mndal*, which carries Arg/Gly and Asp/Tyr polymorphisms. Other genes in the interval with non-synonomous SNPs include *Olfr433, Olfr419, Olfr220, Fmn2, Chml,* and *Exo1*.

4. Discussion

The Chromosome 1 liver cancer modifier *Hcs7* has been localized to a 3.3 Mb region on distal Chromosome 1. In DEN-treated mice, the C3H allele of *Hcs7* bred onto a resistant B6 background confers 3- to 7-fold greater tumor multiplicity, dominantly. Consistent with these results, the B6 allele of *Hcs7* bred onto a susceptible C3H background confers 4-fold resistance, recessively. Importantly, C3H alleles on Chromosome 1 including *Hcs7* confer susceptibility to spontaneous tumorigenesis that is comparable to the susceptibility of inbred C3H mice. The Chr 1 hepatocarcinogenesis susceptibility allele in C57BR/cdJ mice, *Hcif2*, does not appear to correspond to *Hcs7*. B6.BR mice congenic for BR alleles distal of 170 Mb are not more susceptible to liver tumorigenesis than B6 mice.

The initiation of tumors after DEN injection is thought to involve the proliferation of DEN-mutated hepatocytes in response to DEN-induced cell death, within 72 hours of injection (Maeda et al., 2005). We found that *Hcs7* affects neither apoptosis nor mitosis in this time period. We have previously shown that preneoplastic lesions in inbred C3H males grow faster than B6 lesions, and that this differential growth can be seen from prior to 16 weeks until at least 28 weeks of age (Hanigan et al., 1988). Here, we show that *Hcs7* accounts for part of this early growth advantage: the volume of preneoplastic lesions in the B6.C3H congenic lines 1R33 and 2R8 is greater than for B6 lesions by 16 weeks and remains so at 24 weeks. Our results indicate that *Hcs7* begins to affect cell proliferation after the acute reaction to DEN injection and likely tumor initiation, but before 16 weeks, to promote lesion growth.

The 175.35 to 178.64 Mb minimal interval carries 44 genes, of which 12 are related pyrin- and/or p200-domain-containing interferon-gamma response genes such as *Ifi202b*, *Aim2*, and *Mnda*. Two additional genes encode proteins that are known or likely to mediate immune responses (*Exo1* and the *Crp*-like gene 1810030J14Rik). This region also contains the cytoskeletal/cell polarity gene *Fmn2* that is overexpressed in B-cell leukemias, a renal cell cancer tumor suppressor (*Fh1*), four known or likely signaling protein genes, and 14 olfactory receptor genes.

Ifi202b is a strong candidate for the HCC modifier gene in the *Hcs7* locus. It was the only gene significantly differentially expressed on a genome-wide basis between B6.C3H^{Hcs7} congenics and B6 mice at 13 days of age (in the presence and absence of DEN) and in tumors from 32-week-old males. Importantly, CGH analysis indicates that the 5' end of *Ifi202b* is altered in the resistant B6.C3H congenic line 1R5, though the effect of this alteration on the protein or its expression still needs to be established. Finally, *Ifi202b* lies in the minimal susceptibility region determined by congenic lines, between 175.35 and 178.64 Mb. An important test of its candidacy will be to determine whether the CBA inbred strain, closely related to C3H and similarly susceptible to liver tumors, also expresses high levels of *Ifi202b*.

When only genes in the minimal susceptibility region were evaluated for differential expression in tumors, *Aim2* was the only other significantly differentially expressed gene. Aim2 is an interferon-regulated pro-apoptotic protein that is closely related to, can hetero-dimerize with, and affects the expression of *Ifi202b* (Panchanathan et al., 2010; Choubey et al., 2010). Aim2 is a component of inflammasomes that sense cytoplasmic double-stranded DNA and activate caspase 1, which in turn activates IL1-β and induces inflammation (Fernandes-Alnemri et al., 2009; Bürckstümmer et al., 2009).

In transfected macrophage cell lines, *Ifi202b* overexpression reduces *Aim2* expression, and *Aim2* knock-down increases *Ifi202b* expression (Panchanathan et al., 2010). Similarly, *Aim2* null mice overexpress *Ifi202b* in spleen tissue. Absence of *Aim2* expression correlates with cell growth *in vitro* and with cell immortalization *in vitro*, and *Aim2* is inactivated in approximately half of colon cancers with microsatellite instability (Woerner et al., 2007; Choubey et al., 2010). Therefore, high levels of *Ifi202b* may prevent *Aim2* expression and induce growth. Both *Aim2* and *Ifi202b* were overexpressed in line 2R8 tumors relative to B6 tumors. This result may reflect a tumor-specific response, as 13-day-old line 2R8 mice did not express more *Aim2* than B6 mice.

The high expression of *Ifi202b* in line 2R8 mice relative to B6 might reflect promoter and/or enhancer polymorphisms in both *Aim2* and *Ifi202b*. The NZB allele of *Ifi202b* has been shown to be more active than the B6 allele, most likely due to a TATA-box-creating polymorphism in the NZB *Ifi202b* promoter (Choubey et al., 2010). Analysis of congenic lines suggests that B6-specific polymorphisms, conversely, enhance the expression of *Aim2*. Autoimmune-sensitive congenics carrying NZB alleles from 154.7 to ~194 Mb express high levels of *Ifi202b* mRNA and protein relative to B6. However, mice from a line that carries a smaller NZB congenic region between approximately 174.5 to 194 Mb – including the entire *Aim2* gene at 175.2 Mb and the entire *Ifi202b* gene at 175.9 Mb – are not predisposed to autoimmunity. These resistant congenic mice express more *Aim2* mRNA and protein and less *Ifi202b* mRNA and protein than the larger congenic. Indeed, levels of Ifi202b protein are similar to those of B6 mice (Panchanathan et al., 2010). The breakpoint between B6 and NZB alleles in this smaller congenic lies less than one megabase proximal of *Aim2*. The effect of B6 polymorphisms near the 5' end of the *Aim2* gene on *Aim2* expression and, indirectly, *Ifi202b* expression may also explain the resistance to hepatocarcinogenesis of line 2R9. Assessing *Aim2* and *Ifi202b* mRNA and protein levels in lines 2R8, 2R16, 2R9, and 2R7 would address this hypothesis.

Interferon-inducible p200 family members have been shown to interact functionally with p53, MyoD, and Rb and appear to regulate proliferation, differentiation, apoptosis, and senescence (Gariglio et al., 2011). Overexpression of *Ifi202b* in particular has been shown to promote cell survival, while lower levels of expression increase cell death (Roberts et al., 2009; Choubey et al., 2010). The expression of *Ifi202b* is upregulated by IL-6, which has been shown to be virtually required for hepatocarcinogenesis in DEN-treated mice, and *Ifi202b* can stimulate or inhibit the transcription of NFκB target genes depending on cell type (Naugler et al., 2007; Choubey et al., 2010). Given these many cell regulatory functions and its effect on *Aim2* expression, *Ifi202b* could promote lesion growth in multiple ways. Determining whether preneoplastic cells in lines carrying C3H alleles undergo less cell death, an increase in mitosis, or both, will be an important first step in assessing the oncogenicity of *Hcs7*.

Based on genome-wide analysis, no genes other than *Ifi202b* were significantly differentially expressed. However, nine genes were not represented on the expression array. These include several unlikely candidates (olfactory receptors and splicing RNAs that are found throughout the genome), as well as the pyrin/p200 proteins *BC094916*, *Pydc3*, and *Mndal*. The expression of these genes and the effect of amino acid changes in genes in the region will need to be evaluated. Finally, the test of *Ifi202b* as a candidate will require its over-expression (*e.g.*, from a transgene) in B6, or its disruption in C3H.

If Ifi202b is the molecule responsible for promoting hepatocarcinogenesis in mice carrying C3H *Hcs7* alleles, it would make a tempting target for pharmacological intervention. The *Hcs7* region corresponds to parts of human chromosome 1q22-23.1 and 1q43. Chromosome 1q, including these regions, is amplified in 58% to 86% of human hepatocellular carcinomas, independent of stage (Thorgeirsson and Grisham, 2002; Lau and Guan, 2005; Chochi et al., 2009; Zhang et al., 2010). When only parts of 1q are amplified, 1q22-23 is frequently affected. These observations imply that chromosome 1q alterations are an early event in hepatocarcinogenesis. Chromosome 1q is also frequently amplified in other liver cancers such as hepatoblastoma, cholangiocarcinoma, and fibrolamellar carcinoma, as well as cancers of other tissues such as the pancreas and the breast (Buendia, 2002; Climent et al., 2002; Birnbaum et al., 2011; Ward and Waxman, 2011). Humans have four homologs of *Ifi202b* in the 1q22-23.1 region, including an ortholog of *Aim2*, an ortholog of *Mnda*, *Ifi16* and *IfiX/Pyhin1* (www.ensembl.org; 9/2011; Gariglio et al., 2011). All of these genes have been implicated in growth suppression in cell lines and ectopic tumor models; however, *Ifi16* in particular is also associated *in vivo* with rapidly dividing epithelium and with undifferentiated tissue including fetal hepatocytes and hepatocytes following liver transplantation (Gariglio et al., 2011). In an analysis of gene expression in a human tumor carrying a 1q amplification, four chromosome 1 genes were overexpressed. Only two of these correspond to mouse Chromosome 1: *Mnda* and "interferon-gamma inducible gene" at 1q22 (*Ifi16* or *IfiX*; Niketeghad et al., 2001). All four *Ifi* p200 human genes express transcripts that encode both the pyrin cell death and p200 protein interaction domains (www.ensembl.org; 9/2011). Each also expresses transcripts that carry only one of the domains, and *Ifi16* in particular expresses transcripts that carry only the pyrin domain, only the p200 domain, or both. These many alternative transcripts suggest the possibility that one of them is orthologous to *Ifi202b*, which expresses only the p200 domain. An analysis of human tumors should reveal which p200 family transcripts they express. Transgenesis could then be used to test the oncogenicity of these selected transcripts.

C3H alleles from several regions of mouse Chromosome 1 conferred some significant susceptibility to B6 mice. Similarly, several regions on human chromosome 1 are amplified, sometimes simultaneously but separately, in human tumors (Lau and Guan, 2005; Chochi et al., 2009). It seems likely that multiple genes on Chromosome 1 in both mice and humans affect hepatocarcinogenesis.

5. Conclusion

We have mapped the mouse *Hcs7* liver cancer modifier to a 3.3 Mb region on distal Chromosome 1 that carries 44 genes, of which many are involved in responding to immune stimuli. This region corresponds to human chromosome 1q22-23.1, which is amplified in most hepatocellular carcinomas. *Ifi202b* is a strong candidate gene for the *Hcs7* modifier. Further study of the effect of its overexpression or disruption *in vivo* on short-term proliferation or apoptosis and long-term hepatocarcinogenesis will help establish whether its possible functional equivalent on human chromosome 1q is a worthy target for pharmacological intervention.

6. Acknowledgements

The authors would like to thank Drs. Henry Pitot and Ruth Sullivan for liver histopathology training and diagnoses. We thank Bradley Stewart (McArdle) for microarray processing and the Lab Animal Resources technicians for animal care. We thank Christopher Oberley for reading the manuscript and Matt Gigot, Kim Luetkehoelter, Tonia Jorgenson, Manching Leung, Heather Sturm, Katie Halser, Carl Koschmann, Henri Kurniawan, Jessica Linzmeyer, Myrra Windau, Fatima Ashraf, Bridget Borg, and Eric Simpson for their contributions. This work was supported by grants from the U.S. National Institutes of Health (CA22484, CA96654, CA07175, CA09135, and CA14520).

7. References

Bilger, A., Bennett, L.M., Carabeo, R.A., Chiaverotti, T.A., Dvorak, C., Liss, K.M., Schadewald, S.A., Pitot, H.C. & Drinkwater, N.R. (2004). A potent modifier of liver cancer risk on distal mouse chromosome 1: linkage analysis and characterization of congenic lines. *Genetics,* Vol. 167, No. 2, pp. (859–866)

Birnbaum, D.J., Adelaide, J., Mamessier, E., Finetti, P., Lagarde, A., Monges, G., Viret, F., Goncalves, A., Turrini, O., Delpero, J.-P., Iovanna, J., Giovannini, M., Birnbaum, D., & Chaffanet, M. (2011). Genome Profiling of Pancreatic Adenocarcinoma. *Genes, Chromosomes & Cancer,* Vol. 50, pp. (456–465)

Blake, J.A., Bult, C.J., Kadin, J.A., Richardson, J.E., Eppig, J.T., & the Mouse Genome Database Group. (2011). The Mouse Genome Database (MGD): premier model organism resource for mammalian genomics and genetics. *Nucleic Acids Res,* Vol. 39, Suppl. 1, pp. (D842-D848)

Buendia, M.A. (2002). Genetic Alterations in Hepatoblastoma and Hepatocellular Carcinoma: Common and Distinctive Aspects. *Med Pediatr Oncol,* 2002,Vol. 39, pp. (530–535)

Bugni, J.M., Poole, T.M., & Drinkwater, N.R. (2001). The little mutation suppresses DEN-induced hepatocarcinogenesis in mice and abrogates genetic and hormonal modulation of susceptibility. *Carcinogenesis,* Vol. 22, No. 11, pp. (1853-1862)

Bürckstümmer, T., Baumann, C., Blüml, S., Dixit, E., Dürnberger, G., Jahn, H., Planyavsky, M., Bilban, M., Colinge, J., Bennett, K.L., & Superti-Furga, G. (2009) An orthogonal proteomic-genomic screen identifies AIM2 as a cytoplasmic DNA sensor for the inflammasome. *Nature Immunology,* Vol. 10, pp. (266 - 272)

Chochi, Y., Kawauchi, S., Nakao, M., Furuya, T., Hashimoto, K., Oga, A., Oka, M., & Sasaki, K. (2009). A copy number gain of the 6p arm is linked with advanced hepatocellular carcinoma: an array-based comparative genomic hybridization study. *J Pathol,* Vol. 217, No. 5, pp. (677-684)

Choubey, D., Duan, X., Dickerson, E., Ponomareva, L., Panchanathan, R., Shen, H., & Ratika Srivastava. (2010). Interferon-Inducible p200-Family Proteins as Novel Sensors of Cytoplasmic DNA: Role in Inflammation and Autoimmunity. *J Interferon Cytokine Res.,* Vol. 30, No. 6, pp. (371–380)

Climent, J., Martinez-Climent, J. A., Blesa, D., Garcia-Barchino M. J., & Saez R. *et al.* (2002). Genomic loss of 18p predicts an adverse clinical outcome in patients with high-risk breast cancer. *Clin. Cancer Res.,* Vol. 8, pp. (3863–3869)

Dragani, T. A. (2010). Risk of HCC: Genetic heterogeneity and complex genetics. *Journal of Hepatology,* Vol. 52, pp. (252–257)

Drinkwater, N.R., & Ginsler, J.J. (1986). Genetic control of hepatocarcinogenesis in C57BL/6J and C3H/HeJ inbred mice. *Carcinogenesis,* Vol. 7, No. 10, pp. (1701-1707)

Fernandes-Alnemri, T., Yu, J.-W., Datta, P., Wu, J., & Alnemri, E.S. (2009). AIM2 activates the inflammasome and cell death in response to cytoplasmic DNA. *Nature,* Vol. 458, pp. (509-513)

Gariglio, M., Mondini, M., De Andrea, M., & Landolfo, S. (2011). The Multifaceted Interferon-Inducible p200 Family Proteins: From Cell Biology to Human Pathology. *Journal of Interferon & Cytokine Research,* Vol. 31, No. 1, pp. (159-172)

Hanigan, M.H., Kemp, C.J., Ginsler, J.J., & Drinkwater, N.R. (1988). Rapid growth of preneoplastic lesions in hepatocarcinogen-sensitive C3H/HeJ male mice relative to C57BL/6J male mice. *Carcinogenesis,* Vol. 9, No. 6, pp. (885-890)

Kirkpatrick, M. (2010). How and Why Chromosome Inversions Evolve. *PLoS Biol,* Vol. 8, No. 9, (e1000501)

Lau, S.-H., & Guan, X.-Y. (2005). Cytogenetic and molecular genetic alterations in hepatocellular carcinoma. *Acta Pharmacologica Sinica,* Vol. 26, No. 6, pp. (659–665)

Maeda, S., Kamata, H., Luo, J. L., Leffert, H. & Karin, M. (2005). IKK-beta couples hepatocyte death to cytokine-driven compensatory proliferation that promotes chemical hepatocarcinogenesis. *Cell,* Vol. 121, pp. (977–990)

Montalto, G., Cervello, M., Giannitrapani, L., Dantona, F., Terranova, A., & Castagnetta, L.A.M. (2002). Epidemiology, Risk Factors, and Natural History of Hepatocellular Carcinoma. *Ann. N.Y. Acad. Sci.,* Vol. 963, pp. (13–20)

Naugler, W.E., Sakurai, T., Kim, S., Maeda, S., Kim, K,-H., Elsharkawy, A.M., & Karin, M. (2007). Gender Disparity in Liver Cancer Due to Sex Differences in MyD88-Dependent IL-6 Production. *Science,* Vol. 317, No. 5834, pp. (121-124)

Niketeghad, F., Decker, H.J., Caselmann, W.H., Lund, P., Geissler, F., Dienes, H.P., & P Schirmacher. (2001). Frequent genomic imbalances suggest commonly altered tumour genes in human hepatocarcinogenesis. *British Journal of Cancer,* Vol. 85, No. 5, pp. (697–704)

Panchanathan, R., Duan, X., Shen, H., Rathinam, V.A.K., Erickson, L.D., Fitzgerald, K.A., & Choubey, D. (2010). Aim2 deficiency stimulates the expression of IFN-inducible Ifi202, a lupus susceptibility murine gene within the Nba2 autoimmune susceptibility locus. *Journal of Immunology,* Vol. 185, pp. (7385-7393)

Panchanathan., R., Shen, H., Duan, X., Rathinam, V.A., Erickson, L.D., Fitzgerald, K.A., Choubey, D.J. (2011). Aim2 deficiency in mice suppresses the expression of the inhibitory Fcgamma receptor (FcgammaRIIB) through the induction of the IFN-inducible p202, a lupus susceptibility protein. *Immunol,* Vol. 186, No. 12, pp. (6762-6770)

Peychal, S.E., Bilger, A., Pitot, H.C., & Drinkwater, N.R. (2009). Predominant modifier of extreme liver cancer susceptibility in C57BR/cdJ female mice localized to 6 Mb on chromosome 17. *Carcinogenesis,* Vol. 30, No. 5, pp. (879-885)

Poole, T.M., & Drinkwater, N.R. (1996) Two genes abrogate the inhibition of murine hepatocarcinogenesis by ovarian hormones. *Proc Natl Acad Sci U S A,* Vol. 93, No. 12, pp. (5848–5853)

Roberts, T.L., Idris, A., Dunn, J.A., Kelly, G.M., Burnton, C.M., Hodgson, S., Hardy, L.L., Garceau, V., Sweet, M.J., Ross, I.L., Hume, D.A., & Stacey, K.J. (2009). HIN-200 Proteins Regulate Caspase Activation in Response to Foreign Cytoplasmic DNA. *Science,* Vol. 323, No. 5917, pp. (1057-1060)

Santos, G.C., Zielenska, M., Prasad, M., & Squire, J A. (2007). Chromosome 6p amplification and cancer progression. *J Clin Pathol,* Vol. 60, pp. (1–7)

Shih, W.-L., Yu, M.-W., Chen, P.-J., Wu, T.-W., Lin, C.-L., Liu, C.-J., Lin, S.-M., Tai, D.-I., Lee, S.-D. & Liaw, Y.-F. (2009). Evidence for association with hepatocellular carcinoma at the *PAPSS1* locus on chromosome 4q25 in a family-based study. *Eur J Hum Genet,* Vol. 17, No. 10, pp. (1250–1259)

Smyth, G.K. (2004). Linear models and empirical Bayes methods for assessing differential expression in microarray experiments. *Statistical Applications in Genetics and Molecular Biology* 3, No. 1, Article 3.

Szatkiewicz, J.P., Beane, G.L., Ding, Y., Hutchins, L., Pardo-Manuel de Villena, F., & Churchill, G.A. (2008). An Imputed Genotype Resource for the Laboratory Mouse. *Mamm. Genome,* Vol. 19, pp. (199-208)

Thorgeirsson, S.S., & Grisham, J.W. (2002). Molecular pathogenesis of human hepatocellular carcinoma. *Nature Genetics,* Vol. 31, No. 4, pp. (339-346)

Truett, G.E., Heeger, P., Mynatt, R.L., Truett, A.A., Walker, J.A., & Warman, M.L. (2000). Preparation of PCR-quality mouse genomic DNA with hot sodium hydroxide and tris (HotSHOT). *Biotechniques,* Vol. 29, pp. (52–54)

Wan, D., He, M., Wang, J., Qiu, X., Zhou, W., Luo, Z., Chen, J., & Gu, J. (2004). Two Variants of the Human Hepatocellular Carcinoma-Associated *HCAP1* gene and Their Effect on the Growth of the Human Liver Cancer Cell Line Hep3B. *Genes, Chromosomes & Cancer,* Vol. 39, pp. (48–58)

Ward, S.C., & Waxman, S. (2011). Fibrolamellar carcinoma: a review with focus on genetics and comparison to other malignant primary liver tumors. *Semin Liver Dis,* Vol. 31, No. 1, pp. (61-70)

Woerner, S.M., Kloor, M., Schwitalle, Y., Youmans, H., von Knebel Doeberitz, M., Gebert, J., & Dihlmann, S. (2007) The Putative Tumor Suppressor AIM2 is Frequently Affected by Different Genetic Alterations in Microsatellite Unstable Colon Cancers. *Genes, Chromosomes & Cancer,* Vol. 46, No. (1080–1089)

Zhang, S.-G., Song, W.-Q., Gao, Y.-T., Yang, B., & Du, Z. (2010). CD1d gene is a target for a novel amplicon at 1q22–23.1 in human hepatocellular carcinoma. *Molecular Biology Reports,* Vol. 37, No. 1, pp. (381-387)

3

Signaling Pathways in Liver Cancer

Xinle Wu and Yang Li
Amgen Inc.
USA

1. Introduction

Hepatocellular carcinoma (HCC) is the sixth most common type of cancer in the world, with approximately 630,000 new cases each year (Alves et al., 2011). It is also the third most common cause of cancer related mortality (Parkin et al., 2005). Moreover, the incidence of HCC has risen in many countries over the past decade. The greatest risk factor associated with the development of HCC is hepatitis B and C virus infection. Hepatitis infection is believed to increase the risk of developing HCC by 20 fold and is the major etiological factor in more than 80% of HCC cases (Anzola, 2004). Other main risk factors include excessive alcohol consumption, non alcoholic steatohepatitis, exposure to environmental toxins such as aflatoxin B, hemochromatosis, cirrhosis, diabetes and obesity (El-Serag et al., 2006; Hassan et al., 2010; Whittaker et al., 2010).

The standard treatments for early stage HCC, such as surgical resection and liver transplantation, can cure certain population of patients. However, due to the asymptomatic nature of early HCC and lack of effective screening strategies, 80% of patients present with advanced HCC at the time of diagnosis (Thomas and Abbruzzese, 2005). These patients have rather limited treatment options which are mainly palliative. If the patient has developed HCC that is surgical unresectable, systemic treatments are commonly used. However, conventional chemotherapy with cytotoxic agents is not very effective in changing the progress of the tumor growth. Consequently, the mortality rate for advanced stage HCC is quite high, and 5 year survival rate for patients with HCC is only 7% (Bosch et al., 2004; Whittaker et al., 2010). There is clearly an urgent medical need to develop new effective and well-tolerated HCC treatment options.

In recent decades, tremendous progress has been made toward better understanding the molecular mechanisms of oncogenic processes. Many cell signaling pathways involved in tumor pathogenesis have been identified, leading to the identification of new molecular targets for therapeutic development. Unlike conventional chemotherapy which utilizes broad spectrum cytotoxic agents, targeted therapy acts directly and specifically on the components that regulate tumorigenesis. This strategy has shown clinical benefits in various tumor types, such as breast, colorectal and lung cancers (Ansari et al., 2009; Slamon et al., 2001; Takahashi and Nishioka, 2011). Several major cellular signaling pathways have been implicated in HCC, and below we will review those pathways and discuss the potential to target the molecular components within those signaling pathways.

2. Major signaling pathways

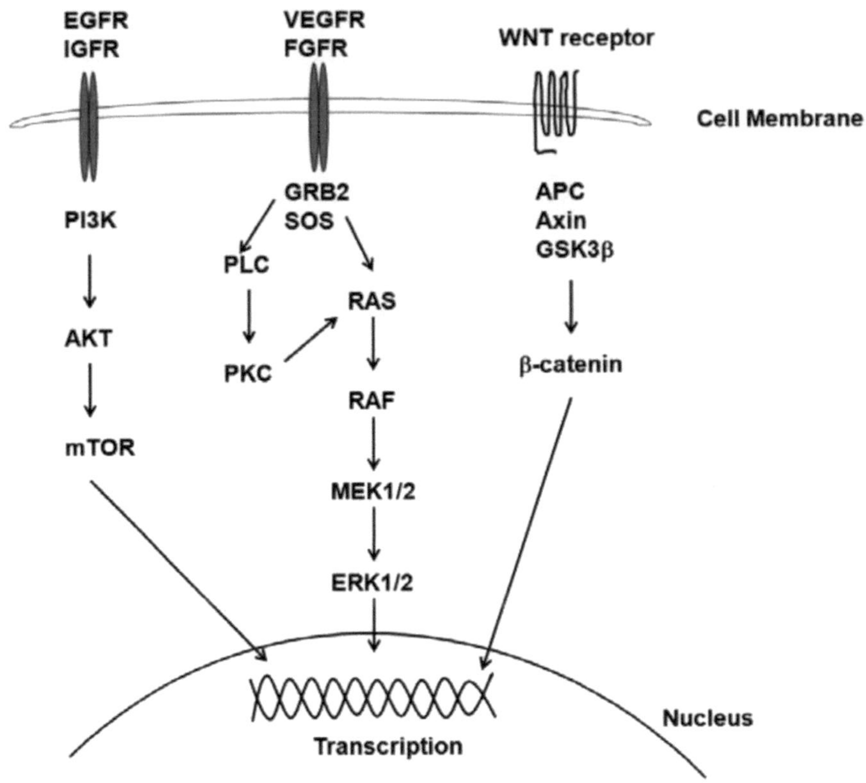

Fig. 1. Major cellular signaling pathways involved in hepatocellular carcinoma tumorigenesis

2.1 Wnt/β-catenin pathway

Wnt signaling pathway involves three main components which include the cell surface, the cytoplasm, and the nucleus (Giles et al., 2003). At the cell membrane, Wnt ligands form complexes with Frizzled receptors and LRP5 or LRP6 co-receptors (Dale, 1998; Wehrli et al., 2000). There are at least 19 known human Wnt family genes and 10 Frizzled family genes, and most Wnt proteins can bind to multiple Frizzled receptors and vice versa (Wang et al., 1996). This ligand receptor interaction can be additionally regulated by other secreted factors and cell surface proteins. For example, soluble forms of Frizzled proteins compete with cell membrane Frizzled receptor for Wnt ligands (Finch et al., 1997). And DKK proteins block Wnt signaling by binding to LRP6 co-receptor (Fedi et al., 1999).

In the cytoplasm, β-catenin associates with a multiprotein complex which includes tumor suppressor proteins APC, axin, and Ser/Thr kinase GSK3β. Axin and APC form a structural scaffold that allows GSK3 β to phosphorylate β-catenin. Phosphorylation of β-catenin targets it for ubiquitination and protein degradation (Clevers, 2006; Gordon and Nusse, 2006). Therefore, under basal conditions, in the absence of Wnt ligands, β-catenin is continuously degraded in the cytosol. Upon Wnt binding, axin is recruited to the membrane to LPR5 and the β-catenin destruction complex is then inactivated. This allows the unphosphorylated β-catenin to accumulate and to translocate into the nucleus (Clevers, 2006; Gordon and Nusse, 2006). The nuclear β-catenin then forms a complex with TCF/LEF family of DNA binding transcription factors to activate TCF/LEF target genes. Many of the target genes are involved in cell proliferation, such as cyclin D1 (Shtutman et al., 1999).

Besides regulating gene transcription, β-catenin also participates in cell–cell adhesion. Cell-cell adhesion and separation are important physiological processes involved in development as well as tumor metastasis. It is known that cadherin mediated adhesion is regulated by β-catenin. The formation of stable cell–cell adhesions depends on the integrity of a core complex including E-cadherin, β-catenin and α-catenin. β-catenin binds directly to the cytoplasmic domain of E-cadherin and such association is regulated by the phosphorylation state of β-catenin (Nelson and Nusse, 2004).

Wnt signaling clearly plays important roles in normal liver function as 8 out of the total 19 Wnt ligands are expressed in hepatocytes (Thompson and Monga, 2007). Both LRP5 and LRP6 and 9 of 10 Frizzled receptors are expressed in normal liver (Fujino et al., 2003; Zeng et al., 2007). Evidence has suggested that the Wnt signaling pathway is critically involved in liver development and postnatal liver homeostasis. In addition, this pathway is also associated with many other important liver functions, such as ammonia and nitrogen metabolism, bile acid homeostasis, drug detoxification and injury recovery (Behari, 2010; Takigawa and Brown, 2008).

Multiple lines of evidence link aberrant Wnt signaling to HCC. Wnt signaling pathway activation is frequently reported in liver carcinoma. It has been demonstrated that there are significant changes in subcellular localization of β-catenin and β-catenin-associated cell adhesion molecules in HCC (Ihara et al., 1996). Studies have shown that 50-70% of liver tumors have increased levels of β-catenin in the cytoplasm and in the nucleus (Wong et al., 2001). Such accumulation can potentially provide tumor cells a growth advantage by promoting proliferation and inhibiting differentiation. A transgenic mouse model overexpressing β-catenin developed severe hepatomegaly (Giles et al., 2003). There are also studies associating β-catenin mutations or activation with worsened HCC outcome such as larger tumor size and increased vascular invasion (Behari, 2010).

Accumulation and stabilization of β-catenin could be a direct result from point mutations or deletions in the β-catenin gene, which is found in 12-26% of HCC (Giles et al., 2003). Such dominant gain-of-function mutations usually occur at the N-terminal phosphorylation sites on β-catenin, including the sites phosphorylated by GSK3β that regulate β-catenin degradation (Takigawa and Brown, 2008). Mutations at these positions disrupt recognition by GSK3β resulting in more stable β-catenin protein. Besides gain of function mutations in positive modulators of Wnt signaling such as β-catenin, the Wnt pathway can also be activated from loss-of function mutations in negative modulators such as Axin and APC (Takigawa and Brown, 2008). However, frequencies of β-catenin accumulation in HCC determined by immunostaining are much higher than the known incidence of Wnt pathway mutations. Thus, other causes of β-catenin accumulation may also exist. Epigenetic changes could be a contributing factor, which leads to higher gene expression without any mutations in the gene (Takigawa and Brown, 2008).

Although there is little doubt about the strong correlation between aberrant Wnt signaling and HCC, the precise role of activated Wnt pathway in the pathogenesis of liver tumor is less well understood. It has been shown that pharmacologic inhibition of β-catenin decreases survival of hepatoma cells (Behari et al., 2007). Inactivation of β-catenin suppressor APC led to spontaneous development of HCC in a mice model, suggesting the direct contribution from activated Wnt signaling to hepatocarcinogenesis (Colnot et al., 2004). However mice overexpressing a gain-of-function β-catenin mutant (exon 3 deletion) only showed increased susceptibility to developing HCC after exposure to carcinogen diethylnitrosamine (DEN), instead of developing spontaneous liver tumor (Harada et al., 2002). These results suggest that the role of the Wnt pathway in the development of liver cancer is highly context-dependent and involves cross-talk with other pathways. Nonetheless, components of the Wnt pathway may represent potential therapeutic intervention points for treating HCC.

Several approaches could be envisioned to target Wnt pathways. Extracellularly, it is possible to design molecules to disrupt Wnt ligand-receptor complexes, preventing initiation of the signaling events. For this approach, Wnt ligands, extracellular Wnt regulators such as DKKs, SFRPs proteins, and members of the receptor complexes can all be targeted. These proteins themselves or variants could be directly considered as candidates for drug developments. Alternatively, antibodies or other modalities that could block ligand receptor interactions may also be explored for therapeutic development. Intracellular components could also be targeted. Small molecule ligands toward kinases of the signaling pathway could also be screened that may regulate Wnt signaling. In addition, small molecule antagonists have been identified to interfere with the binding between β-catenin and TCF/LEF proteins or its coactivator CEBP, blocking downstream gene activation (Dahmani et al., 2011). However, due to the inherent complexity of Wnt signaling in the liver, further research is needed to fully understand the implications of therapeutic inhibition of the pathway in HCC.

2.2 VEGF pathway

Angiogenesis is critical for cancer development. Tumor cells require oxygen and nutrients for survival and proliferation and they need to be located within 100 to 200 μm from blood vessels to obtain an adequate supply of oxygen (Carmeliet and Jain, 2000). Solid tumors smaller than 1 to 2 cubic millimeters are not vascularized (Hawkins, 1995). However, beyond the critical volume of 2 cubic millimeters, new blood vessels need to be recruited to supply oxygen and nutrients and to remove metabolic wastes (Hawkins, 1995). Neovascularization also facilitates the dissemination of cancer cells throughout the entire body eventually leading to metastasis formation.

HCC is a hypervascular tumor and many pro-angiogenic factors are over-expressed in HCC cells and in the surrounding microenvironment (Shen et al., 2010). Among them, VEGF receptor signaling is one of the most well studied. The major VEGF that mediates tumor angiogenesis is VEGF-A, and it has several splicing variants that can be produced simultaneously. The most predominant forms are VEGF-A_{121} and VEGF-A_{165}. Other members in the VEGF family include Placenta growth factor (PlGF), VEGF-B, VEGF-C, and VEGF-D (Kaseb et al., 2009; Roskoski, 2007). VEGF signals through VEGF receptor (tyrosine kinase receptor) on the cell surface. There are three main subtypes of VEGF receptors, numbered 1, 2 and 3 (Kaseb et al., 2009; Roskoski, 2007). They all have an extracellular region consisting of 7 immunoglobulin-like domains, a single transmembrane domain, and an intracellular portion containing a split tyrosine-kinase domain. VEGF ligand binding induces dimerization and autophosphorylation of VEGF receptors. Phosphorylated tyrosine residues in the receptor serve as a docking site for various signal transduction proteins that can eventually activate cellular processes involved in angiogenesis. For example, VEGFR-2 phosphorylation activates PLC-γ which in turn leads to protein kinase C activation (PKC). PKC can activate MAP kinase signaling and promote cell proliferation as well as increase vascular permeability through activation of endothelial nitric oxide synthase (Kaseb et al., 2009; Roskoski, 2007). VEGF also induce activation of Rho GTPase, which plays a crucial role during angiogenesis processes such as vascular permeability, extra cellular matrix degradation, cellular migration and invasion (van der Meel et al., 2011).

Among the three VEGF receptors, VEGFR-2 appears to mediate almost all of the known cellular responses to VEGFs. The activation of VEGFR-2 in endothelial cells results in their proliferation, migration, and increased survival and promotes vascular permeability (Kaseb et al., 2009; Roskoski, 2007). The function of VEGFR-1 is less known. Although it has higher affinity for VEGF than VEFGR-2, it has weak tyrosine kinase phosphorylation activity following ligand stimulation. Activation of VEGFR-1 has no direct proliferative or cytoskeletal effects. It is possibly involved in modulating VEGFR-2 activity. VEGF-C and VEGF-D, but not VEGF-A, are ligands for a third receptor (VEGFR-3), which is important for lymphangiogenesis (Kaseb et al., 2009; Roskoski, 2007).

The VEGF pathway is clearly important for HCC pathogenesis. Expression of VEGF mRNA in liver tumors was found in a majority of HCC patients. And the expression of VEGF steadily increases with the progression of the hepatocarcinogenic process from a normal liver, to a dysplastic nodule, to HCC (Yamaguchi et al., 1998). The levels of VEGF mRNA expression in tumors with tumorous emboli and in poor-encapsulated tumors were higher than those without tumorous emboli and in well-encapsulated tumors. The principle route of HCC dissemination and metastasis is through the portal vein in the liver and VEGF mRNA level correlated well with portal vein tumor thrombus (PVTT) formation of HCC, suggesting VEGF may play an important role in HCC invasion and metastasis (Zhou et al., 2000). Immunohistochemical staining also detected very high VEGF expression in well-differentiated HCC as well as areas surrounding the HCC tissues, where inflammatory cell filtration was apparent. High serum VEGF levels have been shown to correlate with poor response to chemotherapy and poor survival among HCC patients. Increased preoperative serum VEGF may also predict high incidence of tumor recurrence after surgical resection (Whittaker et al., 2010). Furthermore, increased VEGF expression has also been detected in cirrhotic and dysplastic livers, which often lead to liver cancer (El-Assal et al., 1998).

The most direct evidence supporting the role of the VEGF signaling pathway in HCC came from recent progress in molecular targeted therapy inhibiting this pathway. Bevacizumab, an anti-VEGF monoclonal antibody was tested in patients with unresectable HCC and resulted in significant disease-stabilizing effect (Siegel et al., 2008). Clinical effects were assessed by tumor regression and progression-free survival (PFS). Of the 46 patients in the study, 13% had objective response and 65% were progression free at 6 months. The mean PFS time was 6.9 months and median overall survival time is 12.4 months. Overall survival rates were 53% at 1 year, 28% at 2 years and 23% at 3 years. Treatment was associated with significant reductions in tumor arterial enhancement and circulating VEGF-A level. Besides VEGF antibody, small molecule VEGF inhibitors have also been developed and tested in clinic. Sorafenib, an inhibitor targeting the VEGF pathway has been shown to prolong overall survival in patient with advanced HCC (Llovet et al., 2008). In a randomized, placebo-controlled phase III trial, sorafenib prolonged median survival time of advanced HCC patients by 2.8 months, from 7.9 months in the placebo group to 10.7 months in the sorafenib treatment group. Time to radiologic progression was delayed by 2.7 months, from 2.8 months to 5.5 months. This result is quite significant since no effective systemic therapy ever existed for patients with advanced hepatocellular carcinoma before the sorafenib trial. There are several other VEGF small molecule inhibitors that are currently being tested in the clinic for HCC treatment including, sunitinib, vatalanib, cediranib, brivanib, and linifanib (Shen et al., 2010; Whittaker et al., 2010). Studies have also been carried out to assess the benefit of the combined therapy using those compounds.

2.3 FGF pathway

Supported by various mouse genetic models as well as human genetic studies, aberrant FGF/FGFR signaling is clearly associated with tumorigenesis (Beenken and Mohammadi, 2009; Knights and Cook, 2010; Krejci et al., 2009; Turner and Grose, 2010). Signaling is activated upon FGF ligands binding to the FGF receptors on the cell surface. There are more than 20 different FGFs in the FGF family, making it the largest family of growth factors. Fibroblast growth factor receptors consist of an extracellular ligand binding domain, a single transmembrane domain, and an intracellular domain with tyrosine kinase activity. The extracellular domain of the FGF receptor is composed of three immunoglobin-like domains. Alternative splicing of four FGF receptors genes (FGFR1-4) results in over 48 different isoforms of FGFRs, and they have different affinity towards different FGF ligands and have distinct expression patterns (Ornitz and Itoh, 2001; Ornitz et al., 1996). FGFRs are tyrosine kinase receptors that upon ligand binding induce dimerization and kinase activation in the presence of the co-factor, heparan sulfate (Plotnikov et al., 1999). Phosphorylation of the tyrosine residues on the receptor provides docking sites for downstream adaptor proteins, which can couple to the activation of different intracellular signaling pathways. One of the key adaptor proteins of FGF receptors is FGF substrate 2 (FRS2) which can be phosphorylated by FGFR receptors and recruit more adaptor proteins such as son of sevenless (SOS) and growth factor receptor-bound 2 (GRB2) to activate RAS GTPase (Eswarakumar et al., 2005). RAS GTPase promotes several downstream signaling, such as Wnt, MAPK, and PI3K/Akt pathways (Knights and Cook, 2010). These FGF downstream signaling pathways have all been implicated in several aspects of tumorigenesis, such as proliferation, survival, cell migration and invasion, as well as angiogenesis (Balmanno and Cook, 2009; Dailey et al., 2005; Presta et al., 2005; Xian et al., 2005). In HCC, it has been shown that plasma FGF2 level was significantly increased (Hsu et al., 1997) and overexpression of FGFR1 in hepatocytes accelerated the growth of HCC chemically induced by DEN in a mouse model (Huang et al., 2006).

Recently, attention has focused on a unique FGF family member, FGF19, and its involvement in the development of HCC (Nicholes et al., 2002; Wu and Li, 2009). FGF19 belongs to a unique FGF subfamily that has weakened affinity towards heparan sulfate. The reduced affinity liberates FGF19 from tissues where it is expressed, allowing it to act as an endocrine hormone. Furthermore, FGF19 requires βKlotho as a co-receptor in activating FGF receptors. In the presence of βKlotho, FGF19 is able to activate similar downstream signaling through FGF receptors (Kurosu et al., 2007; Wu et al., 2007).

First evidence connecting FGF19 with HCC came from a transgenic FGF19 mice model, where human FGF19 driven by myosin promoters was overexpressed from skeleton muscle, resulting in elevated serum FGF19 protein levels (Nicholes et al., 2002). HCC development was observed in these FGF19 transgenic mice at 8-10 months, while no tumors were observed in wild type control mice. Tumors occurred in different liver lobes and were either solitary or multifocal. Histological staining showed neoplastic cells invasion and replacement of normal hepatocytes (Nicholes et al., 2002). Hepatocytes are normally mitotically quiescent in the liver. However, in case of HCC, hepatocellular proliferation is a prerequisite for transformation. In vivo 5-bromo-2'-deoxyuridine (BrdU) labeling was performed to assess the proliferation in FGF19 transgenic mice. BrdU-labeling index of hepatocytes was eight fold higher in the transgenic mice than age-matched wild type mice at 2 to 4 months of age (Nicholes et al., 2002). Furthermore, recombinant FGF19 protein also induced a significant higher BrdU-labeling index after being injected into normal mice (Nicholes et al., 2002; Wu et al., 2010a; Wu et al., 2010b). These results strongly support the notion that FGF19 can induce hepatocellular proliferation which eventually leads to development of HCC.

FGF19 is able to activate the Wnt pathway in hepatocytes, and 44% of neoplastic hepatocytes in FGF19 transgenic mice have nuclear staining for β-catenin (Nicholes et al., 2002; Pai et al., 2008). Since aberrant Wnt signaling correlates strongly with HCC tumorigenesis, this may be one mechanism whereby FGF19 induces liver tumor formation. To test the hypothesis of whether FGF19 could be a valid target in HCC treatment, a monoclonal anti-FGF19 antibody was generated and tested in tumor inhibition. Anti-FGF19 antibody or control antibody were used to treat DEN accelerated HCC formation in FGF19 transgenic mice (Desnoyers et al., 2008). After six months of antibody treatment, all the animals treated with control antibody developed multifocal, large HCCs throughout the liver lobes while almost none of the mice treated with FGF19 antibody had liver tumors. The same anti-FGF19 antibody was also tested in xenograft mice models (Desnoyers et al., 2008). Mice xenografted with colon cancer cell lines HCT116 and Colo201 were injected with anti-FGF19 antibody twice weekly. At day 35, FGF19 antibody suppressed tumor growth by 57% compared to the control in HCT116 group and 64% growth inhibition was achieved in Colo201 animals treated with the antibody. These data suggest that targeting FGF19 could be a valid strategy for HCC treatment.

The main candidate FGF receptor mediating FGF19 induced tumorigensis in liver is believed to be FGFR4, which is the predominant FGF receptor expressed in the liver. Strong FGFR4 mRNA was detected in hepatocytes adjacent to central vein by in situ hybridization, and the hepatic dysplasia foci and BrdU labeling from FGF19 transgenic livers are also located around central vein. In addition, activation of FGFR4 alone was sufficient to induce hepatocyte proliferation (Wu et al., 2010a; Wu et al., 2010b) and FGF19 induced hepatocytes proliferation was not observed in FGFR4 knockout mice, confirming the role played by FGFR4 in hepatocarcinogenesis (Wu et al., 2011).

FGFR4 has been implicated in HCC in many literature reports (Yang et al., 2011). FGFR4 is frequently overexpressed in patients with hepatocellular carcinoma (Yang et al., 2011). siRNA against FGFR4 in liver cancer lines HuH7 is able to suppress α-fetoprotein production (Yang et al., 2011). However, there have also been reports showing genetic deletion of FGFR4 in mice results in faster progression of DEN-accelerated hepatocellular carcinoma, suggesting that FGFR4 suppresses hepatoma proliferation (Huang et al., 2009). The contribution of FGFR4 in HCC progression requires further clarification.

2.4 MAPK pathway

Mitogen-activated protein kinase (MAPK) is serine-threonine kinase that is involved in a variety of cellular activities. There are three members in the mammalian MAPK family, extracellular signal-regulated kinase (ERK), c-Jun NH2-terminal kinase (JNK), and p38 (Kim and Choi, 2010; Min et al., 2011). Among them, ERK signaling pathway is the most studied for its involvement in promoting cell proliferation, migration, survival, and its association with tumorigenesis and tumor progression (Gollob et al., 2006). Recent data also implicate JNK and p38 as playing important roles during HCC development (Min et al., 2011).

The ERK pathway is ubiquitous and can be activated by various receptors, particularly receptor tyrosine kinases (RTKs). Upon ligand binding, the RTKs dimerize which leads to activation of the intracellular tyrosine kinase domain. Activated kinase results in receptor phosphorylation on tyrosine residues, that then serves as docking sites for adaptor proteins such as GRB2 and SOS (Schulze et al., 2005; Zarich et al., 2006). Upon docking to the receptors, the GRB2 and SOS activate the small GTPase RAS (HRAS, NRAS and KRAS) which in turn will activate the serine/threonine kinase RAF. RAF is a MAPK kinase kinase (MAP3K), and it has three isoforms, ARAF, BRAF and CRAF. Activated RAF will phosphorylate and activate MEK, a MAPK kinase (MAP2K) and MEK is the kinase for ERK (ERK1 and ERK2) (Avruch et al., 2001; Malumbres and Barbacid, 2003).

There are more than 100 substrates downstream of ERK, and many of them are transcription factors. The altered levels and activities of the transcription factors by ERK activation can lead to altered expression levels of genes that are important for cell cycle progression (Davis, 1995). For example, ERK can phosphorylate and activate C-myc, a transcription factor that regulates the expression of many target genes involved in cell growth and proliferation. C-Myc is a strong proto-oncogene and can be found unregulated in many types of cancers (Penn et al., 1990). ERK also directly phosphorylates kinase substrates such as myosin light chain kinase, calpain, and focal adhesion kinase, which promotes cell migration (Huang et al., 2004). Furthermore, the ERK pathway can regulate proteins involved in apoptotic pathway such as BIM and MCL1, promoting survival of cancer cells (Balmanno and Cook, 2009).

Given the contribution of ERK signaling towards cell proliferation, migration and survival, it is not surprising to see constitutive activation of the ERK pathway in many tumors. In fact, genes along the ERK pathway, such as HRAS, KRAS, and CRAF, are often upregulated in HCC. One study has shown that CRAF is overexpresed among all 30 HCC tissue samples tested (Hwang et al., 2004). Immunostaining also showed around 7 fold increase of MEK phosphorylation in HCC tissues compared to surrounding benign liver tissues (Huynh et al., 2003). Other studies also found that phosphorylated ERK level is higher in HCC tissues and ERK activation is associated with aggressive tumor behavior (Schmitz et al., 2008). In addition, negative regulator proteins of MAPK/ERK pathway such as Sprouty and DUSP1 are down-regulated in HCC tumors (Calvisi et al., 2008) (Yoshida et al., 2006). Sustained activation of ERK signaling can also occur due to point mutations in the RAS gene, which leads to constitutive CRAF activation (Downward, 2003; Whittaker et al., 2010). Mutation in the RAS gene has been reported in 10-30% of HCC tumors (Whittaker et al., 2010). The involvement of the ERK pathway in HCC is further confirmed by preclinical studies using the MEK inhibitor, AZD6244, which blocks proliferation and promotes apoptosis in primary HCC cells (Huynh et al., 2007a; Huynh et al., 2007b). AZD6244 also suppresses tumor growth in HCC xenograft model in a dose-dependent manner. And tumor growth inhibition after AZD6244 treatment correlates with inactivation of ERK, up-regulation of apoptotic genes such as caspase-3 and 7 and down-regulation of cell cycle regulators such as cyclin D1. It has also been shown that AZD6244 can induce a synergistic effect in tumor suppression when combined with chemotherapeutic agent doxorubicin (Huynh et al., 2007a; Huynh et al., 2007b).

JNK is another major MAPK signaling pathway. It can be activated by two MAPK kinases, MKK4 and MKK7, and its downstream substrates include c-Jun (Keshet and Seger, 2010). JNK signaling can be activated by various cytokines and environmental factors. It has been demonstrated that JNK1 and JNK2 regulate stress-induced apoptosis, and increased JNK activity has also been shown to enhance proliferation of mouse embryonic fibroblasts (MEFs) (Das et al., 2011). There is strong correlation between activated JNK signaling and HCC. For example, one study has shown that JNK1 is over-activated in 17 out of 31 samples (55%) from Chinese HCC patients (Chang et al., 2009). The activation in JNK1 is associated with increased tumor size and a lack of encapsulation of the tumors. In addition, JNK1 activation also associates with increased histone H3 lysines 4 and 9 tri-methylation, which leads to up-regulation of genes promoting cell growth (Chang et al., 2009).

Direct evidence demonstrating the role of JNK pathway in HCC development comes from studies in mouse models. JNK1 knockout mice had a significant reduction in liver tumorigenesis chemically induced by DEN and hepatocyte proliferation also decreased in those animals (Hui et al., 2008). It was proposed that mice lacking JNK1 have increased expression of p21, a cell cycle inhibitor. Blocking JNK activity using pharmacological inhibitor D-JNKI1 reduced growth of both xenografted human HCC cells and DEN-induced mouse liver cancers, further supporting the role played by JNK pathway in HCC development (Hui et al., 2008).

The activation of p38 is induced by MKK3, 4, and 6, as well as autophosphorylation. Its substrates include transcription factors such as p53 and protein kinases such as MK2 and MK5 (Min et al., 2011). Interestingly, unlike ERK and JNK pathways, p38 seems to play a suppressive role in HCC (Min et al., 2011). It was shown that human embryonic fibroblasts displayed enhanced proliferation upon treatment with a p38 inhibitor (SB203580) (Wang et al., 2002). p38 negatively regulates proliferation partly through suppression of the JNK pathway, which is known to promote cell proliferation. Depending upon the cellular context, p38 can enhance the protein level of JNK phosphatase and repress the activities of JNK kinases (Wagner and Nebreda, 2009). In p38 deficient fetal liver cells and liver tumor cells, the JNK pathway activity was found to be increased. Direct evidence supporting the suppressive role of p38 in HCC came from a study using mice with liver-specific deletion of p38, where enhanced hepatocyte proliferation and tumor development were observed during liver carcinogenesis (Hui et al., 2007). After DEN treatment, p38 deficient mice clearly developed more tumors in the liver and had larger average tumor size compared with control mice. Moreover, inactivation of JNK pathway with Δ-JNKI1 suppressed the hyperproliferation in p38-deficient animals (Hui et al., 2007).

In summary, numerous data have clearly demonstrated the deep involvement of MAPK signaling pathways during liver carcinogenesis. Identifying pharmacological intervention points along these pathways could be considered as a very promising strategy for combating HCC.

2.5 PI3k/AKT/mTOR pathway

Phosphoinositide 3 kinase (PI3K) is an intracellular signal transducer enzyme that can phosphorylate the hydroxyl group of phosphatidylinositol (Vanhaesebroeck and Waterfield, 1999). It belongs to a large family of PI3K-related kinases (Kuruvilla and Schreiber, 1999). PI3K is comprised of a catalytic subunit and a regulatory subunit. The regulatory subunit p85 can interact with phosphotyrosines on activated RTKs that recruit the enzyme to the plasma membrane and activate the enzymatic activities (Paez and Sellers, 2003). PI3K produces the lipid second messenger phosphatidylinosoltriphosphate, which is absent in resting cells but can be acutely produced in response to activated PI3K (Vanhaesebroeck and Waterfield, 1999).

Akt is a serine-threonine kinase downstream of PI3K. It contains a pleckstrin homology (PH) domain in the N-terminus, a central catalytic kinase domain and a C-terminus regulatory domain (Paez and Sellers, 2003). The PH domain will bind to phosphatidylinosoltriphosphate with high affinity. Upon PI3K activation and phosphatidylinosoltriphosphate production, Akt is recruited to the plasma membrane through its PH domain together with another PH domain containing protein, phosphoinositide dependent kinase 1 (PDK1). PDK1 then phosphorylate key residues in the kinase domain activation loop of Akt to activate Akt kinase activity (Paez and Sellers, 2003).

Activated Akt phosphorylates multiple protein substrates and regulates a variety of critical cellular activities (Paez and Sellers, 2003; Whittaker et al., 2010). Mammalian target of rapamycin (mTOR) is one of the most important downstream effectors of Akt. Akt phosphorylates the tuberous sclerosis complex (TSC1/TSC2) which activates the small G protein, Ras homolog enriched in brain (Rheb). Rheb, in its GTP-bound state, can activate mTOR. mTOR is a serine-threonine protein kinase that also belongs to PI3K-related kinase family. It is a large protein consists of tandem HEAT repeats, FAT (FRAP-ATM-TRRAP) and FATC (FAT C-terminus) domains, FKBP12-rapamycin binding domain (FRB), and C-terminus catalytic kinase domain that resembles the catalytic domain of PI3K (Wullschleger et al., 2006). For mTOR to activate its signaling cascade, it must form the ternary complex mTORC1 (mTOR Complex-1) or mTORC2 (mTOR Complex-2), but mTOR is the catalytic subunit of both of these two complexes. mTORC1 complex contains mTOR, RAPTOR (Regulatory Associated Protein of mTOR), mammalian LST8/G-protein β-subunit like protein (mLST8/GβL), PRAS40 and DEPTOR. mTORC2 complex consists of mTOR, rapamycin-insensitive companion of mTOR (Rictor), GβL, and mammalian stress-activated protein kinase interacting protein 1 (mSIN1) (Wullschleger et al., 2006; Paez and Sellers, 2003).

Another very important component of PI3K/Akt/mTOR pathway is PTEN (phosphatase and tensin homolog). It consists of a phosphatase domain which carries out the enzymatic function and a C2 domain which binds the phospholipid membrane. PTEN dephosphorylates phosphatidylinosoltriphosphate and serves as a negative regulator of PI3K/AKT/mTOR pathway (Paez and Sellers, 2003).

mTOR controls several important cellular processes including regulation of protein translation. Abberent protein translation often leads to abnormal cell growth and tumorigenesis (Petroulakis et al., 2006; Wullschleger et al., 2006). mTOR enhances translation initiation via two major targets, the eIF4E binding proteins (4E-BPs) and the ribosomal protein S6 kinases (S6K1 and S6K2). Eukaryotic mRNAs contain a 'cap' structure, m7GpppN at the 5′ end and can be specifically recognized by the initiation factor eIF4E, which associates with eIF4G and eIF4A to form eIF4F complex and initiate cap-dependent translation. 4E-BP binds to eIF4E and inhibits eIF4F complex formation. Upon phosphorylation of 4E-BP by mTOR, eIF4E is released to stimulate translation initiation. S6 kinase is activated by mTOR and phosphorylates 40S ribosomal protein S6, which leads to increased translation of a subset of mRNAs containing 5′ tract of oligopyrimidine (TOP). 5′ TOP mRNAs encode ribosomal proteins, elongation factors, the poly-A binding protein and other components of the translational machinery. Therefore, stimulation of the 5′ TOP mRNA translation by S6 results in up-regulation of the overall cellular translation capacity (Petroulakis et al., 2006).

The PI3K/Akt/mTOR signaling pathway is known to be up-regulated in various carcinoma cell lines, as well as in human ovarian and breast carcinomas (Altomare et al., 2004) (McAuliffe et al., 2010). For HCC, one study has shown overexpression of phospho-mTOR in 15% of liver tumors. Phospho-mTOR also positivity correlated with increased expression of total S6 kinase, which was found in 45% of the cases (Sahin et al., 2004). Elevated Akt phosphorylation was also found in 23% of HCC and implicated early HCC recurrence and poor prognosis (Boyault et al., 2007). There is also a high frequency (35.6%) of somatic PI3K mutations in HCC specimens (Lee et al., 2005). PTEN, the negative component of the PI3K/Akt/mTOR, is mutated in 5% of HCC and its expression is reduced in half of all HCC tumors, leading to the over activation of the pathway (Whittaker et al., 2010). In HCC patients, reduced PTEN expression has been associated with advanced tumor stage, high recurrences rate and poor survival outcome, suggesting inactivation of PTEN is involved in the pathogenesis of HCC (Hu et al., 2003). A study using hepatocyte-specific PTEN deficient mice further supported such a connection, by demonstrating that at 80 weeks of age, 66% of PTEN-deficient mice developed HCC (Horie et al., 2004).

Given the strong association between aberrant PI3K/Akt/mTOR signaling and HCC, pharmacological inhibition of this pathway could be a viable HCC treatment strategy. The mTOR inhibitor everolimus has been shown to decrease the growth of HCC cell line (Villanueva et al., 2008). Everolimus also induced a significant delay of tumor growth in a HCC xenograft mice model (Villanueva et al., 2008). In a separate study, the mTOR inhibitor sirolimus was tested in a rat HCC model and the treatment resulted in significantly longer survival time, smaller tumor size, and fewer extrahepatic metastases in those animals (Semela et al., 2007). Sirolimus has also been tested in human HCC patients, and it induced a partial response in 5% of the patients and tumor stabilization for at least 3 months in 24% of the patients. Another study has shown that 33% of patients partially response to sirolimus treatment (Rizell et al., 2008; Semela et al., 2007). Several new clinical trials are currently testing mTOR inhibitors and its combination with other therapies among HCC patients.

2.6 Other miscellaneous pathways

The EGFR (epidermal growth factor receptor) is a receptor tyrosine kinase which is activated by ligands including epidermal growth factor (EGF) and transforming growth factor α (TGF-α) (Herbst, 2004). Upon activation, EGFR forms a dimer and autophosphorylates the tyrosine residues in its intracellular cytoplasmic domain, which in turn leads to initiation of many downstream signal transduction cascades (Herbst, 2004). The EGFR signaling pathway is one of the most important pathways that regulate growth, survival, proliferation, and differentiation in mammalian cells. Numerous studies have shown that aberrant EGFR signaling plays a vital role in tumor angiogenesis and proliferation and agents that specifically block this pathway showed efficacy in several types of solid tumors (Zhang et al., 2007). For HCC, EGFR overexpression was detected among 40–70% of the tumors and TGF-α level was also elevated in pre-neoplastic HCC (Feitelson et al., 2004). Thus, targeting EGFR may also show beneficial effect for HCC patients. EGFR blocking agents include both small molecule tyrosine kinase inhibitors and monoclonal antibodies targeting the receptor. Erlotinib is a low molecular weight inhibitor of EGFR kinase (Thomas et al., 2007). It is able to suppress the growth of HCC cell lines *in vitro*. Furthermore, during a Phase 2 clinical trial, 17 out of 40 patients with unresectable HCC achieved stable disease at 16 weeks of erlotinib treatment. Progression-free survival at 16 weeks was 43% and median overall survival was 43 weeks, longer than the historical controls. Monoclonal antibody cetuximab which targets the extracelluar domain of EGFR has also been tested in HCC (Zhu et al., 2007). Although cetuximab was able to inhibit cell growth and induce apoptosis in some HCC cell lines, the results from clinical trials testing its efficacy among HCC patients have been inconsistent. Currently, several more anti-EGFR pathway compounds are being tested in clinic, in some cases in combination with other therapeutic methods. The results from those trials might further clarify the benefit of the EGFR blocking agents for HCC.

Deregulation of the insulin-like growth factor (IGF) pathway has also been implicated in the development of HCC (Scharf et al., 2001). IGF-1 and 2 bind to IGF receptor IGF-1R and activate downstream signaling (Alexia et al., 2004). IGF signaling pathway regulates cell proliferation, motility and apoptosis. Pronounced alterations in the expression of components of the IGF pathway have been reported during hepatocarcinogenesis (Whittaker et al., 2010). IGF-2 is overexpressed in 16-40% of HCC and around 30% of HCCs overexpress IFG-1R (Cariani et al., 1988). Neutralizing IGF-2 has been shown to reduce cell proliferation and increase apoptosis in HCC cell lines (Lund et al., 2004). Furthermore, a monoclonal antibody that selectively inhibits IGF-1R was not only able to decrease viability and proliferation of liver cancer cells *in vitro* but also delay tumor growth and prolong survival in HCC xenograft mice model (Tovar et al., 2010). Several small molecules and monoclonal antibodies targeting IGF-1R are now under early clinical development.

In HCC, the transforming growth factor-beta (TGF-β) pathway regulates several steps in tumor progression, including angiogenesis, production of the extracellular matrix and immune suppression (Giannelli et al., 2011). It is also involved in initiating signaling cascade which promotes liver fibrosis, cirrhosis and subsequent progression to HCC (Giannelli et al., 2011). Increased levels of TGF-β in HCC patients' sera and urine are associated with disease progression (Yasmin Anum et al., 2009; Tsai et al., 1997). Specific small molecule inhibitors targeting TGF-β type I receptor (TGF-βRI) kinase LY2109761 reduce migration of HCC cells and blocks invasion of HCC cells into the tissue microenvironment and blood vessels. LY2109761 also is effective in blocking tumor growth in a HCC xenograft chick embryo model and this antitumor activity was associated with anti-angiogenic effect (Mazzocca et al., 2009).

Hepatocyte growth factor (HGF) is a cytokine secreted by mesenchymal cells. It can stimulate mitogenesis, cell motility and has been implicated in tumor invasion. HGF is secreted as a single inactive polypeptide and is cleaved by serine proteases into a 69-kDa alpha-chain and 34-kDa beta-chain (Matsumoto and Nakamura, 1996). Active HGF is a herterodimer between alpha-chain and beta-chain linked by disulfide bond. HGF is homologous to the plasminogen subfamily of S1 peptidases but has no detectable protease activity. The proto oncogene c-Met is a receptor for HGF that is a heterodimer composed of a 50-kDa alpha-chain and a membrane spanning 145-kDa beta-chain with tyrosine kinase activity (Matsumoto and Nakamura, 1996). Activation of c-Met by HGF has been shown to activate MAPK, PI3K and Wnt signaling (Whittaker et al., 2010; Apte et al., 2006). Overexpression of c-Met was noted in 20-48% HCC tissues compared to surrounding non-cancerous liver tissues, and the overexpression levels correlated with worsening behavior of HCC and decreased 5-year survival in HCC patients (Whittaker et al., 2010; Ueki et al., 1997). A preclinical study reported that inhibition of c-Met by small molecule inhibitor SU11274 decreased HCC cell growth (Inagaki et al., 2011).

3. Conclusion

Many critical signaling pathways have been indicated in HCC development and a considerable amount of crosstalk and redundancy among those pathways have been observed. Various strategies targeting these pathways have been explored and have shown varying degrees of success in the clinic. Additional novel strategies are being investigated and raise the hope that more effective therapies may be on the horizon. However, HCC is a complex disease and aberrations in signaling pathways can vary from patient to patient. In addition, defects in multiple pathways may also in combination contribute to the pathogenesis. Uncovering the specific signaling pathways defects in the individual patient and the potential use of combination therapies may be critical for generating effective treatment outcomes in the future.

4. Acknowledgement

We thank Shawn Jeffries and Jeff Reagan for editing this manuscript.

5. References

Alexia, C., Fallot, G., Lasfer, M., Schweizer-Groyer, G., and Groyer, A. (2004). An evaluation of the role of insulin-like growth factors (IGF) and of type-I IGF receptor signalling in hepatocarcinogenesis and in the resistance of hepatocarcinoma cells against drug-induced apoptosis. Biochem Pharmacol *68*, 1003-1015.

Altomare, D.A., Wang, H.Q., Skele, K.L., De Rienzo, A., Klein-Szanto, A.J., Godwin, A.K., and Testa, J.R. (2004). AKT and mTOR phosphorylation is frequently detected in ovarian cancer and can be targeted to disrupt ovarian tumor cell growth. Oncogene *23*, 5853-5857.

Alves, R.C., Alves, D., Guz, B., Matos, C., Viana, M., Harriz, M., Terrabuio, D., Kondo, M., Gampel, O., and Polletti, P. (2011). Advanced hepatocellular carcinoma. Review of targeted molecular drugs. Ann Hepatol *10*, 21-27.

Ansari, J., Palmer, D.H., Rea, D.W., and Hussain, S.A. (2009). Role of tyrosine kinase inhibitors in lung cancer. Anticancer Agents Med Chem *9*, 569-575.

Anzola, M. (2004). Hepatocellular carcinoma: role of hepatitis B and hepatitis C viruses proteins in hepatocarcinogenesis. J Viral Hepat *11*, 383-393.

Apte, U., Zeng, G., Muller, P., Tan, X., Micsenyi, A., Cieply, B., Dai, C., Liu, Y., Kaestner, K.H., and Monga, S.P. (2006). Activation of Wnt/beta-catenin pathway during hepatocyte growth factor-induced hepatomegaly in mice. Hepatology *44*, 992-1002.

Avruch, J., Khokhlatchev, A., Kyriakis, J.M., Luo, Z., Tzivion, G., Vavvas, D., and Zhang, X.F. (2001). Ras activation of the Raf kinase: tyrosine kinase recruitment of the MAP kinase cascade. Recent Prog Horm Res *56*, 127-155.

Balmanno, K., and Cook, S.J. (2009). Tumour cell survival signalling by the ERK1/2 pathway. Cell Death Differ *16*, 368-377.

Beenken, A., and Mohammadi, M. (2009). The FGF family: biology, pathophysiology and therapy. Nat Rev Drug Discov *8*, 235-253.

Behari, J. (2010). The Wnt/beta-catenin signaling pathway in liver biology and disease. Expert Rev Gastroenterol Hepatol *4*, 745-756.

Behari, J., Zeng, G., Otruba, W., Thompson, M.D., Muller, P., Micsenyi, A., Sekhon, S.S., Leoni, L., and Monga, S.P. (2007). R-Etodolac decreases beta-catenin levels along with survival and proliferation of hepatoma cells. J Hepatol *46*, 849-857.

Bosch, F.X., Ribes, J., Diaz, M., and Cleries, R. (2004). Primary liver cancer: worldwide incidence and trends. Gastroenterology *127*, S5-S16.

Boyault, S., Rickman, D.S., de Reynies, A., Balabaud, C., Rebouissou, S., Jeannot, E., Herault, A., Saric, J., Belghiti, J., Franco, D., *et al.* (2007). Transcriptome classification of HCC is related to gene alterations and to new therapeutic targets. Hepatology *45*, 42-52.

Calvisi, D.F., Pinna, F., Meloni, F., Ladu, S., Pellegrino, R., Sini, M., Daino, L., Simile, M.M., De Miglio, M.R., Virdis, P., *et al.* (2008). Dual-specificity phosphatase 1 ubiquitination in extracellular signal-regulated kinase-mediated control of growth in human hepatocellular carcinoma. Cancer Res *68*, 4192-4200.

Cariani, E., Lasserre, C., Seurin, D., Hamelin, B., Kemeny, F., Franco, D., Czech, M.P., Ullrich, A., and Brechot, C. (1988). Differential expression of insulin-like growth factor II mRNA in human primary liver cancers, benign liver tumors, and liver cirrhosis. Cancer Res *48*, 6844-6849.

Carmeliet, P., and Jain, R.K. (2000). Angiogenesis in cancer and other diseases. Nature *407*, 249-257.

Chang, Q., Zhang, Y., Beezhold, K.J., Bhatia, D., Zhao, H., Chen, J., Castranova, V., Shi, X., and Chen, F. (2009). Sustained JNK1 activation is associated with altered histone H3 methylations in human liver cancer. J Hepatol *50*, 323-333.

Clevers, H. (2006). Wnt/beta-catenin signaling in development and disease. Cell *127*, 469-480.

Colnot, S., Decaens, T., Niwa-Kawakita, M., Godard, C., Hamard, G., Kahn, A., Giovannini, M., and Perret, C. (2004). Liver-targeted disruption of Apc in mice activates beta-catenin signaling and leads to hepatocellular carcinomas. Proc Natl Acad Sci U S A *101*, 17216-17221.

Dahmani, R., Just, P.A., and Perret, C. (2011). The Wnt/beta-catenin pathway as a therapeutic target in human hepatocellular carcinoma. Clin Res Hepatol Gastroenterol.

Dailey, L., Ambrosetti, D., Mansukhani, A., and Basilico, C. (2005). Mechanisms underlying differential responses to FGF signaling. Cytokine Growth Factor Rev *16*, 233-247.

Dale, T.C. (1998). Signal transduction by the Wnt family of ligands. Biochem J *329 (Pt 2)*, 209-223.

Das, M., Garlick, D.S., Greiner, D.L., and Davis, R.J. (2011). The role of JNK in the development of hepatocellular carcinoma. Genes & development *25*, 634-645.

Davis, R.J. (1995). Transcriptional regulation by MAP kinases. Mol Reprod Dev *42*, 459-467.

Desnoyers, L.R., Pai, R., Ferrando, R.E., Hotzel, K., Le, T., Ross, J., Carano, R., D'Souza, A., Qing, J., Mohtashemi, I., *et al.* (2008). Targeting FGF19 inhibits tumor growth in colon cancer xenograft and FGF19 transgenic hepatocellular carcinoma models. Oncogene *27*, 85-97.

Downward, J. (2003). Targeting RAS signalling pathways in cancer therapy. Nat Rev Cancer *3*, 11-22.

El-Assal, O.N., Yamanoi, A., Soda, Y., Yamaguchi, M., Igarashi, M., Yamamoto, A., Nabika, T., and Nagasue, N. (1998). Clinical significance of microvessel density and vascular endothelial growth factor expression in hepatocellular carcinoma and surrounding liver: possible involvement of vascular endothelial growth factor in the angiogenesis of cirrhotic liver. Hepatology *27*, 1554-1562.

El-Serag, H.B., Hampel, H., and Javadi, F. (2006). The association between diabetes and hepatocellular carcinoma: a systematic review of epidemiologic evidence. Clin Gastroenterol Hepatol *4*, 369-380.

Eswarakumar, V.P., Lax, I., and Schlessinger, J. (2005). Cellular signaling by fibroblast growth factor receptors. Cytokine Growth Factor Rev *16*, 139-149.

Fedi, P., Bafico, A., Nieto Soria, A., Burgess, W.H., Miki, T., Bottaro, D.P., Kraus, M.H., and Aaronson, S.A. (1999). Isolation and biochemical characterization of the human Dkk-1 homologue, a novel inhibitor of mammalian Wnt signaling. J Biol Chem *274*, 19465-19472.

Feitelson, M.A., Pan, J., and Lian, Z. (2004). Early molecular and genetic determinants of primary liver malignancy. Surg Clin North Am *84*, 339-354.

Finch, P.W., He, X., Kelley, M.J., Uren, A., Schaudies, R.P., Popescu, N.C., Rudikoff, S., Aaronson, S.A., Varmus, H.E., and Rubin, J.S. (1997). Purification and molecular cloning of a secreted, Frizzled-related antagonist of Wnt action. Proc Natl Acad Sci U S A *94*, 6770-6775.

Fujino, T., Asaba, H., Kang, M.J., Ikeda, Y., Sone, H., Takada, S., Kim, D.H., Ioka, R.X., Ono, M., Tomoyori, H., *et al.* (2003). Low-density lipoprotein receptor-related protein 5 (LRP5) is essential for normal cholesterol metabolism and glucose-induced insulin secretion. Proc Natl Acad Sci U S A *100*, 229-234.

Giannelli, G., Mazzocca, A., Fransvea, E., Lahn, M., and Antonaci, S. (2011). Inhibiting TGF-beta signaling in hepatocellular carcinoma. Biochim Biophys Acta *1815*, 214-223.

Giles, R.H., van Es, J.H., and Clevers, H. (2003). Caught up in a Wnt storm: Wnt signaling in cancer. Biochim Biophys Acta *1653*, 1-24.

Gollob, J.A., Wilhelm, S., Carter, C., and Kelley, S.L. (2006). Role of Raf kinase in cancer: therapeutic potential of targeting the Raf/MEK/ERK signal transduction pathway. Semin Oncol *33*, 392-406.

Gordon, M.D., and Nusse, R. (2006). Wnt signaling: multiple pathways, multiple receptors, and multiple transcription factors. J Biol Chem *281*, 22429-22433.

Harada, N., Miyoshi, H., Murai, N., Oshima, H., Tamai, Y., Oshima, M., and Taketo, M.M. (2002). Lack of tumorigenesis in the mouse liver after adenovirus-mediated expression of a dominant stable mutant of beta-catenin. Cancer Res *62*, 1971-1977.

Hassan, M.M., Curley, S.A., Li, D., Kaseb, A., Davila, M., Abdalla, E.K., Javle, M., Moghazy, D.M., Lozano, R.D., Abbruzzese, J.L., *et al.* (2010). Association of diabetes duration and diabetes treatment with the risk of hepatocellular carcinoma. Cancer *116*, 1938-1946.

Hawkins, M.J. (1995). Clinical trials of antiangiogenic agents. Curr Opin Oncol *7*, 90-93.

Herbst, R.S. (2004). Review of epidermal growth factor receptor biology. Int J Radiat Oncol Biol Phys *59*, 21-26.

Horie, Y., Suzuki, A., Kataoka, E., Sasaki, T., Hamada, K., Sasaki, J., Mizuno, K., Hasegawa, G., Kishimoto, H., Iizuka, M., *et al.* (2004). Hepatocyte-specific Pten deficiency results in steatohepatitis and hepatocellular carcinomas. The Journal of clinical investigation *113*, 1774-1783.

Hsu, P.I., Chow, N.H., Lai, K.H., Yang, H.B., Chan, S.H., Lin, X.Z., Cheng, J.S., Huang, J.S., Ger, L.P., Huang, S.M., *et al.* (1997). Implications of serum basic fibroblast growth factor levels in chronic liver diseases and hepatocellular carcinoma. Anticancer research *17*, 2803-2809.

Hu, T.H., Huang, C.C., Lin, P.R., Chang, H.W., Ger, L.P., Lin, Y.W., Changchien, C.S., Lee, C.M., and Tai, M.H. (2003). Expression and prognostic role of tumor suppressor gene PTEN/MMAC1/TEP1 in hepatocellular carcinoma. Cancer *97*, 1929-1940.

Huang, C., Jacobson, K., and Schaller, M.D. (2004). MAP kinases and cell migration. J Cell Sci *117*, 4619-4628.

Huang, X., Yang, C., Jin, C., Luo, Y., Wang, F., and McKeehan, W.L. (2009). Resident hepatocyte fibroblast growth factor receptor 4 limits hepatocarcinogenesis. Molecular carcinogenesis *48*, 553-562.

Huang, X., Yu, C., Jin, C., Kobayashi, M., Bowles, C.A., Wang, F., and McKeehan, W.L. (2006). Ectopic activity of fibroblast growth factor receptor 1 in hepatocytes accelerates hepatocarcinogenesis by driving proliferation and vascular endothelial growth factor-induced angiogenesis. Cancer Res *66*, 1481-1490.

Hui, L., Bakiri, L., Mairhorfer, A., Schweifer, N., Haslinger, C., Kenner, L., Komnenovic, V., Scheuch, H., Beug, H., and Wagner, E.F. (2007). p38alpha suppresses normal and cancer cell proliferation by antagonizing the JNK-c-Jun pathway. Nat Genet *39*, 741-749.

Hui, L., Zatloukal, K., Scheuch, H., Stepniak, E., and Wagner, E.F. (2008). Proliferation of human HCC cells and chemically induced mouse liver cancers requires JNK1-

dependent p21 downregulation. The Journal of clinical investigation *118*, 3943-3953.

Huynh, H., Chow, P.K., and Soo, K.C. (2007a). AZD6244 and doxorubicin induce growth suppression and apoptosis in mouse models of hepatocellular carcinoma. Mol Cancer Ther *6*, 2468-2476.

Huynh, H., Nguyen, T.T., Chow, K.H., Tan, P.H., Soo, K.C., and Tran, E. (2003). Over-expression of the mitogen-activated protein kinase (MAPK) kinase (MEK)-MAPK in hepatocellular carcinoma: its role in tumor progression and apoptosis. BMC Gastroenterol *3*, 19.

Huynh, H., Soo, K.C., Chow, P.K., and Tran, E. (2007b). Targeted inhibition of the extracellular signal-regulated kinase kinase pathway with AZD6244 (ARRY-142886) in the treatment of hepatocellular carcinoma. Mol Cancer Ther *6*, 138-146.

Hwang, Y.H., Choi, J.Y., Kim, S., Chung, E.S., Kim, T., Koh, S.S., Lee, B., Bae, S.H., Kim, J., and Park, Y.M. (2004). Over-expression of c-raf-1 proto-oncogene in liver cirrhosis and hepatocellular carcinoma. Hepatol Res *29*, 113-121.

Ihara, A., Koizumi, H., Hashizume, R., and Uchikoshi, T. (1996). Expression of epithelial cadherin and alpha- and beta-catenins in nontumoral livers and hepatocellular carcinomas. Hepatology *23*, 1441-1447.

Inagaki, Y., Qi, F., Gao, J., Qu, X., Hasegawa, K., Sugawara, Y., Tang, W., and Kokudo, N. (2011). Effect of c-Met inhibitor SU11274 on hepatocellular carcinoma cell growth. Biosci Trends *5*, 52-56.

Kaseb, A.O., Hanbali, A., Cotant, M., Hassan, M.M., Wollner, I., and Philip, P.A. (2009). Vascular endothelial growth factor in the management of hepatocellular carcinoma: a review of literature. Cancer *115*, 4895-4906.

Keshet, Y., and Seger, R. (2010). The MAP kinase signaling cascades: a system of hundreds of components regulates a diverse array of physiological functions. Methods Mol Biol *661*, 3-38.

Kim, E.K., and Choi, E.J. (2010). Pathological roles of MAPK signaling pathways in human diseases. Biochim Biophys Acta *1802*, 396-405.

Knights, V., and Cook, S.J. (2010). De-regulated FGF receptors as therapeutic targets in cancer. Pharmacol Ther *125*, 105-117.

Krejci, P., Prochazkova, J., Bryja, V., Kozubik, A., and Wilcox, W.R. (2009). Molecular pathology of the fibroblast growth factor family. Hum Mutat *30*, 1245-1255.

Kurosu, H., Choi, M., Ogawa, Y., Dickson, A.S., Goetz, R., Eliseenkova, A.V., Mohammadi, M., Rosenblatt, K.P., Kliewer, S.A., and Kuro-o, M. (2007). Tissue-specific expression of betaKlotho and fibroblast growth factor (FGF) receptor isoforms determines metabolic activity of FGF19 and FGF21. J Biol Chem *282*, 26687-26695.

Kuruvilla, F.G., and Schreiber, S.L. (1999). The PIK-related kinases intercept conventional signaling pathways. Chem Biol *6*, R129-136.

Lee, J.W., Soung, Y.H., Kim, S.Y., Lee, H.W., Park, W.S., Nam, S.W., Kim, S.H., Lee, J.Y., Yoo, N.J., and Lee, S.H. (2005). PIK3CA gene is frequently mutated in breast carcinomas and hepatocellular carcinomas. Oncogene *24*, 1477-1480.

Llovet, J.M., Ricci, S., Mazzaferro, V., Hilgard, P., Gane, E., Blanc, J.F., de Oliveira, A.C., Santoro, A., Raoul, J.L., Forner, A., *et al.* (2008). Sorafenib in advanced hepatocellular carcinoma. N Engl J Med *359*, 378-390.

Lund, P., Schubert, D., Niketeghad, F., and Schirmacher, P. (2004). Autocrine inhibition of chemotherapy response in human liver tumor cells by insulin-like growth factor-II. Cancer Lett *206*, 85-96.

Malumbres, M., and Barbacid, M. (2003). RAS oncogenes: the first 30 years. Nat Rev Cancer *3*, 459-465.

Matsumoto, K., and Nakamura, T. (1996). Emerging multipotent aspects of hepatocyte growth factor. J Biochem *119*, 591-600.

Mazzocca, A., Fransvea, E., Lavezzari, G., Antonaci, S., and Giannelli, G. (2009). Inhibition of transforming growth factor beta receptor I kinase blocks hepatocellular carcinoma growth through neo-angiogenesis regulation. Hepatology *50*, 1140-1151.

McAuliffe, P.F., Meric-Bernstam, F., Mills, G.B., and Gonzalez-Angulo, A.M. (2010). Deciphering the role of PI3K/Akt/mTOR pathway in breast cancer biology and pathogenesis. Clin Breast Cancer *10 Suppl 3*, S59-65.

Min, L., He, B., and Hui, L. (2011). Mitogen-activated protein kinases in hepatocellular carcinoma development. Semin Cancer Biol *21*, 10-20.

Nelson, W.J., and Nusse, R. (2004). Convergence of Wnt, beta-catenin, and cadherin pathways. Science *303*, 1483-1487.

Nicholes, K., Guillet, S., Tomlinson, E., Hillan, K., Wright, B., Frantz, G.D., Pham, T.A., Dillard-Telm, L., Tsai, S.P., Stephan, J.P., *et al.* (2002). A mouse model of hepatocellular carcinoma: ectopic expression of fibroblast growth factor 19 in skeletal muscle of transgenic mice. The American journal of pathology *160*, 2295-2307.

Ornitz, D.M., and Itoh, N. (2001). Fibroblast growth factors. Genome biology *2*, REVIEWS3005.

Ornitz, D.M., Xu, J., Colvin, J.S., McEwen, D.G., MacArthur, C.A., Coulier, F., Gao, G., and Goldfarb, M. (1996). Receptor specificity of the fibroblast growth factor family. J Biol Chem *271*, 15292-15297.

Paez, J., and Sellers, W.R. (2003). PI3K/PTEN/AKT pathway. A critical mediator of oncogenic signaling. Cancer Treat Res *115*, 145-167.

Pai, R., Dunlap, D., Qing, J., Mohtashemi, I., Hotzel, K., and French, D.M. (2008). Inhibition of fibroblast growth factor 19 reduces tumor growth by modulating beta-catenin signaling. Cancer Res *68*, 5086-5095.

Parkin, D.M., Bray, F., Ferlay, J., and Pisani, P. (2005). Global cancer statistics, 2002. CA Cancer J Clin *55*, 74-108.

Penn, L.J., Laufer, E.M., and Land, H. (1990). C-MYC: evidence for multiple regulatory functions. Semin Cancer Biol *1*, 69-80.

Petroulakis, E., Mamane, Y., Le Bacquer, O., Shahbazian, D., and Sonenberg, N. (2006). mTOR signaling: implications for cancer and anticancer therapy. Br J Cancer *94*, 195-199.

Plotnikov, A.N., Schlessinger, J., Hubbard, S.R., and Mohammadi, M. (1999). Structural basis for FGF receptor dimerization and activation. Cell *98*, 641-650.

Presta, M., Dell'Era, P., Mitola, S., Moroni, E., Ronca, R., and Rusnati, M. (2005). Fibroblast growth factor/fibroblast growth factor receptor system in angiogenesis. Cytokine Growth Factor Rev *16*, 159-178.

Rizell, M., Andersson, M., Cahlin, C., Hafstrom, L., Olausson, M., and Lindner, P. (2008). Effects of the mTOR inhibitor sirolimus in patients with hepatocellular and cholangiocellular cancer. Int J Clin Oncol *13*, 66-70.

Roskoski, R., Jr. (2007). Vascular endothelial growth factor (VEGF) signaling in tumor progression. Crit Rev Oncol Hematol *62*, 179-213.

Sahin, F., Kannangai, R., Adegbola, O., Wang, J., Su, G., and Torbenson, M. (2004). mTOR and P70 S6 kinase expression in primary liver neoplasms. Clin Cancer Res *10*, 8421-8425.

Scharf, J.G., Dombrowski, F., and Ramadori, G. (2001). The IGF axis and hepatocarcinogenesis. Mol Pathol *54*, 138-144.

Schmitz, K.J., Wohlschlaeger, J., Lang, H., Sotiropoulos, G.C., Malago, M., Steveling, K., Reis, H., Cicinnati, V.R., Schmid, K.W., and Baba, H.A. (2008). Activation of the ERK and AKT signalling pathway predicts poor prognosis in hepatocellular carcinoma and ERK activation in cancer tissue is associated with hepatitis C virus infection. J Hepatol *48*, 83-90.

Schulze, W.X., Deng, L., and Mann, M. (2005). Phosphotyrosine interactome of the ErbB-receptor kinase family. Mol Syst Biol *1*, 2005 0008.

Semela, D., Piguet, A.C., Kolev, M., Schmitter, K., Hlushchuk, R., Djonov, V., Stoupis, C., and Dufour, J.F. (2007). Vascular remodeling and antitumoral effects of mTOR inhibition in a rat model of hepatocellular carcinoma. J Hepatol *46*, 840-848.

Shen, Y.C., Hsu, C., and Cheng, A.L. (2010). Molecular targeted therapy for advanced hepatocellular carcinoma: current status and future perspectives. J Gastroenterol *45*, 794-807.

Shtutman, M., Zhurinsky, J., Simcha, I., Albanese, C., D'Amico, M., Pestell, R., and Ben-Ze'ev, A. (1999). The cyclin D1 gene is a target of the beta-catenin/LEF-1 pathway. Proc Natl Acad Sci U S A *96*, 5522-5527.

Siegel, A.B., Cohen, E.I., Ocean, A., Lehrer, D., Goldenberg, A., Knox, J.J., Chen, H., Clark-Garvey, S., Weinberg, A., Mandeli, J., *et al.* (2008). Phase II trial evaluating the clinical and biologic effects of bevacizumab in unresectable hepatocellular carcinoma. J Clin Oncol *26*, 2992-2998.

Slamon, D.J., Leyland-Jones, B., Shak, S., Fuchs, H., Paton, V., Bajamonde, A., Fleming, T., Eiermann, W., Wolter, J., Pegram, M., *et al.* (2001). Use of chemotherapy plus a monoclonal antibody against HER2 for metastatic breast cancer that overexpresses HER2. N Engl J Med *344*, 783-792.

Takahashi, Y., and Nishioka, K. (2011). Therapeutic approaches targeting tumor vasculature in gastrointestinal cancers. Front Biosci (Elite Ed) *3*, 541-548.

Takigawa, Y., and Brown, A.M. (2008). Wnt signaling in liver cancer. Curr Drug Targets *9*, 1013-1024.

Thomas, M.B., and Abbruzzese, J.L. (2005). Opportunities for targeted therapies in hepatocellular carcinoma. J Clin Oncol *23*, 8093-8108.

Thomas, M.B., Chadha, R., Glover, K., Wang, X., Morris, J., Brown, T., Rashid, A., Dancey, J., and Abbruzzese, J.L. (2007). Phase 2 study of erlotinib in patients with unresectable hepatocellular carcinoma. Cancer *110*, 1059-1067.

Thompson, M.D., and Monga, S.P. (2007). WNT/beta-catenin signaling in liver health and disease. Hepatology *45*, 1298-1305.

Tovar, V., Alsinet, C., Villanueva, A., Hoshida, Y., Chiang, D.Y., Sole, M., Thung, S., Moyano, S., Toffanin, S., Minguez, B., *et al.* (2010). IGF activation in a molecular subclass of hepatocellular carcinoma and pre-clinical efficacy of IGF-1R blockage. J Hepatol *52*, 550-559.

Tsai, J.F., Chuang, L.Y., Jeng, J.E., Yang, M.L., Chang, W.Y., Hsieh, M.Y., Lin, Z.Y., and Tsai, J.H. (1997). Clinical relevance of transforming growth factor-beta 1 in the urine of patients with hepatocellular carcinoma. Medicine (Baltimore) *76*, 213-226.

Turner, N., and Grose, R. (2010). Fibroblast growth factor signalling: from development to cancer. Nat Rev Cancer *10*, 116-129.

Ueki, T., Fujimoto, J., Suzuki, T., Yamamoto, H., and Okamoto, E. (1997). Expression of hepatocyte growth factor and its receptor, the c-met proto-oncogene, in hepatocellular carcinoma. Hepatology *25*, 619-623.

van der Meel, R., Symons, M.H., Kudernatsch, R., Kok, R.J., Schiffelers, R.M., Storm, G., Gallagher, W.M., and Byrne, A.T. (2011). The VEGF/Rho GTPase signalling pathway: a promising target for anti-angiogenic/anti-invasion therapy. Drug Discov Today *16*, 219-228.

Vanhaesebroeck, B., and Waterfield, M.D. (1999). Signaling by distinct classes of phosphoinositide 3-kinases. Exp Cell Res *253*, 239-254.

Villanueva, A., Chiang, D.Y., Newell, P., Peix, J., Thung, S., Alsinet, C., Tovar, V., Roayaie, S., Minguez, B., Sole, M., *et al.* (2008). Pivotal role of mTOR signaling in hepatocellular carcinoma. Gastroenterology *135*, 1972-1983, 1983 e1971-1911.

Wagner, E.F., and Nebreda, A.R. (2009). Signal integration by JNK and p38 MAPK pathways in cancer development. Nat Rev Cancer *9*, 537-549.

Wang, W., Chen, J.X., Liao, R., Deng, Q., Zhou, J.J., Huang, S., and Sun, P. (2002). Sequential activation of the MEK-extracellular signal-regulated kinase and MKK3/6-p38 mitogen-activated protein kinase pathways mediates oncogenic ras-induced premature senescence. Mol Cell Biol *22*, 3389-3403.

Wang, Y., Macke, J.P., Abella, B.S., Andreasson, K., Worley, P., Gilbert, D.J., Copeland, N.G., Jenkins, N.A., and Nathans, J. (1996). A large family of putative transmembrane receptors homologous to the product of the Drosophila tissue polarity gene frizzled. J Biol Chem *271*, 4468-4476.

Wehrli, M., Dougan, S.T., Caldwell, K., O'Keefe, L., Schwartz, S., Vaizel-Ohayon, D., Schejter, E., Tomlinson, A., and DiNardo, S. (2000). arrow encodes an LDL-receptor-related protein essential for Wingless signalling. Nature *407*, 527-530.

Whittaker, S., Marais, R., and Zhu, A.X. (2010). The role of signaling pathways in the development and treatment of hepatocellular carcinoma. Oncogene *29*, 4989-5005.

Wong, C.M., Fan, S.T., and Ng, I.O. (2001). beta-Catenin mutation and overexpression in hepatocellular carcinoma: clinicopathologic and prognostic significance. Cancer *92*, 136-145.

Wu, A.L., Coulter, S., Liddle, C., Wong, A., Eastham-Anderson, J., French, D.M., Peterson, A.S., and Sonoda, J. (2011). FGF19 regulates cell proliferation, glucose and bile acid metabolism via FGFR4-dependent and independent pathways. PLoS One *6*, e17868.

Wu, X., Ge, H., Gupte, J., Weiszmann, J., Shimamoto, G., Stevens, J., Hawkins, N., Lemon, B., Shen, W., Xu, J., *et al.* (2007). Co-receptor requirements for fibroblast growth factor-19 signaling. J Biol Chem *282*, 29069-29072.

Wu, X., Ge, H., Lemon, B., Vonderfecht, S., Baribault, H., Weiszmann, J., Gupte, J., Gardner, J., Lindberg, R., Wang, Z., *et al.* (2010a). Separating mitogenic and metabolic activities of fibroblast growth factor 19 (FGF19). Proc Natl Acad Sci U S A *107*, 14158-14163.

Wu, X., Ge, H., Lemon, B., Vonderfecht, S., Weiszmann, J., Hecht, R., Gupte, J., Hager, T., Wang, Z., Lindberg, R., *et al.* (2010b). FGF19-induced hepatocyte proliferation is mediated through FGFR4 activation. J Biol Chem *285*, 5165-5170.

Wu, X., and Li, Y. (2009). Role of FGF19 induced FGFR4 activation in the regulation of glucose homeostasis. Aging *1*, 1023.

Wullschleger, S., Loewith, R., and Hall, M.N. (2006). TOR signaling in growth and metabolism. Cell *124*, 471-484.

Xian, W., Schwertfeger, K.L., Vargo-Gogola, T., and Rosen, J.M. (2005). Pleiotropic effects of FGFR1 on cell proliferation, survival, and migration in a 3D mammary epithelial cell model. J Cell Biol *171*, 663-673.

Yamaguchi, R., Yano, H., Iemura, A., Ogasawara, S., Haramaki, M., and Kojiro, M. (1998). Expression of vascular endothelial growth factor in human hepatocellular carcinoma. Hepatology *28*, 68-77.

Yang, Y., Zhou, Y., Lu, M., An, Y., Li, R., Chen, Y., Lu, D.R., Jin, L., Zhou, W.P., Qian, J., *et al.* (2011). Association between fibroblast growth factor receptor 4 polymorphisms and risk of hepatocellular carcinoma. Molecular carcinogenesis.

Yasmin Anum, M.Y., Looi, M.L., Nor Aini, A.H., Merican, I., Wahidah, A., Mohd Radzi, A.H., Nor Azizah, A., and Othman, N.H. (2009). Combined assessment of TGF-beta-1 and alpha-fetoprotein values improves specificity in the diagnosis of hepatocellular carcinoma and other chronic liver diseases in Malaysia. Med J Malaysia *64*, 223-227.

Yoshida, T., Hisamoto, T., Akiba, J., Koga, H., Nakamura, K., Tokunaga, Y., Hanada, S., Kumemura, H., Maeyama, M., Harada, M., *et al.* (2006). Spreds, inhibitors of the Ras/ERK signal transduction, are dysregulated in human hepatocellular carcinoma and linked to the malignant phenotype of tumors. Oncogene *25*, 6056-6066.

Zarich, N., Oliva, J.L., Martinez, N., Jorge, R., Ballester, A., Gutierrez-Eisman, S., Garcia-Vargas, S., and Rojas, J.M. (2006). Grb2 is a negative modulator of the intrinsic Ras-GEF activity of hSos1. Mol Biol Cell *17*, 3591-3597.

Zeng, G., Awan, F., Otruba, W., Muller, P., Apte, U., Tan, X., Gandhi, C., Demetris, A.J., and Monga, S.P. (2007). Wnt'er in liver: expression of Wnt and frizzled genes in mouse. Hepatology *45*, 195-204.

Zhang, H., Berezov, A., Wang, Q., Zhang, G., Drebin, J., Murali, R., and Greene, M.I. (2007). ErbB receptors: from oncogenes to targeted cancer therapies. The Journal of clinical investigation *117*, 2051-2058.

Zhou, J., Tang, Z.Y., Fan, J., Wu, Z.Q., Li, X.M., Liu, Y.K., Liu, F., Sun, H.C., and Ye, S.L. (2000). Expression of platelet-derived endothelial cell growth factor and vascular endothelial growth factor in hepatocellular carcinoma and portal vein tumor thrombus. J Cancer Res Clin Oncol *126*, 57-61.

Zhu, A.X., Stuart, K., Blaszkowsky, L.S., Muzikansky, A., Reitberg, D.P., Clark, J.W., Enzinger, P.C., Bhargava, P., Meyerhardt, J.A., Horgan, K., *et al.* (2007). Phase 2 study of cetuximab in patients with advanced hepatocellular carcinoma. Cancer *110*, 581-589.

4

The Role of the Tumor Microenvironment in the Pathogenesis of Cholangiocarcinoma

Matthew Quinn, Matthew McMillin, Gabriel Frampton, Syeda Humayra Afroze, Li Huang and Sharon DeMorrow
Digestive Disease Research Center, Department of Internal Medicine
Scott & White Hospital and Texas A&M Health Science Center
Research Service, Central Texas Veterans Health Care System
Temple, Texas,
USA

1. Introduction

Cholangiocarcinoma is a type of liver cancer arising from the neoplastic transformation of the epithelial cells that line the intra- and extrahepatic bile ducts. Symptoms are usually evident only after blockage of the bile duct by the tumor. This is an extremely aggressive tumor, which has very poor prognosis and limited treatment options. Cholangiocarcinoma is relatively resistant to chemotherapy and radiation therapy leaving conventional treatment like surgery as the only option. Therefore, further understanding into the factors that are involved in tumor initiation, promotion and progression is required for designing alternate therapies to combat this devastating disease.

The tumor microenvironment is one of the most important factors regulating tumor angiogenesis, tumor invasion and metastasis. The microenvironment is a well-recognized system that plays a key role in tumor progression. However, the mechanism through which tumor microenvironment regulates tumor progression and invasion is largely unknown. In this review, we discuss the current knowledge about the role of the tumor microenvironment in the pathogenesis of cholangiocarcinoma, the role of the tumor microenvironment in the classification of cholangiocarcinoma and efforts to develop treatments targeting the tumor microenvironment.

2. Background

Cholangiocarcinoma arises from the neoplastic transformation of cholangiocytes and can exist as either intrahepatic, perihilar or distal extrahepatic tumors (Alpini et al. 2001). Typically, cholangiocarcinomas are adenocarcinomas and have a poor prognosis and limited treatment options. This is due, at least in part, to the late presentation of symptoms and the relative resistance to current treatment options (Sirica 2005).

The incidence of both intra- and extra-hepatic cholangiocarcinoma is typically more prevalent in Asian countries (Patel 2002). The mortality rates for intrahepatic cholangiocarcinoma have increased since the 1970s, whereas deaths from extrahepatic cholangiocarcinoma have declined in most countries (Patel 2002). There is a slight preponderance for cholangiocarcinoma in males (Tominaga and Kuroishi 1994) and the incidence in both sexes increases with age (Patel 2002).

2.1 Risk factors

Cholangiocarcinoma occurs with varying frequency in different regions of the world. This can be explained in part by the distribution of risk factors in geographic regions and ethnic groups (Ben-Menachem 2007). The common link between these regional risk factors seems to involve chronic inflammation and biliary irritation (Gores 2003).

The prevalence of cholangiocarcinoma in Asian countries shares a relationship with infections such as liver flukes, Hepatitis B and Hepatitis C (Ben-Menachem 2007). In contrast, approximately 90% of patients diagnosed with cholangiocarcinoma in Western countries do not have any recognized risk factors (Ben-Menachem 2007). However, the remaining 10% of cases are associated with certain risk factors. Apart from factors related to chronic inflammation, both intra- and extrahepatic cholangiocarcinomas are well-known complications of primary sclerosing cholangitis (de Groen et al. 1999). Other known risk factors include obesity, hepatolithiasis, bacterial infection and/or bile stasis-related chronic cholangitis (Chen 1999; de Groen et al. 1999; Catalano et al. 2009).

3. Tumor microenvironment

Neoplastic epithelial cells coexist with a biologically complex stroma composed of various types of stromal cells as well as the extracellular matrix, both of which create the complexity of the tumor microenvironment (Orimo and Weinberg 2006). Mouse models of tumorigenesis have revealed that stromal cells, in particular inflammatory cells, vascular endothelial cells and fibroblasts actively support tumor growth (Olumi et al. 1999; Tlsty 2001; Cunha et al. 2003; Bhowmick et al. 2004). In addition, the microenvironment is now well recognized as playing a role in neoplastic transformation, malignant progression and metastasis and invasion of cancer cells (Tlsty 2001; Bhowmick et al. 2004). Furthermore, the interaction between the cancer cells and the tumor microenvironment is a major factor influencing cancer treatment resistance to radiotherapy and chemotherapy (de Visser and Jonkers 2009; Shinohara and Maity 2009). Research indicates that the interplay between the cancer cells and the stromal cells of the microenvironment is bi-directional and dynamic. For example, neoplastic cells often secrete factors that work in a paracrine manner to recruit and activate a number of types of stromal cells into the tumor microenvironment as required (Rasanen and Vaheri 2010; Rojas et al. 2010; Onimaru and Yonemitsu 2011). Conversely, stromal cells, once recruited and activated, release factors into the extracellular milieu that can either stimulate or inhibit growth of the tumor (Rasanen and Vaheri 2010; Rojas et al. 2010; Onimaru and Yonemitsu 2011). The effects of the components of the tumor microenvironment on tumor growth are summarized in Figure 1. In particular, the proliferation and recruitment of vascular endothelial cells and subsequent formation of new blood vessels brings a nutrient supply thereby allowing growth and metastasis of the tumor. Cancer associated fibroblasts, on the other hand, can stimulate angiogenesis as well promote tumor growth and invasion. The presence of immune cells, in particular tumor-associated macrophages, in the microenvironment, confers resistance to toxic insults and also promotes growth. Lastly, proliferation of lymph endothelial cells and subsequent increase in lymphatic vessel density promotes tumor metastasis.

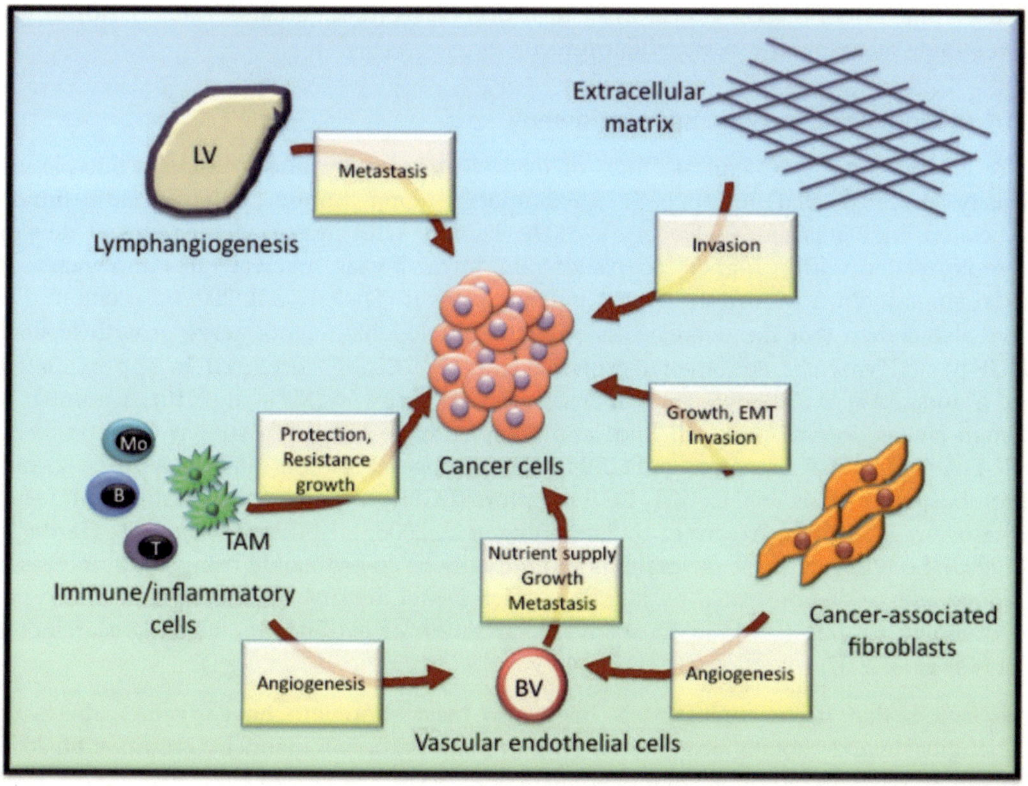

Fig. 1. Schematic representation of the effects of stromal support cells on tumor growth and metastasis. Abbreviations: B, B cell; BV, Blood vessel; EMT, Epithelial-mesenchymal transition; LV, lymph vessel; M, monocyte; T, T cell; TAM, Tumor associated macrophage.

3.1 Angiogenesis

The physiological process of the formation of new blood vessels from pre-existing blood vessels is termed angiogenesis. Tumors require the formation of new blood vessels to supply oxygen and other essential nutrients, without which their growth would be severely restricted (McDougall et al. 2006). Generally, the process of angiogenesis involves a sequence of co-ordinated events that is initiated with the expression and release of various angiogenic factors from the tumor cells, such as vascular endothelial growth factor (VEGF), epidermal growth factor (EGF) and fibroblast growth factor (FGF). Once these angiogenic factors bind to their corresponding receptors on the cell surface of the endothelial cells, there is an increase in vascular permeability, leading to extravasation of plasma proteins and dissociation of pericyte coverage (Roberts and Palade 1997; Dvorak 2005). This is followed by proliferation and migration of the endothelial cells to initiate new vessel formation (Ausprunk and Folkman 1977). For new vessel formation to occur, there also needs to be localized degradation of the extracellular matrix, which is performed by the matrix metalloproteinases, cathepsin B and other degradation enzymes, as well as the expression of matrix proteins such as fibronectin and laminin (Mikkelsen et al. 1995; Gladson 1999; Ljubimova et al. 2006). The expression of these essential extracellular matrix proteins largely occurs in the tumor cells or cancer associated fibroblasts (Rasanen and Vaheri 2010), which then secrete them into the extracellular milieu.

3.1.1 Angiogenesis in cholangiocarcinoma

A recent immunohistochemical study of microvessel density and lymphatic microvessel density revealed that intrahepatic cholangiocarcinoma tumors demonstrated tumor-associated angiogenesis (Thelen et al. 2009). Tumors with increased microvessel density were correlated with a higher recurrence rate, lower 5-year survival rates and increased nodal spread which in turn influences patient survival (Thelen et al. 2009). Recent studies have also shown that the overexpression of the angiogenic factors nerve growth factor-β (NGF-β) and vascular endothelial growth factor-C (VEGF-C) occurred in approximately 57.1% and 46.4% of cholangiocarcinoma samples, respectively (Xu et al. 2010). A number of human cholangiocarcinoma cell lines and samples have also been shown to overexpress VEGF-A and VEGF receptors (VEGFRs), the angiogenic factors angiopoietin-1, -2, and thrombospondin-1, as well as EGF, EGF receptors (EGFR) and basic fibroblast growth factor (Ogasawara et al. 2001; Alvaro et al. 2006; Tang et al. 2006; Yoshikawa et al. 2008; Harder et al. 2009). Secretion of these factors may individually or co-ordinately bring about increased angiogenesis as demonstrated by increased microvessel density. For example, VEGF-A has been shown to play a role in the neovascularization of extrahepatic cholangiocarcinoma (Mobius et al. 2007).

The factors that drive angiogenesis have also been shown to have distinct effects on cholangiocyte and cholangiocarcinoma growth in an autocrine manner (Gaudio et al. 2006; Tang et al. 2006; Mobius et al. 2007; Yabuuchi et al. 2009; Yoshikawa et al. 2009; Glaser et al. 2010). Indeed, the proliferative effects of estrogen on cholangiocarcinoma cell lines have been attributed to a mechanism involving the upregulation of VEGF expression, as blocking VEGF ameliorates the estrogenic effects on proliferation (Mancino et al. 2009).

Taken together, these data suggest that agents that block angiogenesis (by blocking VEGF expression, for example) may also have a direct effect on cholangiocarcinoma cell proliferation in addition to their anti-angiogenic effects. In support of this notion, inhibition of VEGFR and EGFR signaling with vandetanib (ZD6474, a tyrosine kinase inhibitor) can be an important approach for the management of the subset of cholangiocarcinoma that lack KRAS mutations and/or have EGFR amplification (Yoshikawa et al. 2009). Furthermore, ZD1839 (IRESSA), an orally active, selective inhibitor of EGFR tyrosine kinase has clinical activity against cholangiocarcinoma by stabilizing the cell cycle inhibitor, p27Kip1 and enhancing radiosensitivity in cholangiocarcinoma cell lines (Yabuuchi et al. 2009). Curcumin, a natural phenol found in tumeric has recently been shown to suppress the expression of VEGF and decrease the microvessel density in a hamster model of cholangiocarcinoma (Prakobwong et al. 2011a). In parallel, curcumin also exerts antiproliferative and proapoptotic effects on cholangiocarcinoma cells independent of the effects on angiogenesis (Prakobwong et al. 2011a; Prakobwong et al. 2011b). Similar effects have been shown with inhibitors of histamine synthesis (Francis et al. 2011), H3 histamine receptor agonists (Francis et al. 2009), and Endothelin-1 (Fava et al. 2009) just to name a few. The interaction between angiogenesis, angiogenic factors and cholangiocarcinoma growth and progression is summarized in Figure 2.

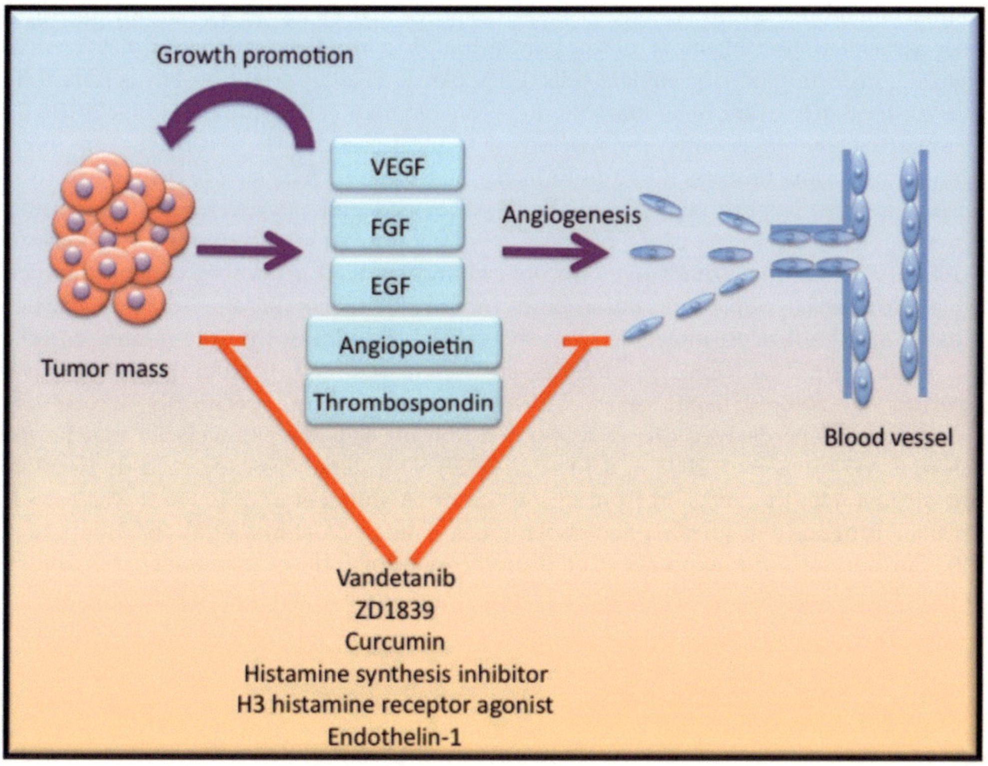

Fig. 2. Schematic representation of the interactions between cholangiocarcinoma and angiogenic factors regulating cell proliferation and angiogenesis

3.2 Cancer associated fibroblasts

Under normal physiological conditions, fibroblasts have a low proliferative index and only secrete factors needed to maintain normal tissue homeostasis (Tuxhorn et al. 2001; Beacham and Cukierman 2005). Indeed, normal fibroblasts provide biochemical cues that constrain epithelial tumor cells within their basement membrane (Tuxhorn et al. 2001; Beacham and Cukierman 2005). In contrast, when homeostasis is disrupted during tissue injury, stromal cells rapidly and reversibly alter their phenotype and proliferation rate (Tuxhorn et al. 2001). However, during tumorigenesis, the fibroblastic wound healing machinery lacks the regulatory mechanisms to revert to normal homeostasis (Tuxhorn et al. 2001). The inability to down-regulate the wound healing response affects stromal dynamics. Tumor-dependent changes in signaling and plasticity of the stroma trigger a continuum of alterations yielding a 'primed' stroma that can support and incite tumor initiation or progression (Tuxhorn et al. 2001).

3.2.1 Cancer-associated fibroblasts in cholangiocarcinoma

Cancer-associated fibroblasts are the predominant cell type in the stroma of cholangiocarcinoma tumors (Sirica et al. 2009). Increased α-smooth muscle actin-positive fibroblasts were correlated with shorter survival times and larger tumor sizes in resected cholangiocarcinoma tissue (Chuaysri et al. 2009; Okabe et al. 2009). The origin of these cancer-associated fibroblasts is unknown, although a number of possibilities have been suggested, including hepatic stellate cells (Okabe et al. 2009), portal fibroblasts (Dranoff and Wells 2010) or circulating bone marrow-derived precursor cells (Shimoda et al. 2010). Given the apparent heterogeneous population of cancer-associated fibroblasts observed in cholangiocarcinoma tumors, it is highly likely that these fibroblasts are derived from more than one source. Recently, researchers have performed genetic screening to determine the differences in gene expression between cholangiocarcinoma-derived cancer-associated fibroblasts and non-malignant liver fibroblasts and showed a number of genes associated with angiogenesis, cell proliferation and motility (Utispan et al. 2010). In particular, periostin, a cell adhesion molecule, was shown to be significantly upregulated correlating with shorter survival time in patients and increased cell proliferation and invasive properties *in vitro* (Utispan et al. 2010). Another gene specifically expressed by cholangiocarcinoma-derived cancer-associated fibroblasts is the extracellular matrix protein tenascin-C (Aishima et al. 2003; Iguchi et al. 2009). This gene was expressed predominantly in the stroma near the invasion front of the tumor (Aishima et al. 2003) and was associated with poor prognosis in intrahepatic cholangiocarcinoma (Aishima et al. 2003; Iguchi et al. 2009). Furthermore, the expression of thrombospondin-1 by cancer-associated fibroblasts correlated with increased metastatsis (Kawahara et al. 1998; Tang et al. 2006).

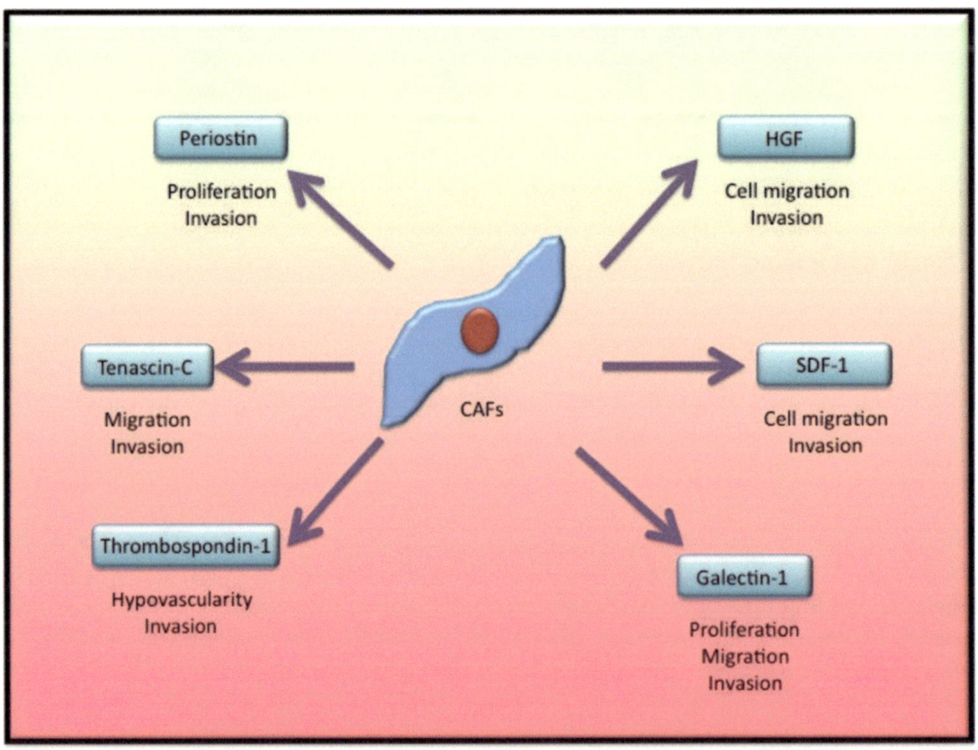

Fig. 3. Summary of the signalling molecules released by cholangiocarcinoma-derived cancer-associated fibroblasts and their known effects on cholangiocarcinoma progression. CAFs; cancer-associated fibroblasts, HGF; hepatocyte growth factor, SDF-1; stromal derived factor-1.

One last cancer-associated fibroblast gene of note is the expression of the chemokine, stromal-derived factor 1, which is released from stromal fibroblasts and stimulates the invasion and migration of cholangiocarcinoma cells via interaction with the chemokine receptor, CXCR4 (Ohira et al. 2006). A summary of these and other cholangiocarcinoma-derived cancer-associated fibroblasts can be found in Figure 3.

The preponderance of data demonstrating a role for cancer-associated fibroblasts in the growth and invasion of cholangiocarcinoma suggest that targeting molecular signals released from cancer-associated fibroblasts may be a viable option, in addition to strategies for suppressing cholangiocarcinoma cell proliferation, for the treatment of cholangiocarcinoma.

3.3 Tumor-associated macrophages

Inflammation and the immune system share a long-standing relationship with tumor initiation and progression. Indeed, the primary risk factor for the development of a number of different tumor types is chronic inflammation of the target organ (Sica 2010). Once a tumor is initiated, tumor-associated macrophages (TAMs) are the major immune cell found within tumors. Macrophages generally have the potential to express and secrete pro- and anti-inflammatory molecules, and as such, may have pro- and anti-tumor activities depending upon the activation stimulus (Sica 2010). For example, macrophages activated with tumor necrosis factor α, (considered M1 activation), have anti-tumor activity and signal tissue destruction (Mantovani et al. 2002). Alternatively, in response to interleukin-4, macrophages undergo M2 activation and are involved in tissue repair, remodelling and tumor promotion (Mantovani et al. 2002).

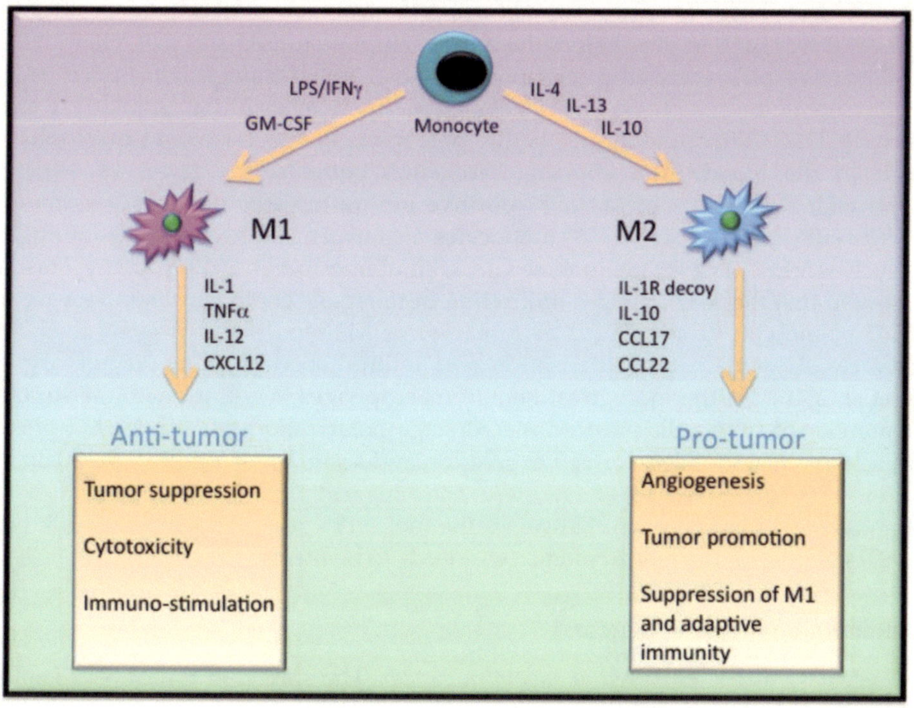

Fig. 4. Schematic representation of the pro- (M1) and anti-(M2) inflammatory activation of macrophages and their effect on tumor growth.

Logically, most TAMs have an M2-like phenotype (Mantovani and Sica 2010) thought to be brought about by various signals expressed within the tumor microenvironment, including interleukin-10, transforming growth factor-β and colony stimulating factor-1 (Sica 2010). These signals responsible for the M2-activation of macrophages have been reported to come from myeloid-derived suppressor cells, IL-10+ B lymphocytes, Th2 subtype of T helper cells and the tumor cells themselves (Sica 2010). Once alternatively activated, TAMs exhibit reduced anti-tumor activities, while increasing the production of mediators of angiogenesis such as VEGF and IL-10 (Mantovani and Sica 2010), as well as M2-specific genes that are known to be involved in promoting cell proliferation (Mantovani and Sica 2010). These events are summarized in Figure 4.

It has been proposed that strategies to inhibit the M2- and activation of the M1-inducing signals may lead to the restoration of the anti-tumor functions of TAM and help to remove the protective signals originating from the M2 TAM (Sica and Bronte 2007), which may trigger an innate immune response, thereby reducing tumor size (Sica 2010).

3.3.1 Tumor-associated macrophages in cholangiocarcinoma

As mentioned previously, cholangiocarcinoma shares a long-standing relationship with chronic inflammation (Gores 2003). Indeed, cholangiocarcinoma cells are known to over-produce many inflammatory cytokines, with IL-6 being the most studied (Isomoto et al. 2007). The role of TAMs in the development and progression of cholangiocarcinoma is poorly understood. However, recent studies have demonstrated that the density of infiltrating macrophages (as demonstrated using the MAC387 antibody to specifically stain macrophages) was high in over half of the tumor samples studied and that a high density of MAC387-positive cells correlated to a poor survival rate although conclusive proof that these cells were of the M2-phenotype is lacking (Subimerb et al. 2010a). Similarly, a subset of monocytes ($CD14^{+}CD16^{+}$) thought to be the precursors of tissue-resident macrophages are increased in the blood from cholangiocarcinoma patients, the levels of which were correlated with the density of MAC387-positive infiltrating macrophages (Subimerb et al. 2010b). The circulating $CD14^{+}CD16^{+}$ monocytes also expressed higher levels of angiogenic factors such as VEGF and the chemokine CXCL3 (Subimerb et al. 2010b). Lastly, Hasita et al. demonstrated that the macrophages infiltrating intrahepatic cholangiocarcinoma are mainly of the M2 phenotype (using CD163 as a marker of M2-type macrophages); their number correlates closely with neovascularization and infiltration of FOXP3+ regulatory T cells (Hasita et al. 2010). Furthermore, treatment of macrophages in culture with the supernatant from a number of CCA cells induced macrophage polarization toward the M2 phenotype and induced the macrophage-derived expression and secretion of VEGF-A, IL-10 and TGFβ (Hasita et al. 2010). Taken together, these data suggest that TAMs may play a role in cholangiocarcinoma progression. However, the molecules regulating the crosstalk between M2-type TAMs and cholangiocarcinoma cells needs to be further clarified.

3.4 Lymphangiogenesis in cancer

Tumor metastasis is the most lethal aspect of cancer. The spread of tumor cells is often via the lymphatic vasculature and the presence of tumor foci in lymph nodes is considered an adverse prognostic factor in most carcinomas (Achen and Stacker 2008). Metastatic spread of tumor cells via the lymphatic system was previously thought to be via a passive process by which detached tumor cells enter pre-existing lymphatic vessels in the vicinity of the tumor (Achen and Stacker 2008). However, recent studies suggest that the formation of new lymphatic vessels in the tumor microenvironment correlates with lymphatic metastasis (Achen et al. 2005).

To date, the growth factors recognized to be associated with the control of lymphangiogenesis are similar to those that control angiogenesis. That is, the most characterized factors are VEGF-C and VEGF-D, which are secreted from the tumors, and then activate VEGFR-3 expressed on lymphatic endothelium (Lymboussaki et al. 1998). Activation of VEGFR-3 induces the proliferation of lymphatic endothelial cells *in vitro* (Makinen et al. 2001) and the formation of new lymphatic vessels *in vivo* (Veikkola et al. 2001). Other identified lymphangiogenic factors include VEGF-A (Nagy et al. 2002), fibroblast growth factor-2 (Kubo et al. 2002), angiopoietin-2 (Gale et al. 2002) and platelet-derived growth factor-BB (Cao et al. 2004).

Because of the overlap in angiogenic and lymphangiogenic activity of the above-mentioned factors, agents designed to block angiogenesis may also be effective in blocking lymphangiogenesis. For example, inhibitors that block the VEGF-C/VEGF-D/VEGFR3 signalling mechanism might have the potential to not only block angiogenesis, but to also block lymphangiogenesis and hence to block lymphogenous metastatic spread (Baldwin et al. 2002; Stacker et al. 2002a; Stacker et al. 2002b). Indeed, a neutralizing VEGF-D monoclonal antibody designed to block the interaction between VEGF-D and its receptors, inhibited angiogenesis, lymphangiogenesis and metastatic spread via the lymphatics in a mouse tumor model (Stacker et al. 2001). Further studies into therapeutic strategies designed to block lymphangiogenesis are required in an attempt to stop the metastatic spread of tumors.

3.4.1 Lymphangiogenesis in cholangiocarcinoma

The role of lymphangiogenesis in cholangiocarcinoma metastasis and progression is largely unknown and controversial. However, recent studies suggest that there is a correlation between lymphangiogenesis and lymph node metastases and prognosis; patients diagnosed with cholangiocarcinoma tumors exhibiting low lymphatic vessel density have a longer survival rate than those with higher lymphatic vessel density (Thelen et al. 2008). In addition, in intrahepatic cholangiocarcinoma tumors, high lymphatic vessel density correlated with increased nodal spread and higher recurrence rate (Thelen et al. 2009). Conversely, other researchers demonstrated that in intrahepatic cholangiocarcinoma tumors, lymph node metastasis did not correlate with lymphangiogenesis, but did correlate with VEGF-C expression and the presence of a subset of myofibroblasts expressing the same markers as lymphendothelial cells (Aishima et al. 2008), which may explain the discrepancy in conclusions.

NGF has previously been linked to tumor progression and growth (Sortino et al. 2000; Descamps et al. 2001a; Descamps et al. 2001b) as well as VEGF expression (Lazarovici et al. 2006a; Lazarovici et al. 2006b) in a number of other cell types. Therefore, Xu et al. assessed the correlation of NGF-β expression with lymphangiogenesis, lymph node metastasis or VEGF-C expression in hilar cholangiocarcinoma tissue (Xu et al. 2010). Indeed, high NGF expression was correlated with VEGF-C overexpression, lymphatic vessel density, and lymph node metastasis suggesting that NGF may also be responsible for stimulating lymphangiogenesis in cholangiocarcinoma tumors.

4. Conclusions

The work highlighted in this review clearly demonstrates a role for the tumor microenvironment in the growth, progression and metastatic invasion of cholangiocarcinoma. There is obviously a strong interplay between the cells found in the stroma and cholangiocarcinoma cells with signaling molecules passing back and forth between the cell types to co-ordinately support an environment that nurtures tumor growth and suppresses innate immunity while conferring resistance to cytotoxic insults (both endogenous and chemotherapeutic). The mechanism by which each of the support cells found in the stroma of cholangiocarcinoma tumors are recruited and activated is still largely unknown. Therapeutic strategies designed to target the microenvironment rather than specifically targeting the cholangiocarcinoma cells might prove fruitful in the quest to combat this devastating cancer.

5. Acknowledgements

Portions of these studies were supported by an American Cancer Society Research Scholar award (RSC118760), an NIH K01 award (DK078532) and an NIH R03 award (DK088012) to Dr DeMorrow. This material is the result of work supported with resources and the use of facilities at the Central Texas Veterans Health Care System, Temple, Texas

6. References

Achen, M., McColl, B., & Stacker, S. (2005). Focus on lymphangiogenesis in tumor metastasis. *Cancer Cell* Vol. 7 Issue 2 (Feb 2005). pp 121-7. ISSN 1535-6108

Achen, M. & Stacker, S (2008). Molecular control of lymphatic metastasis. *Ann N Y Acad Sci* Vol. 1131 (May 2008), pp 225-34. ISSN 0077-8923

Aishima, S., Nishihara, Y., Iguchi, T., Taguchi, K., Taketomi, A., Maehara, Y., & Tsuneyoshi, M. (2008). Lymphatic spread is related to VEGF-C expression and D2-40-positive myofibroblasts in intrahepatic cholangiocarcinoma. *Mod Pathol* Vol 21, Issue 3(Mar 2008), pp 256-64. ISSN 0893-3952.

Aishima, S., Taguchi, K., Terashi, T., Matsuura, S., Shimada, M., & Tsuneyoshi, M. (2003). Tenascin expression at the invasive front is associated with poor prognosis in intrahepatic cholangiocarcinoma. *Mod Pathol* Vol 16, issue 10 (Oct 2003). pp 1019-27. ISSN 0893-3952

Alpini, G., Prall, R., & LaRusso, NF. (2001). The pathobiology of biliary epithelia. *The Liver; Biology & Pathobiology*, 4E: pp 421-435.

Alvaro, D., Barbaro, B., Franchitto, A., Onori, P., Glaser, S., Alpini, G., Francis, H., Marucci, L., Sterpetti, P., Ginanni-Corradini, S., Onetti Muda, A., Dostal, D., De Santis, A., Atilli, A., Benedetti, A., & Gaudio, E. (2006). Estrogens and insulin-like growth factor 1 modulate neoplastic cell growth in human cholangiocarcinoma. *Am J Pathol* Vol 169, Issue 3 (Sep 2006), pp 877-88. ISSN 0002-9440.

Ausprunk, D. H. & Folkman J. (1977). Migration and proliferation of endothelial cells in preformed and newly formed blood vessels during tumor angiogenesis. *Microvasc Res* Vol 14, Issue 1 (Jul 1977) pp 53-65. ISSN 0026-2862.

Baldwin, M. E., Stacker, S.A & Achen, M.G. (2002). Molecular control of lymphangiogenesis. *Bioessays* Vol 24, issue 11 (Nov 2002) pp 1030-40. ISSN 0265-9247.

Beacham, D. A. & Cukierman E. (2005). Stromagenesis: the changing face of fibroblastic microenvironments during tumor progression. *Semin Cancer Biol* Vol 15, Issue 5 (Oct, 2005), pp 329-41. ISSN 1044-579X.

Ben-Menachem, T. (2007). Risk factors for cholangiocarcinoma. *Eur J Gastroenterol Hepatol* Vol 19, Issue 8 (Aug 2007), pp 615-7. ISSN 0954-691X

Bhowmick, N. A., Neilson, E. G. & Moses H.L (2004). Stromal fibroblasts in cancer initiation and progression. *Nature* Vol 432, Issue 7015 (Nov 2004) pp 332-7. ISSN 1476-4687

Cao, R., Bjorndahl, M.A., Religa, P., Clasper, S., Garvin, S., Galter, D., Meister, B., Ikomi, F., Tritsaris, K., Dissing, S., Ohhashi, T., Jackson, D.G., & Cao Y (2004). PDGF-BB induces intratumoral lymphangiogenesis and promotes lymphatic metastasis. *Cancer Cell* Vol 6, Issue 4 (Oct 2004), pp 333-45. ISSN 1535-6108.

Catalano, O.A., Sahani, D.V., Forcione, D.G., Czermak, B., Liu, C.H., Soricelli, A., Arellano, R.S., Muller, P.R., &Hahn, P.F. (2009). Biliary infections: spectrum of imaging findings and management. *Radiographics* Vol 29, Issue 7 (Nov 2009), pp 2059-80. ISSN 1527-1323.

Chen, M. F. (1999). Peripheral cholangiocarcinoma (cholangiocellular carcinoma): clinical features, diagnosis and treatment. *J Gastroenterol Hepatol* Vol 14 Issue 12 (Dec 1999) pp 1144-9. ISSN 0815-9319.

Chuaysri, C., Thuwajit P., Paupairoj, A., Chau-In, S., Suthiphongchai, T., & Thuwajit, C. (2009). Alpha-smooth muscle actin-positive fibroblasts promote biliary cell proliferation and correlate with poor survival in cholangiocarcinoma. *Oncol Rep* Vol 21, Issue 4 (Apr 2009) pp 957-69. ISSN 1021-335X.

Cunha, G. R., Hayward S. W., Wang, Y.Z., & Ricke, W.A. (2003). Role of the stromal microenvironment in carcinogenesis of the prostate. *Int J Cancer* Vol 107 Issue 1(Oct 2003), pp 1-10. ISSN 0020-7136.

de Groen, P. C., Gores G. J., LaRusso, N.F., Gunderson, L.L., & Nagorney, D.M. (1999). Biliary tract cancers. *N Engl J Med* Vol 341, Issue 18 (Oct 1999) pp 1368-78. ISSN 0028-4793.

de Visser, K. E. & Jonkers, J. (2009). Towards understanding the role of cancer-associated inflammation in chemoresistance. *Curr Pharm Des* Vol 15 Issue 16 (Jun 2009) pp 1844-53. ISSN 1873-4286.

Descamps, S., Pawlowski V., Revillion, F., Hornez, L., Hebbar, M., Boilly, B., Hondermarck, H., & Peyrat, J.P. (2001a). Expression of nerve growth factor receptors and their prognostic value in human breast cancer. *Cancer Res* Vol 61, Issue 11 (Jun 2001), pp 4337-40. ISSN 0008-5472.

Descamps, S., Toillon R. A., Adriaenssens, E., Pawlowski, V., Cool, S.M., Nurcombe, V., Le Bourhis, X., Boilly, B., Peyrat, J.P., & Hondermarck, H. (2001b). Nerve growth factor stimulates proliferation and survival of human breast cancer cells through two distinct signaling pathways. *J Biol Chem* Vol 276 Issue 21 (May 2001) pp 17864-70. ISSN 0021-9258.

Dranoff, J. A. & Wells, R.G. (2010). Portal fibroblasts: Underappreciated mediators of biliary fibrosis. *Hepatology* Vol 51 Issue 4 (Apr 2010), pp 1438-44. ISSN 1527-3350.

Dvorak, H. F. (2005). Angiogenesis: update 2005. *J Thromb Haemost* Vol 3, Issue 8 (Aug 2005) pp 1835-42. ISSN 1538-7933.

Fava, G., DeMorrow S., Gaudio, E., Franchitto, A., Onori, P., Carpino, G., Glaser, S., Francis, H., Coufal, M., Marucci, L., Alvaro, D., Marzioni, M., Horst, T., Mancielli, R., Benedetti, A., & Alpini, G. (2009). Endothelin inhibits cholangiocarcinoma growth by a decrease in the vascular endothelial growth factor expression. *Liver Int* Vol 29 Issue 7 (August 2009), pp 1031-42. ISSN 1478-3231.

Francis, H., DeMorrow S., Venter, J., Onori, P., White, M., Gaudio, E., Francis, T., Greene, J., Tran, S., Meininger, C., & Alpini, G. (2011). Inhibition of histidine decarboxylase ablates the autocrine tumorigenic effects of histamine in human cholangiocarcinoma. *Gut* In press.

Francis, H., Onori P., Gaudio, E., Franchitto, A., DeMorrow, S., Venter, J., Kopriva, S., Carpino, G., Mancinelli, R., White, M., Meng, F., Vetuschi, A., Sferra, R., & Alpini, G. (2009). H3 histamine receptor-mediated activation of protein kinase Calpha inhibits the growth of cholangiocarcinoma in vitro and in vivo. *Mol Cancer Res* Vol 7 Issue 10 (Oct 2009), pp 1704-13. ISSN 1557-3125.

Gale, N. W., Thurston G., Hackett, S.f., Renard, R., Wang, Q., McClain, J., Martin, C., Witte, C., Witte, M.H., Jackson, D., Suri, C., Campochiaro, P.A., Wiegand, S.J., & Yancopoulos, G.D. (2002). Angiopoietin-2 is required for postnatal angiogenesis and lymphatic patterning, and only the latter role is rescued by Angiopoietin-1. *Dev Cell* Vol 3, Issue 3 (Sept 2002), pp 411-23. ISSN 1534-5807.

Gaudio, E., Barbaro B., Alvaro, D., Glaser, S., Francis, H., Ueno, Y., Meininger, C.J., Franchitto, A., Onori, P., Marzioni, M., Taffetani, S., Fava, G., Stoica, G., Venter, J., Reichenbach, R., DeMorrow, S., Summers, R., & Alpini, G. (2006). Vascular endothelial growth factor stimulates rat cholangiocyte proliferation via an autocrine mechanism. *Gastroenterology* Vol 130, Issue 4 (Apr 2006) pp 1270-82. ISSN 0016-5085.

Gladson, C. L. (1999). The extracellular matrix of gliomas: modulation of cell function. *J Neuropathol Exp Neurol* Vol 58, Issue 10 (Oct 1999), pp 1029-40. ISSN 0022-3069.

Glaser, S. S., Gaudio E., & Alpini, G. (2010). Vascular factors, angiogenesis and biliary tract disease. *Curr Opin Gastroenterol.* Vol 26, Issue 3 (Jan 2010) pp 246-50. ISSN 1531-7056.

Gores, G. J. (2003). Cholangiocarcinoma: current concepts and insights. *Hepatology* Vol 37, Issue 5 (May 2003), pp 961-9. ISSN 0270-9139.

Harder, J., Waiz O.,Otto, F., Geissler, M., Olschewski, M., Winhold, B., Blum, H.E., Schmitt0Graeff, A., & Opitz, O.G. (2009). EGFR and HER2 expression in advanced biliary tract cancer. *World J Gastroenterol* Vol 15 Issue 36 (Sep 2009), pp 4511-7. ISSN 1007-9327.

Hasita, H., Komohara Y., Okabe, H., Masuda, T., Ohnishi, K., Lei, X.F., Beppu, T., Baba, H., & Takeya, M. (2010). Significance of alternatively activated macrophages in patients with intrahepatic cholangiocarcinoma. *Cancer Sci* Vol 101, Issue 8 (Aug 2010) pp 1913-9. ISSN 1349-7006.

Iguchi, T., Yamashita N., Aishima, S., Kuroda, Y., Terashi, T., Sugimachi, K., Taguchi, K., Taketomi, A., Maehara, Y., & Tsuneyoshi, M. (2009). A comprehensive analysis of immunohistochemical studies in intrahepatic cholangiocarcinoma using the survival tree model. *Oncology* Vol 76 Issue 4 (Sep 2009) pp 293-300. ISSN 1423-0232.

Isomoto, H., Mott, J.L., Kobayashi, S., Werneburg, N.W., Bronk, S.F., Haan, S., & Gores, G.J. (2007). Sustained IL-6/STAT-3 signaling in cholangiocarcinoma cells due to SOCS-3 epigenetic silencing. *Gastroenterology* Vol 132, Issue 1 (Jan 2007), pp 384-96.

Kawahara, N., Ono, M., Taguchi, K., Okamoto, M., Shimada, M., Takenaka, K., Hayashi, K., Mosher, D.F., Sugimachi, K., Tsuneyoshi, M., & Kuwano, M. (1998). Enhanced expression of thrombospondin-1 and hypovascularity in human cholangiocarcinoma. *Hepatology* Vol 28 Issue 6 (Dec 1998), pp 1512-7. ISSN 0270-9139.

Kubo, H., Cao, R., Brakenhielm, E., Makinen, T., Cao, Y., & Alitalo, K. (2002). Blockade of vascular endothelial growth factor receptor-3 signaling inhibits fibroblast growth factor-2-induced lymphangiogenesis in mouse cornea. *Proc Natl Acad Sci U S A* Vol 99, Issue 13 (Jun 2002), pp 8868-73. ISSN 0027-8424.

Lazarovici, P., Gazit, A., Staniszewska, I., Marcinkiewicz, C., & Lelkes, P.I. (2006a). Nerve growth factor (NGF) promotes angiogenesis in the quail chorioallantoic membrane. *Endothelium* Vol 13 Issue 1 (Jan-Feb 2006) pp 51-9. ISSN 1062-3329.

Lazarovici, P., Marcinkiewicz C., & Lelkes, P.I. (2006b). Cross talk between the cardiovascular and nervous systems: neurotrophic effects of vascular endothelial growth factor (VEGF) and angiogenic effects of nerve growth factor (NGF)-implications in drug development. *Curr Pharm Des* Vol 12 Issue 21 (Nov 2006) pp 2609-22. ISSN 1381-6128.

Ljubimova, J. Y., Fujita M., Khazenzon, N.M., Ljubimov, A.V., & Black, K.L. (2006). Changes in laminin isoforms associated with brain tumor invasion and angiogenesis. *Front Biosci* Vol 11 (Nov 2006) pp 81-8. ISSN 1093-4715.

Lymboussaki, A., Partanen T. A., Olofsson, B., Thomas-Crusells, J., Fletcher, C.D., de Waal, R.M., Kaipainen, A., & Alitalo, K. (1998). Expression of the vascular endothelial growth factor C receptor VEGFR-3 in lymphatic endothelium of the skin and in vascular tumors. *Am J Pathol* Vol 153, Issue 2 (Aug 1998) pp 395-403. ISSN 0002-9440.

Makinen, T., Veikkola T., Mustjoki, S., Karpanen, T., Catimel, B., Nice, E.C., Wise, L., Mercer, A., Kowalski, H., Kerjaschki, D., Stacker, S.A., Achen, M.G., & Alitalo, K. (2001). Isolated lymphatic endothelial cells transduce growth, survival and migratory signals via the VEGF-C/D receptor VEGFR-3. *EMBO J* Vol 20, Issue 17, (Sept 2001), pp 4762-73. ISSN 0261-4189.

Mancino, A., Mancino M. G., Glaser, S.S., Alpini, G., Bolognese, A., Izzo, L., Francis, H., Onori, P., Franchitto, A., Ginanni-Corradini, S., Gaudio, E., & Alvaro, D. (2009). Estrogens stimulate the proliferation of human cholangiocarcinoma by inducing the expression and secretion of vascular endothelial growth factor. *Dig Liver Dis* Vol 41, Issue 2 (Feb 2009), pp 156-63. ISSN 1878-3562.

Mantovani, A. and Sica A. (2010). Macrophages, innate immunity and cancer: balance, tolerance, and diversity. *Curr Opin Immunol* Vol 22, Issue 2 (Apr 2010) pp 231-7. ISSN 1879-0372.

Mantovani, A., Sozzani S., Locati, M., Allavena, P., & Sica, A. (2002). Macrophage polarization: tumor-associated macrophages as a paradigm for polarized M2 mononuclear phagocytes. *Trends Immunol* Vol 23, Issue 11 (Nov 2002), pp 549-55. ISSN 1471-4906.

McDougall, S. R., Anderson A. R., & Chaplain, M.A. (2006). Mathematical modelling of dynamic adaptive tumour-induced angiogenesis: clinical implications and therapeutic targeting strategies. *J Theor Biol* Vol 241, Issue 3 (Aug 2006), pp 564-89. ISSN 0022-5193.

Mikkelsen, T., Yan P. S., Ho, K.L., Sameni, M., Sloane, B.F., & Rosenblum, M.L. (1995). Immunolocalization of cathepsin B in human glioma: implications for tumor invasion and angiogenesis. *J Neurosurg* Vol 83, Issue 2 (Aug 1995), pp 285-90. ISSN 0022-3085.

Mobius, C., Demuth C., Aigner, T., Wiedmann, M., Wittekind, C., Mossner, J., Hauss, J., & Witzigmann, H. (2007). Evaluation of VEGF A expression and microvascular density as prognostic factors in extrahepatic cholangiocarcinoma. *Eur J Surg Oncol* Vol 33, Issue 8 (Oct 2007), pp 1025-9. ISSN 0748-7983.

Nagy, J. A., Vasile E., Feng, D., Sundberg, C., Brown, L.F., Detmar, M.J., Lawitts, J.A., Benjamin, L., Tan, X., Manseau, E.J., Dvorak, A.M., & Dvorak, H.F.(2002). Vascular permeability factor/vascular endothelial growth factor induces lymphangiogenesis as well as angiogenesis. *J Exp Med* Vol 196, Issue 11 (Dec 2002), pp 1497-506. ISSN 0022-1007.

Ogasawara, S., Yano H., Higaki, K., Takayama, A., Akiba, J., Shiota, K., & Kojiro, M. (2001). Expression of angiogenic factors, basic fibroblast growth factor and vascular endothelial growth factor, in human biliary tract carcinoma cell lines. *Hepatol Res* Vol 20, Issue 1 (May 2001), pp 97-113. ISSN 1386-6346.

Ohira, S., Sasaki M., Harada, K., Sato, Y., Zen, Y., Isse, K., Kozaka, K., Ishikawa, A., Oda, DK., Nimura, Y., & Nakanuma, Y. (2006). Possible regulation of migration of intrahepatic cholangiocarcinoma cells by interaction of CXCR4 expressed in carcinoma cells with tumor necrosis factor-alpha and stromal-derived factor-1 released in stroma. *Am J Pathol* Vol 168, Issue 4 (Apr 2006), pp 1155-68. ISSN 0002-9440.

Okabe, H., Beppu T., Hayashi, H., Horino, K., Masuda, T., Komori, H., Ishikawa, S., Watanabe, M., Takamori, H., Iyama, K., & Baba, H. (2009). Hepatic stellate cells may relate to progression of intrahepatic cholangiocarcinoma. *Ann Surg Oncol* Vol 16 Issue 9 (Sep 2009), pp 2555-64. ISSN 1534-4681.

Olumi, A. F., Grossfeld G. D., Hayward, S.W., Carroll, P.R., Tisty, T.D., & Cunha, G.R. (1999). Carcinoma-associated fibroblasts direct tumor progression of initiated human prostatic epithelium. *Cancer Res* Vol 59, Issue 19 (Oct 1999), pp 5002-11. ISSN 0008-5472.

Onimaru, M. and Yonemitsu Y. (2011). Angiogenic and lymphangiogenic cascades in the tumor microenvironment. *Front Biosci (Schol Ed)* Vol 3, pp 216-25. ISSN 1945-0524.

Orimo, A. and Weinberg R. A. (2006). Stromal fibroblasts in cancer: a novel tumor-promoting cell type. *Cell Cycle* Vol 5, Issue 15 (Aug 2006) pp 1597-601. ISSN 1551-4005.

Patel, T. (2002). Worldwide trends in mortality from biliary tract malignancies. *BMC Cancer* Vol 2 (May 2002), pp 10. ISSN 1471-2407.

Prakobwong, S., Gupta S. C., Kim, J.H., Sung, B., Pinlaor, P., Hiraku, Y., Wongkham, S., Sripa, B., Pinlaor, S., & Aggarwal, B.B. (2011). Curcumin suppresses proliferation and induces apoptosis in human biliary cancer cells through modulation of multiple cell signaling pathways. *Carcinogenesis.* In press ISSN 1460-2180.

Prakobwong, S., Khoontawad, J., Yongvanit, P., Pairojkul, C., Hiraku, Y., Sithithaworn, P., Pinlaor, P., Aggarwal, B.B., & Pinlaor, S. (2011). Curcumin decreases cholangiocarcinogenesis in hamsters by suppressing inflammation-mediated molecular events related to multistep carcinogenesis. *Int J Cancer* Vol 129 Issue 1 (Jul 2011), pp 88-100. ISSN 1097-0215.

Rasanen, K. and Vaheri A. (2010). Activation of fibroblasts in cancer stroma. *Exp Cell Res* Vol 316, Issue 17 (Oct 2010), pp 2713-22. ISSN 1090-2422.

Roberts, W. G. and Palade G. E. (1997). Neovasculature induced by vascular endothelial growth factor is fenestrated. *Cancer Res* Vol 57, Issue 4 (Feb 1997), pp 765-72. ISSN 0008-5472.

Rojas, A., Figueroa H., & Morales, E. (2010). Fueling inflammation at tumor microenvironment: the role of multiligand/RAGE axis. *Carcinogenesis* Vol 31 Issue 3 (Mar 2010), pp 334-41. ISSN 1460-2180.

Shimoda, M., Mellody K. T., & Orimo, A. (2010). Carcinoma-associated fibroblasts are a rate-limiting determinant for tumour progression. *Semin Cell Dev Biol* Vol 21, Issue 1 (Feb 2010), pp 19-25. ISSN 1096-3634.

Shinohara, E. T. and Maity A. (2009). Increasing sensitivity to radiotherapy and chemotherapy by using novel biological agents that alter the tumor microenvironment. *Curr Mol Med* Vol 9, Issue 9 (Dec 2009), pp 1034-45. ISSN 1875-5666.

Sica, A. (2010). Role of tumour-associated macrophages in cancer-related inflammation. *Exp Oncol* Vol 32, Issue 3 (Sep 2010), pp 153-8. ISSN 1812-9269.

Sica, A. and Bronte V. (2007). Altered macrophage differentiation and immune dysfunction in tumor development. *J Clin Invest* Vol 117 Issue 5 (May 2007) pp 1155-66. ISSN 0021-9738.

Sirica, A. E. (2005). Cholangiocarcinoma: molecular targeting strategies for chemoprevention and therapy. *Hepatology* Vol 41, Issue 1 (Jan 2005), pp 5-15.

Sirica, A. E., Dumur C. I., Campbell, D.J., Almenara, J.A., Ogunwobi, O.O., & Dewitt, J.L. (2009). Intrahepatic cholangiocarcinoma progression: prognostic factors and basic mechanisms. *Clin Gastroenterol Hepatol* Vol 7 Issue 11 Suppl (Nov 2009), pp S68-78. ISSN 1542-7714.

Sortino, M. A., Condorelli F., Vancheri, C., Chiarenza, A., Bernardini, R., Consoli, U., & Canonico, P.L. (2000). Mitogenic effect of nerve growth factor (NGF) in LNCaP prostate adenocarcinoma cells: role of the high- and low-affinity NGF receptors. *Mol Endocrinol* Vol 14 Issue 1 (Jan 2000), pp 124-36. ISSN 0888-8809.

Stacker, S. A., Achen M. G., Jussila, L., Baldwin, M.E., & Alitalo, K. (2002a). Lymphangiogenesis and cancer metastasis. *Nat Rev Cancer* Vol 2 Issue 8 (Aug 2002) pp 573-83. ISSN 1474-175X

Stacker, S. A., Baldwin M. E., & Achen, M.G.. (2002b). The role of tumor lymphangiogenesis in metastatic spread. *FASEB J* Vol 16, Issue 9 (Jul 2002), pp 922-34. ISSN 1530-6860.

Stacker, S. A., Caesar C., Baldwin, M.E., Thornton, G.E., Williams, R.A., Prevo, R., Jackson, D.G., Nishikawa, S., Kubo, H., & Achen, M.G. (2001). VEGF-D promotes the metastatic spread of tumor cells via the lymphatics. *Nat Med* Vol 7, Issue 2 (Feb 2001) pp 186-91. ISSN 1078-8956.

Subimerb, C., Pinlaor S., Khuntikeo, N., Leelayuwat, C., Morris, A., McGrath, M.S., & Wongkham, S. (2010a). Tissue invasive macrophage density is correlated with prognosis in cholangiocarcinoma. *Mol Med Report* Vol 3 Issue 4 (Jul-Aug 2010) pp 597-605. ISSN 1791-3004.

Subimerb, C., Pinlaor S., Lulitanond, V., Khuntikeo, N., Okada, S., McGrath, M.S., & Wongkham, S. (2010b). Circulating CD14(+) CD16(+) monocyte levels predict tissue invasive character of cholangiocarcinoma. *Clin Exp Immunol* Vol 161 Issue 3 (Sep 2010) pp 471-9. ISSN 1365-2249.

Tang, D., Nagano H., Yamamoto, H., Wada, H., Nakamura, M., Kondo, M., Ota, H., Yoshioka, S., Kato, H., Damdinsuren, B., Marubashi, S., Miyamoto, A., Takeda, Y.,

Umeshita, K., Dono, K., Wakasa, K., & Monden, M. (2006). Angiogenesis in cholangiocellular carcinoma: expression of vascular endothelial growth factor, angiopoietin-1/2, thrombospondin-1 and clinicopathological significance. *Oncol Rep* Vol 15 Issue 3 (Mar 2006), pp 525-32. ISSN 1021-335X.

Thelen, A., A. Scholz, et al. (2008). Tumor-associated lymphangiogenesis correlates with lymph node metastases and prognosis in hilar cholangiocarcinoma. *Ann Surg Oncol* Vol 15 Issue 3 (Mar 2008), pp 791-9.

Thelen, A., Scholz A., Benckert, C., Weichert, W., Dietz, E., Wiedenmann, B., Neuhaus, P., & Jonas, S. (2010). Tumor-Associated Angiogenesis and Lymphangiogenesis Correlate With Progression of Intrahepatic Cholangiocarcinoma. *Am J Gastroenterol.* Vol 105, Issue 5 (Mar 2010) pp 1123-32. ISSN 1534-4681.

Tlsty, T. D. (2001). Stromal cells can contribute oncogenic signals. *Semin Cancer Biol* Vol 11 Issue 2 (Apr 2001) pp 97-104. ISSN 1044-579X.

Tominaga, S. and Kuroishi T. (1994). Biliary tract cancer. *Cancer Surv* Vol 19-20, pp 125-37. ISSN 0261-2429.

Tuxhorn, J. A., Ayala G. E., & Rowley, D.R. (2001). Reactive stroma in prostate cancer progression. *J Urol* Vol 166, Issue 6 (Dec 2001), pp 2472-83. ISSN 0022-5347.

Utispan, K., Thuwajit P., Abiko, Y., Charngkaew, K., Paupairoj, A., Chau-in, S., & Thuwajit, C. (2010). Gene expression profiling of cholangiocarcinoma-derived fibroblast reveals alterations related to tumor progression and indicates periostin as a poor prognostic marker. *Mol Cancer* Vol 9, pp 13. ISSN 1476-4598.

Veikkola, T., Jussila L., Makinen, T., Karpanen, T., Jeltsch, M., Petrova, T.V., Kubo, H., Thurston, G., McDonald, D.M., Achen, M.G., Stacker, S.A., & Alitalo, K. (2001). Signalling via vascular endothelial growth factor receptor-3 is sufficient for lymphangiogenesis in transgenic mice. *EMBO J* Vol 20 Issue 6 (Mar 2001), pp 1223-31. ISSN 0261-4189.

Xu, L. B., Liu C., Gao, G.Q., Yu, X.H., Zhang, R., & Wang, J. (2010). Nerve growth factor-beta expression is associated with lymph node metastasis and nerve infiltration in human hilar cholangiocarcinoma. *World J Surg* Vol 34, Issue 5 (May 2010), pp 1039-45. ISSN 1432-2323.

Yabuuchi, S., Katayose Y., Oda, A., Mizuma, M., Shirasou, S., Sasaki, T., Yamamoto, K., Oikawa, M., Rikiyama, T., Onogawa, T., Yoshia, H., Ohtuska, H., Motoi, F., Egawa, S., & Unno, M. (2009). ZD1839 (IRESSA) stabilizes p27Kip1 and enhances radiosensitivity in cholangiocarcinoma cell lines. *Anticancer Res* Vol 29 Issue 4 (Apr 2009) pp 1169-80. ISSN 0250-7005.

Yoshikawa, D., Ojima H., Iwasaki, M., Hiraoka, N., Kosuge, T., Kasai, S., Hirohashi, S., & Shibata, T. (2008). Clinicopathological and prognostic significance of EGFR, VEGF, and HER2 expression in cholangiocarcinoma. *Br J Cancer* Vol 98, Issue 2 (Jan 2008), pp 418-25. ISSN 0007-0920.

Yoshikawa, D., Ojima H., Kokubu, A., Ochiya, T., Kasai, S., Hirohashi, S., & Shibata, T. (2009). Vandetanib (ZD6474), an inhibitor of VEGFR and EGFR signalling, as a novel molecular-targeted therapy against cholangiocarcinoma. *Br J Cancer* Vol 100, Issue 8 (Apr 2009), pp 1257-66. ISSN 1532-1827.

5

Ultrasound Imaging of Liver Tumors – Current Clinical Applications

R. Badea[1] and Simona Ioanitescu[2]
[1]*Ultrasound Dept., Institute of Gastroenterology and Hepatology, Univ. of Medicine & Pharmacy "Iuliu Hatieganu" Cluj-Napoca*
[2]*Center of Internal Medicine, Fundeni Clinical Institute, Bucharest*
Romania

1. Introduction

1.1 Definition of ultrasonographic method

Ultrasound exploration (ultrasonography) is a very common diagnostic method. It is part of imaging procedures, without using ionizing radiations but ultrasounds (US) with usual frequencies of 2 - 5 - 12 MHz. Ultrasounds cross biological environments and are reflected at the demarcation limit between structures of different consistencies. The current procedure of ultrasound examination called "scanning" is based on the analysis of every plane from a region of interest in the human body. Each plane contains a high number of points with different brightness (within the limit of the gray scale used by the equipment) and their sum makes a defining "echostructure" for each organ. Ultrasound diagnosis is based on changes in tissue density due to pathological changes, resulting in echostructure transformation. Ultrasonography is an anatomical, hemodynamic and functional exploration.

1.2 Brief history

Since the 1940s there have been pioneers (physicians, biologists, physicists) who intuited that acoustic energy, at that time used only in war industry to detect submarines, could have applications in medical diagnosis. The first ultrasound images contained information about the density of tissues displayed along an axis ("A- mode" ultrasound). Later, "sectional" ultrasound was invented, which detailed echoes in a plane ("B-mode" ultrasound with applications in obstetrics). In the '60s the procedure had an accelerated development by diversifying examination techniques, identifying more clinical applications and increasing access to a large number of specialties. In the '70s clinical specialties such as obstetrics and cardiology "claimed" the method, using as the main argument its clinical character arising from the direct relationship between the examining physician and the patient. After the '90s, emergency physicians requested the presence of miniature, portable ultrasound equipment in the emergency room proving that ultrasound, using accordingly well defined algorithms, contributed to saving lives. Today, ultrasonography is used by clinicians in more than 50% of cases. Although there is still an ongoing "battle" between clinicians and radiologists for the monopoly over the ultrasound method, the final outcome is an exceptional dynamic of the method, considered today the most common diagnostic imaging procedure in the world (Derchi & Claudon, 2009). In the near future the ultrasound examination will be unrestrictedly generalized with the introduction of the procedure as basic training for medical students, as part of clinical examination.

1.3 Advantages and disadvantages of the ultrasound method

Ultrasound is useful for the practitioner as a first imaging procedure in direct correlation to the clinical examination. The method has a very good cost/quality ratio, the image is very accurate and precise and the information has a dynamic character ("real time imaging"). It is important to note that ultrasound has its limitations which the examining physician must take into account. Thus, the ultrasound image contains a number of artifacts and is mainly limited by phenomena such as US attenuation related to distance and density. Ultrasound is an operator-dependent method, thus its reproducibility is reduced.

1.4 Ultrasound techniques and procedures

The principles of ultrasonography are complex. The US picture is generated by ultrasound penetration into the human body. US are reflected as echoes and converted by the transducer into signals. The ultrasound image is multimodal. There are multiple US procedures systematized into "clinical applications" and the information obtained is tissular ("morphometric" type) and vascular ("hemodynamic "type). Finally, US examination is a "real time" procedure which reflects the movements of the organs. It is mandatory to connect the US information to the clinical and functional-biochemical data in order to obtain the final diagnosis.

1.4.1 Tissue investigation

The conventional US currently used in practice is called "2D, gray scale" sonography. The technique is based on US property with frequencies > 20 kHz and constant acoustic power to cross tissues with an average speed of 1540 cm/sec. US are returned with different acoustic power at a variable timeframe depending on the acoustic density of the crossed environment and on the position of the reflecting element. There is a proportional relationship between the intensity of the echo and the density of a crossed biological environment; therefore, ultrasound is a noninvasive tissue density assessment procedure. There are two categories of echoes according to their frequency: basic (similar to the incident beam, i.e. 3 MHz) and "harmonic" (multiples of the emission frequency, i.e. 6 MHz). Harmonic echoes arise from the non-linear vibration of the tissues. Due to their high frequency, the result is a high quality image. Harmonic ultrasound technique ("coded harmonics" or "tissue harmonic imaging," THI) combined with the pulse inversion procedure ("pulse inversion harmonic imaging") allows to obtain information regardless of the depth where the region of interest lies and is available on most commercial equipment (Choudhry et al, 2000).

Image resolution (minimum size at which a reflected structure is distinctly shown on the screen) is essential for tumor detection. The number of crystals included into the transducer and the nominal frequency of the ultrasound beam (the higher the frequency the better the resolution) also contribute to the ultrasound image quality. The gain of echoes ("gain" function) and the time compensation of echoes gain ("time gain compensation" function) measured in decibels, image depth and the number of focuses, echoes acquisition and their representation rate are other elements that allow information rendering with the same quality at an approximate ultrasound penetration of 20 to 25 cm. All these phenomena contribute to image the tissue echostructure. The sonography has a very good capacity to discriminate lesions depending on their consistency (a parenchymal cyst is detectable at a 2-3 mm size!; a solid nodule is distinctly shown at sizes of 5 - 6 mm). In addition, the method allows accurate assessment of the lesion size and the evaluation of organ motility (gastrointestinal tract, heart, main vessels).

The ultrasound image is planar, two-dimensional (2D ultrasound). In recent years equipments have been developed, allowing 3D reconstruction of ultrasound images. The resulting images are not planes but volumes that can be static (3D) or dynamic (4D). 3D/4D exploration has recognized obstetrical applications but other areas of application of this method have been identified in recent years, mainly in oncology. 3D/4D ultrasound provides accurate information in connection with the space, shape, size and tumors texture. This procedure may be useful to measure the real tumor volume as well as the healthy surrounding parenchyma which should to be removed in case of surgery. Combining this procedure with intratumoral circulation assessment methods allows more accurate diagnosis of the tumor nature (Badea et al, 2007).

1.4.2 Blood flow and microcirculation investigation

Blood flow can be explored by ultrasound using various techniques. Some are based on Doppler principle (or derivatives) and others on the use of intravenous contrast agents (CA).

1.4.2.1 Doppler ultrasound

It is an established method for the assessment of blood flow based on the frequency variation of a US beam hitting a target (in our case, groups of red blood cells) in motion. The difference in frequency and its positive or negative character are elements that allow vectorial representation of blood speed and direction of movement against the transducer. Doppler ultrasound has several technical options: spectral and color coded, each of them with their advantages and disadvantages. Thus: spectral ultrasound describes the flow type (arterial or venous) and allows measurements. Color flow mode (CFM) ultrasound encodes speed vectors related to red blood cells groups thus detecting blood flows. Evaluation of tumor vasculature will be made first using the CFM module and then spectral Doppler module by positioning the Doppler sample on reference regions. On CFM investigation tumor vessels have tortuous paths, aberrant spatial ramifications, they intercommunicate and can abruptly end in "glove finger" (Cherrington et al, 2000). Spatial positioning of intratumoral vessels can also be illustrated by 3D/4D reconstruction procedures and quantitative assessment can be achieved with techniques using color pixel count per unit area. Spectral investigation measurements into the tumor vessels lumen show either low values (RI<0.65; S/D <2.5) suggesting the absence of arterial precapillary sphincter and the presence of arterio-venous shunts or high values secondary to increased interstitial pressure. Accelerated flow speed can be identified in the input vessels from the tumor hilum suggesting a circulatory bed avid for blood (Cosgrove & Eckersley, 1997).

1.4.2.2 Contrast Enhanced Ultrasound (CEUS)

The introduction of intravenous (i.v.) contrast agents (CAs) is a great step forward for ultrasound. The first attempts to contrast ultrasound emerged in the '60s and had applications in interventional cardiology. After the 90s, first generation contrast agents were introduced into the clinical practice (the most used product is Levovist, Schering AG). These are air containing microbubbles, wrapped in a stabilizing membrane with the property to enhance the intensity of the echoes received from the blood flow thus making the Doppler signal more evident. This type of CAs has the disadvantage of a "blooming" effect of the color on CFM examination which masks the information derived from the microcirculation. With the development of transducer technology and the introduction of intermittent pulses emission with high mechanical index (MI> 0.2) it was possible to detect slow flows by identifying signals resulting from "breaking" microbubbles. This technique, called "destructive" contrast ultrasound is similar to that of contrast CT or MRI. Its disadvantage is that information cannot be obtained in "real time". After the year 2000, second generation contrast agents were introduced in clinical practice [SonoVue® in Europe, Sonazoid™ in Japan, Definity in Canada, Optison™). They consist of microbubbles filled with different gases other than air, with stability and elasticity in the bloodstream higher than that of the first generation CAs. The exposure of these CAs to low mechanical index (MI <0.1 to 0.2) US generates harmonics echoes resulting from non linear microbubble oscillation (table 1).

Particularity	Importance
They do not cross vessel walls, being strictly confined to the circulatory bed.	They are real angiospecific tracers useful for quantification of circulation in a region of interest.
Characterized by repeated recirculation from the large to small circulation until complete clearance	High persistence and prolonged investigation
Elimination of contrast agent is made through respiration and breakage	Can be used in renal and hepatic failure
They show a non-linear oscillation when exposed to low MI ultrasounds	Ultrasound information is found in harmonic echoes Ultrasound exploration is dynamic, "in real time"

Table 1. Characteristics of second generation contrast agents. Particularities and importance.

As low acoustic power US are used, this procedure does not break the microbubbles, which allows "real time" blood flow examination during several minutes (Burns & Wilson, 2006).

Harmonic contrast US examination, using second generation CAs requires special software equipment which suppresses 2D ultrasound image derived from the tissues by inverted phase ultrasound emission (the technique is called "pulse inversion"). In this way the information on the screen will correlate only to harmonic echoes generated by the microbubbles (Burns et al, 2000).

CEUS examination is a qualitative examination. As it is a continuous exploration, CEUS allows successive identification of vascular phases: arterial (approximately 10 - 15 sec. from the time of injection in the peripherals up to approx. 30-40 seconds) and venous. Some circulation areas (liver, spleen) have a "late" phase due to the "capture" of microbubbles into the reticulo-histiocyte system (RHS). In addition, the investigation also allows the assessment of vascular morphology which provides information similar to angiography. CEUS investigation has a high temporal resolution, superior to CT or MRI explorations.

CEUS liver investigation has two important elements that make it distinct (Cosgrove, 2007; Claudon et al, 2008):

a. the liver has a complex vascularization: for input (arterial and portal phase, the first can be identified in approx. 10 - 30 seconds after injection and the second in approx. 30 - 90 seconds after i.v. CA injection) and for elimination (sinusoidal phase, progressively occurs in approx. 120 seconds after injection and has a total duration of approx. 4-5 minutes);
b. liver tumors have a characteristic vasculature according to their nature, e.g. hepatocellular carcinoma is highly arterialized; metastases have a mixed input vasculature; benign tumors have a variable circulatory bed (hemangioma is highly capillarized). Tumor characterization using CEUS procedure is based on the contrast agent crossing the region of interest (dynamic, particularities) and on the vascular bed characteristics (presence, spatial distribution, vascular morphology, areas lacking signal which means scar or necrosis). This analysis is separately carried out in the arterial, portal venous and late phases. Algorithms are currently available that help liver mass discrimination (Bolondi et al, 2007). The procedure can be combined with 3D reconstruction techniques, which confers additional utility to the method (Luo et al, 2009).

A useful procedure to obtain more quantitative details is contrast curves analysis. These consist of graphical representation of the CA dynamics while crossing a region of interest. The method is useful for assessing chemotherapy efficacy in various malignancies.

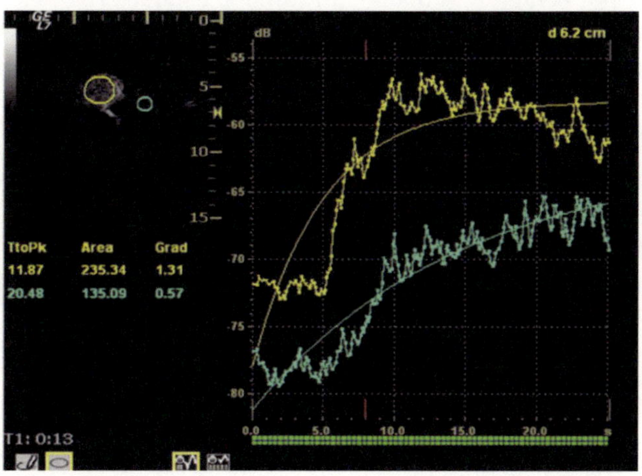

Fig. 1. Contrast dynamic analysis curves in the region of interest - TIC. Tracer dynamics in the region of reference is marked with blue and with yellow in the region of interest (tumor). It can be seen that the tumor has a more abundant circulation than the surrounding liver parenchyma.

Limitations of CEUS examination. Harmonic contrast examination has some limitations including: a) the procedure is indicated only correlated with good 2D image; b) it has a relatively high cost; c) it is operator dependent examination.

2. 2D and harmonic ultrasonography in detecting and characterizing liver tumors

2.1 Characteristics of ultrasound diagnosis

Ultrasound diagnosis of liver tumors involves two stages: detection and characterization.

Tumor detection is based on the performance of the method as already presented and should include morphometric information (three axes dimensions, volume) and topographic information (number, location specifying liver segment and lobe/lobes). The specification of these data is important for staging liver tumors and prognosis.

Tumor characterization is a complex process based on a sum of criteria leading towards tumor nature definition. Often, other diagnostic procedures, especially interventional ones are no longer necessary. Ultrasound examination has the same morphological and hemodynamic criteria as those of CT and MRI imaging procedures. However, semiology will be adjusted to the specifics of this method. Tumor characterization using the ultrasound method will be based on the following elements: consistency (solid, liquid, mixed), echogenity, structure appearance (homogeneous or heterogeneous), delineation from adjacent liver parenchyma (capsular, imprecise), elasticity, posterior acoustic enhancement effect, the relation with neighboring organs or structures (displacement, invasion), vasculature (presence, Doppler and CEUS characteristics). The substrate on which the tumor condition develops (if the liver is normal or if there is evidence of diffuse liver disease) and the developing context (oncology, septic) are also added. Particular attention should be paid to the analysis of the circulatory bed. Microcirculation investigation allows for discrimination between benign and malignant tumors. Characteristic elements of malignant circulation are vascular density, presence of vessels with irregular paths and size, some of them intercommunicating, some others blocked in the end with "glove finger" appearance, the presence of arterio-arterial and arterio-venous shunts, lack or incompetence of arterial precapillary sphincter made up of smooth musculatures (Weidener et al, 1991).

Diagnosis and characterization of liver tumors require a distinct approach for each group of conditions, using the available procedures discussed above for each of them. The correlation with the medical history, the patient's clinical and functional (biochemical and hematological) status are important elements that should also be considered.

2.2 Benign liver tumors

They generally develop on normal or fatty liver, are single or multiple (generally paucilocular), have distinct delineation, with increased echogenity (hemangiomas, benign focal nodular hyperplasia) or absent, with posterior acoustic enhancement effect (cysts), have distinct delineation (hydatid cyst), lack of vascularization or show a characteristic circulatory pattern, displace normal liver structures and even neighboring organs (in case of large sizes), are quite elastic and do not invade liver vessels. The patient has a good general status, as tumors are often asymptomatic, being incidentally discovered.

2.2.1 Liver cysts

They can be single or multiple, with variable size, generally less than 20 mm (congenital). Rarely, sizes can reach several centimeters, leading up to the substitution of a whole liver lobe (acquired, parasitic). They may be associated with renal cysts; in this case the disease has a hereditary, autosomal dominant transmission (von Hippel Lindau disease). The ultrasound appearance is a well defined lesion, with very thin, almost unapparent walls, without circulatory signal at Doppler or CEUS investigation. The content is transonic suggesting fluid composition. The presence of membranes, abundant sediment or cysts inside is suggestive for parasitic, hydatid nature. Posterior from the lesion the "acoustic enhancement" phenomenon is seen, which strengthens the suspicion of fluid mass. They typically displace normal liver vessels but no vascular or biliary invasion occurs.

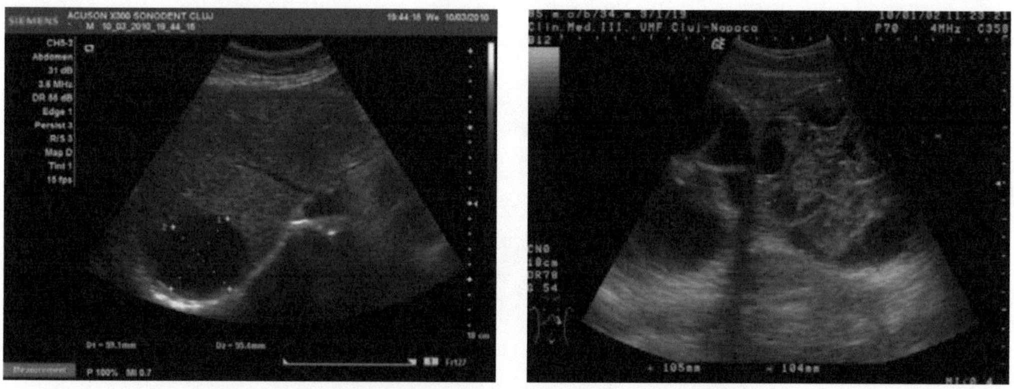

Fig. 2. Liver cyst – left image. Hydatid liver cyst (2D exam) – right image. Diagnostic criteria are the presence of membranes and sediment inside.

2.2.2 Hemangioma

It is the most common liver tumor with a prevalence of 0.4 - 7.4%. It is generally asymptomatic but also can be associated with pain complaints or cytopenia and/or anemia when it is very bulky. It is unique or paucilocular. It can be associated with other types of benign liver tumors. Characteristic 2D ultrasound appearance is that of a very well defined lesion, with sizes of 2-3 cm or less, showing increased echogenity and, when located in contact with the diaphragm, a "mirror image" phenomenon can be seen. When palpating the liver with the transducer the hemangioma is compressible sending reverberations backwards. Doppler exploration reveals no circulatory signal due to very slow flow speed. CEUS investigation has real diagnosis value due to the typical behavior of progressive CA enhancement of the tumor from the periphery towards the center. The enhancement is slow, during several minutes, depending on the size of hemangioma and on the presence (or absence) of internal thrombosis. During late (sinusoidal) phase, if totally "filled" with CA, hemangioma appears isoechoic to the liver. Deviations from the above described behavior can occur in arterialized hemangiomas or those containing arterio-venous shunts. In these cases differentiation from a malignant tumor is difficult and requires other imaging procedures, follow up and measurements of the tumor at short time intervals.

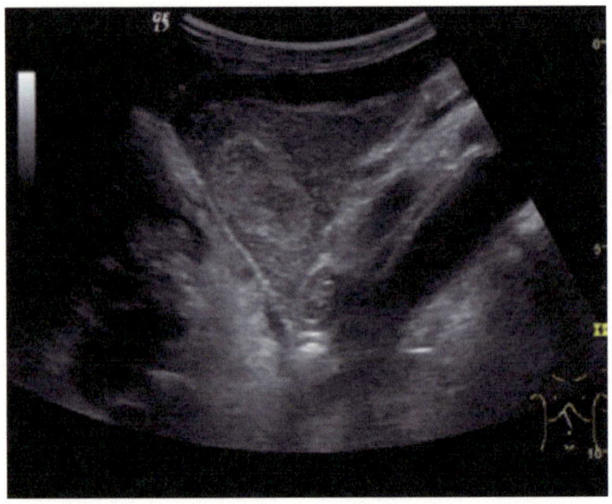

Fig. 3. Hepatic hemangioma (2D). The lesion is located in the left hepatic lobe. Note precise delineation, their increased echogenity and the heterogeneous internal structure.

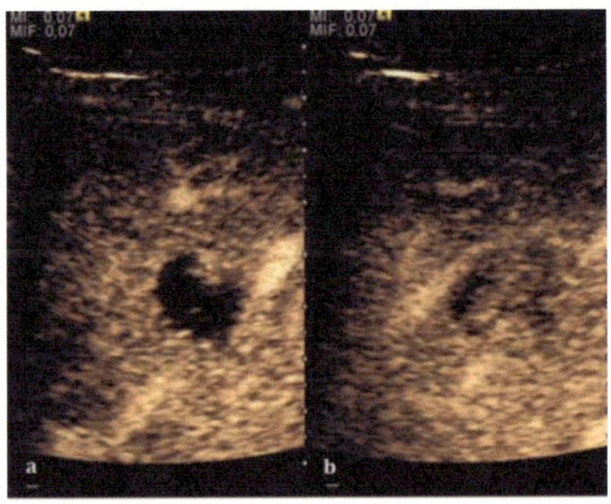

Fig. 4. Hepatic hemangioma (CEUS). Progression of CA from the periphery toward the center of the lesion is evidenced by examination at various time intervals (a - arterial phase; b - late phase).

2.2.3 Focal nodular hyperplasia

It is a tumor developed secondary to a circulatory abnormality with abundant arterial vessels having a characteristic location in the center of the tumor, within a fibrotic scar. A radial vessels network develops from this level with peripheral orientation. The tumor's circulatory bed is rich in microcirculatory and portal venous elements. The incidence is higher in younger women and tumor development is accelerated by oral contraceptives intake. 2D ultrasound appearance is a fairly well-defined mass, with variable sizes, usually single, solid consistency with inhomogeneous structure. Rarely the central scar can be distinguished. Spectral Doppler examination detects central arterial vessels and CFM exploration reveals their radial position. CEUS examination shows central tumor filling of the circulatory bed during arterial phase and completely enhancement during portal venous phase. During this phase the center of the lesion becomes hypoechoic, enhancing the tumor scar. During the late phase the tumor remains isoechoic to the liver, which strengthens the diagnosis of benign lesion.

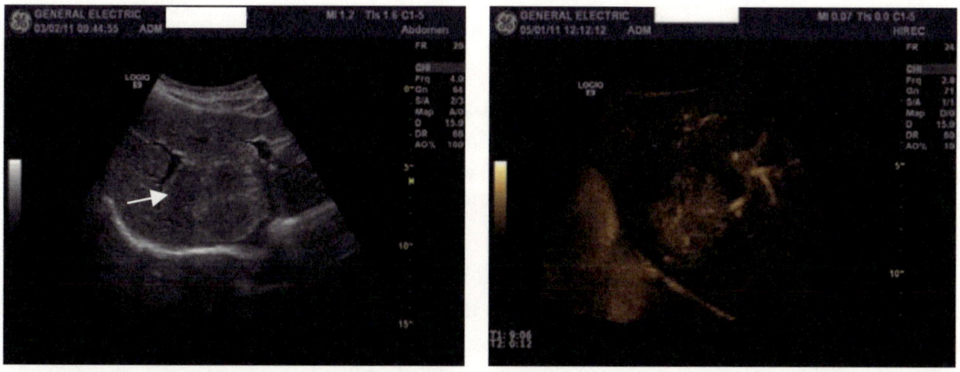

Fig. 5. Benign focal nodular hyperplasia (CEUS). Gray scale examination (left) detects the lesion. CEUS examination (right) allows characterization of tumor nature based on central contrast enhancement and centrifugal dispersion.

2.2.4 Adenoma

It is a benign tumor made up of normal or atypical hepatocytes. It has an incidence of 0.03%. Its development is induced by intake of anabolic hormones and oral contraceptives. The tumor is asymptomatic, but may be associated with right upper quadrant pain in case of internal bleeding. 2D ultrasound shows a well-defined, un-encapsulated, solid mass. It may have a heterogeneous structure in case of intratumoral hemorrhage. Doppler examination shows no circulatory signal. CEUS exploration is quite ambiguous and cannot always establish a differential diagnosis with hepatocellular carcinoma. Thus, during the arterial phase there is a centripetal and inhomogeneous enhancement. During the portal venous phase there is a moderate wash out. During late phase the appearance is isoechoic or hypoechoic, due to lack of Kupffer cells.

2.3 Malignant liver tumors

Malignant liver tumors develop on cirrhotic liver (hepatocellular carcinoma, HCC) or normal liver (metastases). They are single or multiple (especially metastases), have a variable, generally imprecise delineation, may have a very pronounced circulatory signal (hepatocellular carcinoma and some types of metastases), have a heterogeneous structure (the result of intratumoral circulatory disorders, consequence of hemorrhage or necrosis) and are firm to touch, even rigid. The patient's general status correlates with the underlying disease (vascular and parenchymal decompensation for liver cirrhosis, weight loss, lack of appetite and anemia with cancer).

2.3.1 Hepatocellular carcinoma (HCC)

It is the most common liver malignancy (Parkin et al, 2005). It develops secondary to cirrhosis (in approx. 80% of cases) (Llovet et al, 2003) therefore, ultrasound examination every 6 months combined with alpha fetoprotein (AFP) determination is an effective method for early detection and treatment monitoring for this type of tumor (Bruix & Sherman 2005; Llovet & Bruix 2008). Clinically, HCC overlaps with advanced liver cirrhosis (long evolution, repeated vascular and parenchymal decompensation, sometimes bleeding due to variceal leakage) in addition to accelerated weight loss in the recent past and lack of appetite.

HCC appearance on 2D ultrasound is that of a solid tumor, with imprecise delineation, with heterogeneous structure, uni- or multilocular (encephaloid form). An "infiltrative" type is also described which is difficult to discriminate from liver nodular reconstruction in cirrhosis. Typically HCC invades liver vessels, primarily the portal veins but also the hepatic veins (Badea R. & Badea Gh, 1991). Doppler examination detects a high speed arterial flow and low impedance index (correlated with described changes in tumor angiogenesis). The spatial distribution of the vessels is irregular, disordered. CEUS examination shows hyperenhancement of the lesion during the arterial phase. During the portal venous phase there is a specific "wash out" of ultrasound contrast agent (UCA) and the tumor appears hypoechoic during the late phase. Poorly differentiated tumors may have a stronger wash out leading to an isoechoic appearance to the liver parenchyma during portal venous phase. This appearance was found in approx. 30% of cases (Nicolau et al, 2004). The described changes have diagnostic value in liver nodules larger than 2 cm.

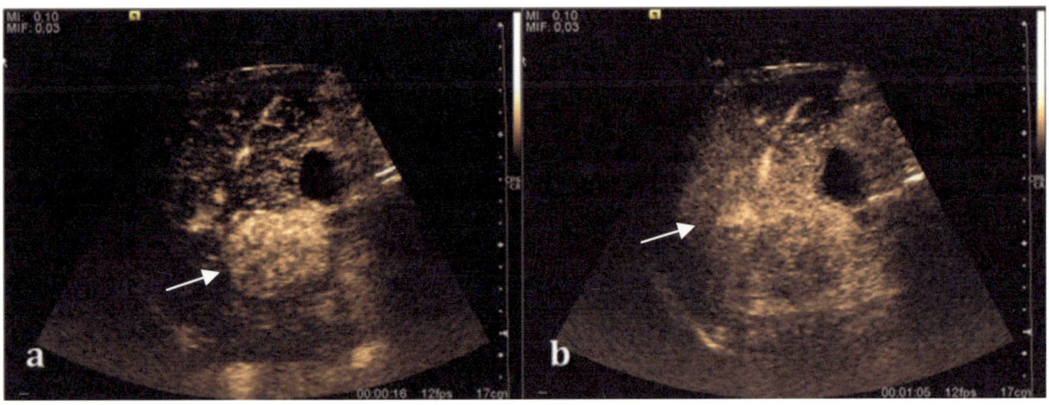

Fig. 6. Encephaloid hepatocellular carcinoma (CEUS). Contrast tumor enhancement is observed on the left during arterial phase. The "wash-out" phenomenon can be seen on the right, during portal venous phase.

Ultrasound is useful in HCC detection, stadialization and assessing therapeutic efficacy. In terms of staging related to therapy effectiveness, the Barcelona classification is used (Llovet et al, 1999) which identifies five HCC stages. Curative therapy is indicated in early stages, which include very early stage (single nodule <2 cm), curable by surgical resection (survival 50-70% five years after surgical resection) (Llovet et al, 2003) and early stage (single nodule of 2-5 cm, or up to 3 nodules <3 cm) which can be treated by radiofrequency ablation (RFA) and liver transplantation. Intermediate stage (polinodular, without portal invasion) and advanced stage (N1, M1, with portal invasion) undergo palliative therapies (TACE and sorafenib systemic therapy) and in the end stage only symptomatic therapy applies.

2.3.2 Cholangiocarcinoma

It develops on non cirrhotic liver. 2D ultrasound appearance is uncharacteristic - solid mass with heterogeneous structure, poorly delineated, often with peripheral location and weak Doppler circulation signal. CEUS examination reveals a moderate enhancement of the tumor periphery during arterial phase followed by wash-out during portal venous phase and hypoechoic appearance during late phase.

2.3.3 Liver metastases

US examination is required to detect liver metastases in patients with oncologic history. In addition, the method can incidentally detect metastases in asymptomatic patients. Early identification (small sizes, small number) is important to establish an optimal course of treatment which can be complex (chemotherapy, radiofrequency ablation, surgical resection) but welcomed. In addition, discrimination of synchronous lesions that have a different nature is also important knowing that up to 25-50% of liver lesions less than 2 cm detected in cancer patients may be benign (Kreft et al, 2001). US sensitivity for metastases detection varies depending on the examiner's experience and the equipment used and ranges between 40-80% (Wernecke et al, 1991). Sensitivity is conditioned by the size and acoustic impedance of the nodules. For a lesion diameter below 10 mm US accuracy is greatly reduced, reaching approx. 20%. Other elements contributing to lower US performance are: excessive obesity, fatty liver disease, hypomobility of the diaphragm, and certain patterns of hyperechoic or isoechoic metastases that can be overlooked or can mimic benign conditions. Conventional US appearance of metastases is uncharacteristic, consisting of circumscribed lesions, with clear, imprecise or "halo" delineation, with homogeneous or heterogeneous echo pattern. They can be single (often liver metastases from colonic neoplasm) or multiple. Echogenity is variable. When increased, they can compress the bile ducts (which may be dilated) and the liver vessels. Liver involvement can be segmental, lobar or generalized. In this situation a pronounced hepatomegaly occurs. Generally, metastases have non-characteristic Doppler vascular pattern, with few exceptions (carcinoid metastases). Cyst-adenocarcinoma metastases due to semifluid content may have a transonic appearance. When increasing, they can result in central necrosis. CEUS examination is a real breakthrough for detection and characterization of liver metastases. Increased performance is based on identifying specific vascular patterns during the arterial phase and seeing metastases in contrast to normal liver parenchyma during the sinusoidal phase. CEUS increased accuracy is due to the different behavior of normal liver parenchyma (captures CA in Kuppfer cells) against tumor parenchyma (does not contain Kuppfer cells, therefore CEUS appearance is hypoechoic). To this adds the particularities of intratumoral circulation represented by a reduced arterial bed compared to that of the surrounding normal liver and the absence of the portal vessels (Cosgrove & Blomley 2004). In terms of vascularity, metastases can be hypovascular (in gastric, colonic, pancreatic or ovarian adenocarcinomas) with hypoechoic pattern during arterial phase, and similar during portal venous and late phases, respectively hypervascular (neuroendocrine tumors, malignant melanoma, sarcomas, renal, breast or thyroid tumors) with hyperechoic appearance during arterial phase, with washout during the portal venous phase and hypoechoic pattern 30 seconds after injection (Larsen, 2010).

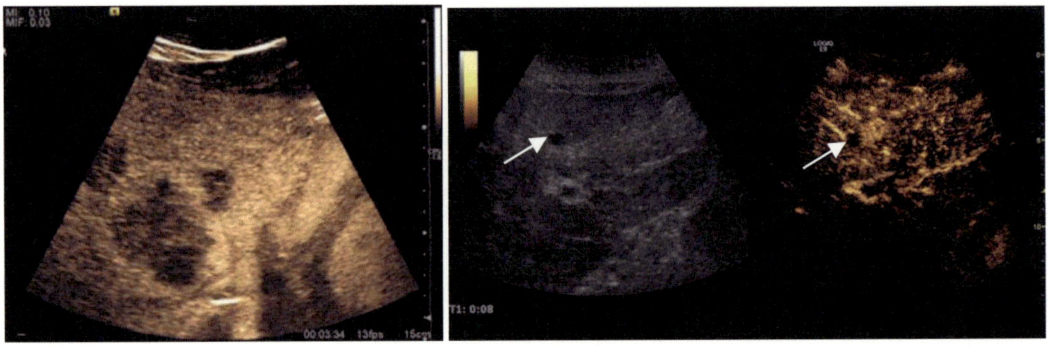

Fig. 7. Liver metastases (CEUS). Peripheral vascular pattern of the lesion is observed on the left in colon cancer metastasis. Lesion hyperenhancement in ovarian cancer liver metastasis is seen on the right during the arterial phase.

Using CEUS examination to detect metastases a sensitivity of 80-95% is obtained, similar to that of contrast CT and MRI (Quaia et al, 2006 ; Piscaglia et al, 2007). Intraoperative use of the procedure increases its performance even if it does not have a decisive contribution to change the therapeutic behavior (Konopke et al, 2005). Limitations of the method are those related to US penetration (pronounced fatty liver disease, deep lesion, excessive obesity) and to the experience of the examiner. To this the risk of confusion between hypervascular metastases, hepatocellular carcinoma and hemangioma and the confusion between hypovascular metastases and small liver cysts is added. Routine use of CEUS examination to detect liver metastases is recommended when conventional US examination is not conclusive, when precise information on some injuries (number, location) is necessary in conjunction with contrast CT/MRI and to assess the effectiveness of treatment when using a antiangiogenic therapy for hypervascular metastases (Claudon et al, 2008). The method cannot replace CT/MRI examinations which have well established indications in oncology (Larsen, 2010).

2.4 Pseudotumors and inflammatory masses of the liver

Besides the entities listed above inflammatory masses or even pseudo-masses can occur. Their diagnosis is quite difficult and the criteria used for differentiation are often insufficient, requiring morphologic diagnostic procedures, use of other diagnostic imaging methods or patient reevaluation from time to time. This includes lesions developed on liver parenchyma reconstruction, as occurs in cirrhosis, steatosis accumulation or in case of acute or chronic inflammatory diseases.

2.4.1 Focal steatosis

It consists of localized accumulation of fat-rich liver cells. In some cases this accumulation can mimic a liver tumor. Sometimes the opposite phenomenon can be seen, that is an "island" of normal parenchyma in a "shining" liver. In both cases ultrasound examination identifies a well defined, un-encapsulated area, with echostructure and vasculature similar to those of normal liver parenchyma. The lesion can have different forms, most cases being oval and located in the IVth segment, anterior from the hepatic hilum. It occurs in dyslipidemic or alcohol intake patients with normal physical and biological status. Benign diagnosis confirmation is made using CEUS examination which proves a normal circulatory bed similar to adjacent liver parenchyma in all three phases of investigation (Molins et al, 2010).

2.4.2 Liver abscess

Liver abscess have heteromorphic ultrasound appearance, the most typical being that of a mass with irregular shapes, fringed, with fluid or semifluid content, with or without air inside. Doppler examination shows the lack of vessels within the lesion. CEUS exploration shows hyperenhancement during arterial phase close to the lesion, this being suggestive of a liver parenchymal hyperemia. During venous and sinusoidal phase the pattern is hypoechoic, and the central fluid is contrast enhanced. CEUS examination is useful because it confirms the clinical suspicion of abscess. In addition, it allows for an accurate measurement of the collection size and an indication regarding its topography inside the liver (lobe, segment).

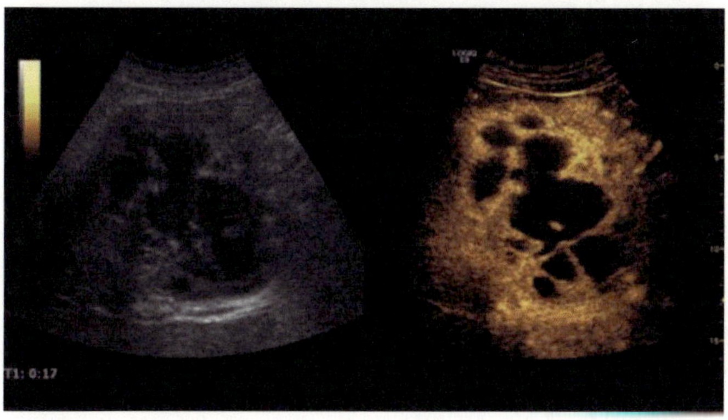

Fig. 8. Liver abscess (2D and CEUS). 2D Examination reveals the fluid nature of the mass and imprecise delineation. CEUS examination shows congestion in the surrounding liver parenchyma and excludes a vascular tumor.

3. Preneoplastic status. Cirrhotic liver monitoring

Cirrhotic liver is characterized by the occurrence of nodules with different sizes and evolution degrees, so that regenerative nodules, dysplastic nodules and even early hepatocellular carcinoma can coexist at some moment during disease progression. There are studies showing that between 59-94% of newly diagnosed liver nodules in cirrhotic patients have malignant histology and up to 50% of hyperechoic lesions, with ultrasound appearance of hemangioma, ultimately prove to be hepatocellular carcinoma. Therefore, current practice in many centers considers that any new lesion revealed in a cirrhotic patient should be regarded as malignant until otherwise proven (Andreana et al, 2009). There are three categories of cirrhotic liver nodules: regenerative, dysplastic (considered as premalignant conditions) and tumoral (HCC) (Int WP, 1995).

3.1 Regenerative nodules (RN)

These lesions are well defined, with isoechoic or hypoechoic appearance and sizes less than 1 cm. They are high in numbers and have a more or less uniform distribution, involving all liver segments. They can crowd resulting in large pseudo tumors. At Doppler examination, these nodules have no circulatory signal. CEUS exploration is indicated when a nodule is different against the general pattern of restructured liver either by different echogenity or by a different size than the majority of nodules. During the arterial phase, the signal is weak or absent. During the portal venous and late phase, the appearance is persistently isoechoic. Generally, RN is not distinct from the surrounding parenchyma. CEUS examination is useful to exclude an active lesion at the moment of exploration but does not have absolute prognostic value; therefore the patient should be periodically examined at short intervals (Kojiro, 2004; Bolondi et al, 2005). Correlation with clinical status and AFP measurements is required.

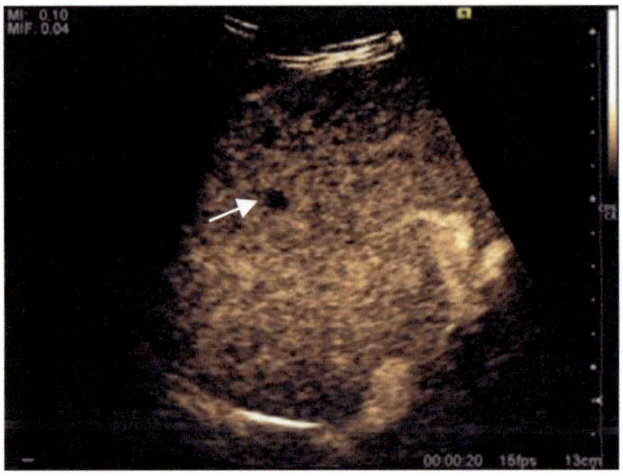

Fig. 9. Regenerative nodule (CEUS). One can see the hypovascular pattern of the solid nodule, with a size <10 mm.

3.2 Dysplastic nodules (DN)

These lesions have various patterns (hypo or hyperechoic) with at least 1 cm diameter. They are hepatocytes with dysplastic changes, but without clear histological criteria for malignancy. They are divided into low-grade dysplastic nodules, where cellular atypia are mild and high-grade dysplastic nodules with moderate or severe cellular atypia, but without any established signs of malignancy. Occasionally, well-differentiated HCC foci can be identified in high-grade dysplastic nodules (appearance called "nodule in nodule") (Minami & Kudo, 2010). Most authors accept the carcinogenesis process as a progressive transformation of DN from low-grade to high-grade and into HCC. The nodule's vasculature changes progressively, correlated with the degree of malignancy, and it is characterized by decrease until absence of portal venous input and by increase of arterial intratumoral input. Neoformation vessels occur with increasing degree of dysplasia. Arterial neovascularization is enhanced in a chaotic and explosive way, while normal, arterial and portal vasculature continues to decline. High-grade dysplastic nodules are hypo-vascularized both arterial and portal phases, while early HCC nodules may have similar arterial pattern with the surrounding parenchyma or exacerbated, and portal hypo-vascularization. In moderate or poorly differentiated HCC (classic HCC) tumor nutrition is performed only by neoformation vessels (abundant), the normal arterial and portal vasculature completely disappearing (Matsui 2004). This behavior of intratumoral vascularization is typical for HCC and is the key to imaging diagnosis (Lencioni et al 2008).

B-mode ultrasonography is unable to distinguish between regenerative nodules and "borderline" lesions such as dysplastic nodules and even early HCC. Doppler examination also has a low sensitivity in differentiating dysplastic nodules from early HCC. Doppler signal may be absent in both regenerative and dysplastic nodules. Some authors indicate the presence of venous type Doppler flow which reflects the portal venous nutrition of the nodule as a characteristic feature of dysplastic nodules and early HCC (Minami & Kudo, 2010). Other authors noticed the presence of an arterial flow with small frequency variations and a normal resistivity index (RI) (Lencioni et al 2008).

On CEUS examination both RN and DN may have quite a variable enhancement pattern. Generally, both nodules enhances identically with the surrounding liver parenchyma after UCAs injection. Dysplastic nodules are hypovascular in the arterial phase. In case of high-grade dysplastic nodule sometimes a hypervascularization can be detected, but without associating "wash out" during portal and late CEUS phases. In these cases, biopsy may clarify the diagnosis.

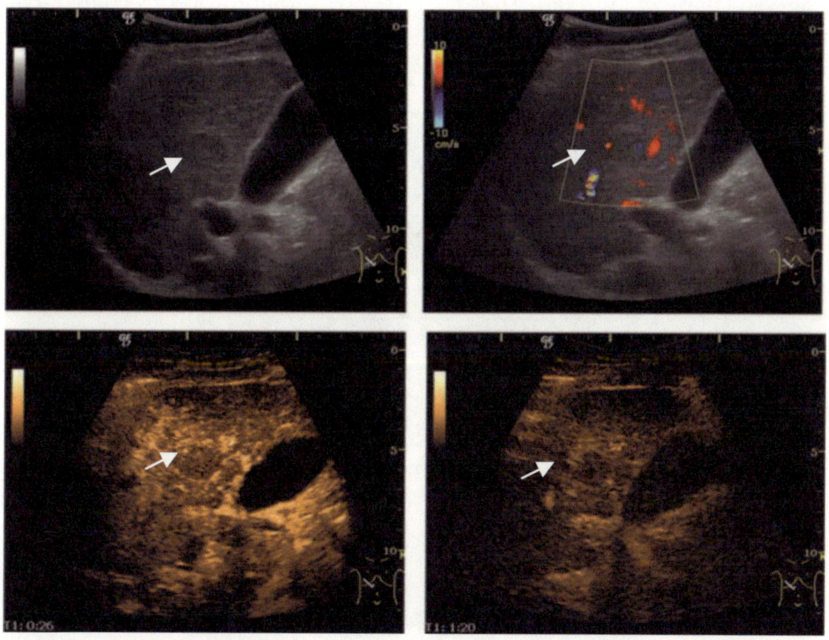

Fig. 10. Dysplastic nodule (2D, CFM, CEUS). The nodule is well-defined with a size between 10- 20 mm, lacks vessels in CFM and CEUS exploration.

3.3 Early hepatocellular carcinoma (Early HCC)

The suggestive appearance of early HCC on 2D ultrasound examination is that of hypo-echoic nodule, with distinct pattern, developed on cirrhotic liver. Hypoechoic appearance is characteristic of moderate/poorly differentiated HCC, with low or absent fatty changes. Rarely, HCC may appear isoechoic, consist of a tumor type with a higher degree of differentiation and therefore with slower development. Another common aspect is "bright loop" or "nodule-in-nodule" appearance, hypoechoic nodules in a hyperechoic tumor. (Minami & Kudo, 2010).

Spectral Doppler characteristics of early HCC overlap those of the dysplastic nodule, as they are represented by the presence of portal venous signal type or arterial type with normal RI (well differentiated HCC) or increased RI (moderately or poorly differentiated HCC). The CFM exploration identifies a chaotic vessels pattern.

On CEUS examination, early HCC has an iso- or hypervascular appearance during the arterial phase followed by wash out during portal venous and late phase. There are studies showing that the wash out process is directly correlated with the size and features of neoplastic circulatory bed. Thus, highly differentiated HCC illustrates the phenomenon of late or even very late "wash out" while poorly differentiated HCC has an accelerated wash out at the end of arterial phase (Strobel et al, 2005; von Herbay et al, 2009; Jang et al, 2009). It is therefore mandatory to analyze all these three phases of CEUS examination for a proper characterization of liver nodules. Tumor wash out at the end of the arterial phase allows the HCC diagnosis with a predictability of 89.5%. Some authors consider that early pronounced contrast enhancement of a nodule within 1-2 cm developed on a cirrhotic liver is sufficient for HCC diagnosis (Jang et al, 2009). These results prove that for a correct characterization of the lesions it is necessary to extend the examination time to 5 minutes or even longer (von Herbay et al, 2009).

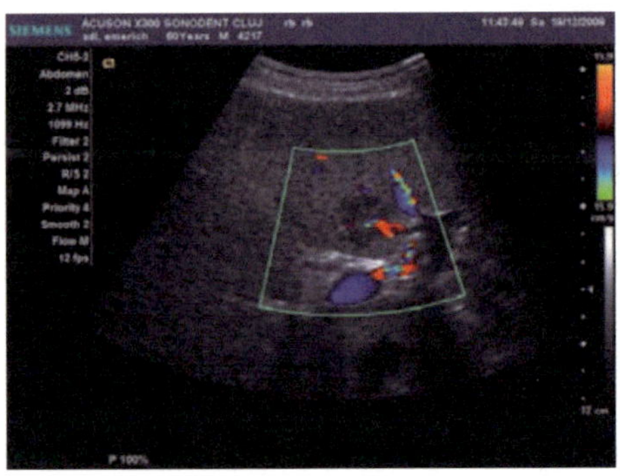

Fig. 11. Early hepatocellular carcinoma (2D, CFM). The 2D examination reveals a solid, hypoechoic nodule in IVth liver segment, without encapsulation. CFM shows a central vessel with ramifications to the periphery. The underlying liver is cirrhotic.

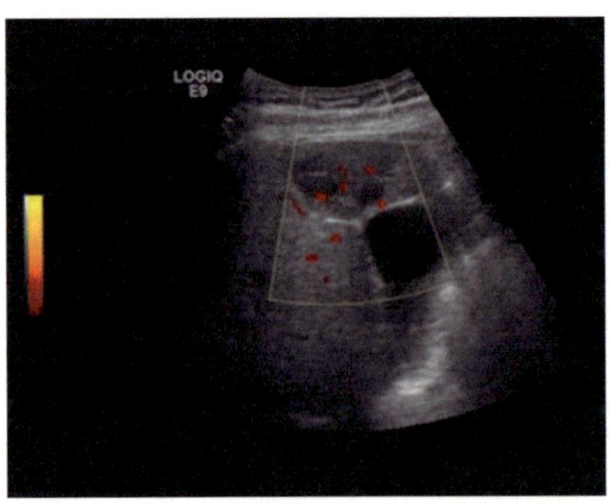

Fig. 12. Early hepatocellular carcinoma (2D, CFM). "Nodule in nodule" image: small hypoechoic early HCC inside monitored dysplastic nodule.

3.4 The ultrasound value in HCC "screening"

Baseline 2D ultrasound has an important role in surveillance programs for patients at risk to develop HCC (Bruix & Sherman, 2011). The examination has an acceptable sensitivity which increases with the tumor size. Sensitivity varies between 42% for lesions <1 cm and 95% for tumors larger than 1 cm, and specificity can reach 90% (Andreana et al, 2009). Optimal time interval for ultrasound screening of "at risk" population is 6 months as it results from clinical trials that investigated the tumor size doubling time (Bruix, 2005; Maruyama et al, 2008). For a recently developed nodule the dimensional criteria will be taken into account. Thus, for a nodule with a size of less than 10 mm the patient will be reevaluated by ultrasound every 3 months, as the growth trend is an indication for completion of investigations with other diagnostic procedures; at a size between 10 - 20 mm two concordant imaging procedures are necessary, supplemented if necessary by an ultrasound guided biopsy; at a size over 20 mm one single dynamic imaging technique with characteristic appearance is enough for positive diagnostic. In uncertain cases complementary dynamic imaging techniques or biopsy should be performed. When Doppler exploration is not enough, CEUS examination will be performed (Gaiani et al, 2001). One should always keep in mind the risk of false positive results for HCC in case of cholangiocarcinomas so complementary diagnostic procedures should be considered (Bruix & Sherman, 2011).

The effectiveness of screening programs is proved by an increase in detection rate of HCC <2 cm (from <5% in the 90s in Europe to > 30% today in Japan) with curative therapy options (Llovet & Bruix 2008). The main problem of ultrasound screening is that, in order to be cost-effective, it should be applied to the general population and not in tertiary hospitals. This raises the importance of the operator and equipment dependent part of the ultrasound examination (Bruix et al, 2001). The efficiency of such a program is linked to the functional liver parenchyma of the cirrhotic patient. Therefore, some authors argue that screening should be excluded in patients with etiologies that prevent curative treatment or in patients with advanced liver disease (Child-Pugh class C) (Zapata et al, 2010).

After curative therapies (surgical resection, local ablative therapies) continuing ultrasound screening is recommended first at 1 month then at 3 months intervals after the therapy to assess the effectiveness of therapy and to detect other nodules.

4. Antitumor therapies

Ultrasound exploration can be an effective procedure for the assessment of liver tumors response to treatment. Over the years, different criteria for assessing the effectiveness of curative or palliative therapies have been considered. Now it has been proved that the degree of tumor necrosis is not correlated with tumor diameter, therefore simple measurement of the tumor diameter (RECIST criteria) is not enough for therapy assessment. Currently, local response to treatment is focused on tumor necrosis diagnosed by contrast dynamic imaging techniques and recognized by the presence of intratumoral non-enhanced areas. Local response to treatment is defined as:

a. complete response, defined as complete disappearance of all known lesions (absence of tumor enhanced areas, reflecting total tumor necrosis) and absence of other new lesions determined by two observations not less than 4 weeks apart;

b. partial response, defined as more than 50% reduction in total tumor enhancement in all measurable lesions, determined by two observations not less than 4 weeks apart
c. stable disease (is not described by a, b, or d)
d. progressive disease, defined as 25% increase in size of one or more measurable lesions or the appearance of new lesions (Bruix et al, 2001).

4.1 Techniques for evaluating the efficiency of therapy

The efficiency of 2D ultrasound is low in assessing the effects of HCC or metastasis therapy, as it is unable to differentiate viable tumor tissue from post-therapy tumor necrosis. However, it is able to detect the appearance of new lesions and to assess the occurrence of any complications of disease progression (ascites or portal vein thrombosis). Color Doppler ultrasound can be useful sometimes being able to show the presence of intratumoral vasculature as a sign of incomplete therapy or intratumoral recurrence. The absence of Doppler signal does not exclude the presence of viable tumor tissue. CEUS exploration, by its ability to enhance intra-lesion microcirculation, has proved its utility in monitoring therapeutic efficacy. Its indications are defined for HCC ablative treatments (pre, intra and post-therapy), while monitoring of systemic therapies of HCC and metastases are not validated indications at this time, but with proved efficacy in extensive clinical trials (Claudon et al, 2008). CEUS examination cannot completely replace the other imaging diagnostic methods currently in use because of the known limitations of the ultrasound method (operator/ equipment dependent, ultrasound examination limitations). In addition to bloating, in cancer patients post-therapy steatosis occurs, which prevent deep visibility. Spiral CT scan remains the method of choice in monitoring cancer therapies because it provides an overview of tumor extension and it is not limited by bloating or steatosis (Bartolozzi et al, 1999).

Gadolinium MRI examination is a procedure used more and more often, and its advantages are the absence of irradiation and its high sensitivity in tumor vasculature detection, especially in smaller tumors (Dromain et al, 2002). However it remains an expensive and not a very accessible procedure, although it has a high specificity. Currently, CEUS and MRI are considered complementary methods to CT scan.

4.2 Ultrasound monitoring ablative therapies (alcoholization - PEI, radiofrequency ablation - RFA)

Ablative therapies are considered curative treatments for HCC together with surgical resection and liver transplantation and they are indicated for early tumor stages in patients with good liver function (Bruix & Sherman, 2005; Bruix & Sherman, 2011). Also they are successfully applied in the treatment of liver metastases, where surgical resection is contraindicated. They are chemical (intratumoral ethanol injection) or thermal (radiofrequency, laser or microwave ablation). They are applied in order to obtain a full therapeutic response, without affecting liver function. Complete response is locally proved by complete tumor necrosis with a safety margin around the tumor.

2D ultrasound, Doppler ultrasound and especially CEUS can play an important role in pre-therapeutic staging, particularly when sectional imaging investigations (CT, MRI) provide uncertain results or are contraindicated. During the interventional procedure, ultrasound allows guidance of the needle into the tumor. CEUS allows guidance in areas of viable tissue and avoids intratumoral necrotic areas. CEUS also allows assessment of therapeutic effect immediately post-procedure (with the possibility of reintervention in case of partial response) (Claudon et al, 2008). To accurately assess the effectiveness of treatment it is mandatory to compare the tumor diameter before therapy with the ablation area. The volume of damaged tissue must be higher than the initial tumor volume. CEUS appearance is that of central non-enhanced area showing a peripheral homogeneous hyperenhanced rim due to post-procedure inflammation. 24 hours after the procedure the inflammatory peripheral rim is thinning and the necrotic area appears larger than at the previous examination. Thus, a possible residual tumor may appear more evident. Residual tumor has poorly defined edges, irregular shape, and the tumor diameter is unchanged. Residual tumor tissue is evidenced at the periphery of the tumor as an eccentric area behaving as the original tumor at CEUS examination, with arterial hyperenhancement and portal and late wash-out. Ultrasound examination 24 hours after the procedure, including CEUS, can show apart from the character of the lesion any potential post-intervention complications (e.g. active bleeding).

In the first days after RFA both CEUS and spiral CT have low sensitivity in assessing therapeutic efficacy. CT sensitivity 24 hours post-therapy is reported to be even lower than CEUS (Vilana et al, 2006). Difficulties in CEUS examination result from post-lesion hyperemia, presence of intratumoral air, ultrasound limitations (too deep lesion or the presence of fatty liver) or lack of patient's cooperation (immediately after therapy). For this reasons contrast imaging (CT or CEUS) control should be performed one month after ablation to confirm the result of the therapy (Spârchez et al, 2009).

Local recurrence is defined as recurrence of a hyperenhanced area at tumor periphery in the arterial phase, with portal and late wash-out. Sometimes, especially for HCC treated by alcoholization (PEI) hyperenhanced septa or vessels can be shown inside the lesion (Spârchez et al, 2009).

In case of successful treatment, US monitoring using CEUS is performed every three months. Although CE-CT and/or MRI are considered the method of choice in post-therapy monitoring, CEUS can be used in follow-up protocols (Claudon et al, 2008), its diagnostic accuracy being equivalent to that of CE-CT or MRI (Frieser et al, 2011).

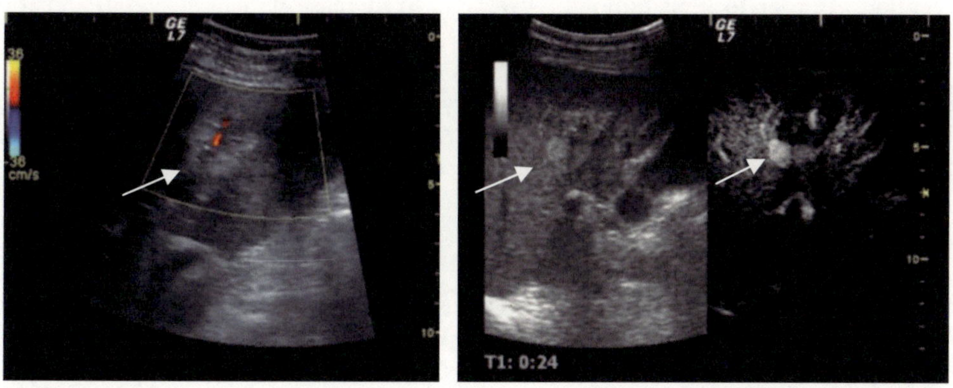

Fig. 13. Assessment of therapeutic efficacy on ultrasound (2D, CFM, CEUS). US exam shows vascular Doppler signal at CFM (left) and CEUS examination reveals incomplete therapy (right).

4.3 Ultrasound monitoring of TACE therapy (transarterial chemoembolization)

Transarterial chemoembolization (TACE) is part of palliative therapies for HCC used in intermediate stages of the disease. It consists of selective angiographic catheterization of the hepatic artery and injection of chemotherapeutic agents (usually adriamycin, but other molecules are currently the subject of clinical trials), followed by embolization of hepatic artery with gelfoam, alcohol or metal rings (Bruix & Sherman, 2005). A similar procedure is transarterial embolization but without chemotherapeutic agents injection, used in the treatment of hypervascular liver metastases. These therapies are based on the predominantly arterial vasculature of HCC and hypervascular metastases, while the remaining liver parenchyma has a dual vascular intake, predominantly portal. Their efficacy is high only for lesions who are hyperenhanced during arterial phase. The role of US is limited in the first few days after the procedure, and refers only to its complications, due to Lipiodol retention mainly intratumoral, but also diffusely intrahepatic. On ultrasound, Lipiodol appears intensely hyperechoic inside the tumor, with significant posterior attenuation which make US examination more difficult. On the other hand, CE-CT is also limited by the presence of Lipiodol (iodine oil), therefore the evaluation of therapeutic efficiency is currently made by indirect assessing Lipiodol binding to the tumor using non-enhanced CT (Maruyama et al, 2008). CE-MRI is not influenced by the presence of Lipiodol, but it is an expensive method and still difficult to reach. Several studies have proved similar efficacy, even superior, of CEUS compared to CE-CT and CE-MRI for the evaluation of post-TACE treatment results, while other studies have shown the limitations of CEUS especially for deep or small lesions. Given the CEUS limitations, currently some authors consider CT as standard method for the evaluation of TACE and local ablative therapies and CEUS and CE-MRI as complementary methods (Lim et al, 2006, Maruyama et al, 2008). Monitoring TACE therapeutic results by contrast imaging techniques is performed as for ablative therapies initially after one month then after every 3 months post-TACE.

Given that TACE is indicated only for hyperenhanced lesions during arterial phase, CEUS plays a very important role in monitoring the dysplastic nodules to identify the moment when changes occur in arterial vasculature, being able to have an early therapeutic intervention in order to limit tumor progression, to increase patient survival, and thus to create a bridge to liver transplantation.

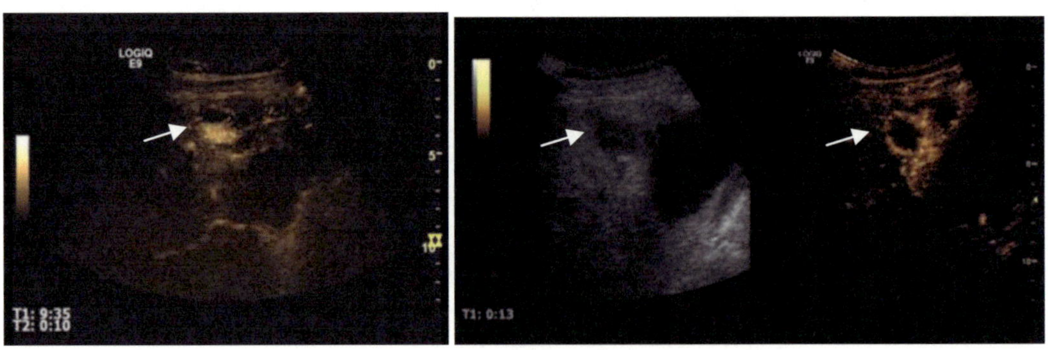

Fig. 14. Small HCC is seen on the left (nodule in nodule). Efficient chemoembolization of the nodule (right). CEUS examination shows no circulatory signal within the nodule.

4.4 Ultrasound monitoring of systemic therapies

Systemic therapies are procedures based on the affinity of certain molecules to inhibit either tumor cell replication or multiplication of neoplastic vasculature (antiangiogenic therapies). They are intravenously administered and are indicated in advanced stages of liver tumor diseases, when there are no other effective therapeutic solutions. Among ultrasound techniques, CEUS is the one that brought a significant benefit not only by increasing the sensitivity and specificity of ultrasound in detecting liver metastases, but also by assessing the efficacy of systemic therapy for HCC and metastases. The method has been adopted by oncologists since 2003, because it involves no irradiation and has no hepatic or renal toxicity, and it is now currently used in tumor therapeutic evaluation (Lassau et al, 2011). It is currently used in large clinical trials aimed at determining the efficacy of different types of anti-angiogenic molecules by quantifying intratumoral perfusion based on the statistical analysis performed using specific software during post-processing in order to assess therapeutic efficacy as early as possible.

4.5 Ultrasound monitoring of post-surgical resection status

Surgical resection is the treatment of choice for non-cirrhotic or cirrhotic patients with well preserved liver function with single liver lesion. After resection, recurrence rate exceeds 70% at 5 years and is mainly due to primary tumor dissemination. The strongest predictors of tumor recurrence are the development of other tumors near the primary tumor scar and vascular microinvasion (Bruix & Sherman, 2005). 2D ultrasound is used within screening programs. CEUS efficacy has not been proven so far in monitoring post-resection patients.

5. Other applications of ultrasound in liver tumor pathology. Technical progress

Ultrasound has known a great development arising from the need to increase patient access to advanced investigations while avoiding procedures using radiation (CT), contrast agents with allergic potential (iodine substances) and hepatic or renal toxic agents.

Interventional and intraoperative ultrasound. Ultrasound exploration by maneuverability of the equipment and dynamic character of the image allows guided interventional procedures or intraoperative examination. Combining ultrasound with such procedures is necessary due to the lack of specificity of the method in case of tumors. Even if tumor markers for defining the nature of some masses are available, their accuracy is not good enough; therefore biological samples from the nodules detected by imaging is often required. Accuracy of ultrasound guided puncture in the diagnosis of liver tumors is dependent on the operator's experience and can reach up to 87.5 - 99% (Horigome et al, 1999). The extracted material can be either a histology fragment or cytology aspiration; in both cases the credibility of the method is sufficient to ensure optimal cancer therapies (Badea R & Badea Gh 1991). Intraoperative ultrasound is also a complementary investigation that allows detection of very small nodules. In addition it allows the characterization of tumor using Doppler and CEUS procedure as well as guided interventional procedures such as intraoperative PEI or RFA.

Targeted therapy using contrast agents. The introduction of second generation contrast agents has been a great progress. Diagnostic performance is already proven. A step forward is tumor targeted therapy under ultrasound guidance. The principle is that of transporting chemotherapeutic agents to the target using microbubbles as vectors. Experiments have been made for binding different substances and/or genes to the lesion, with local release by "breaking" and intracellular penetration using the phenomenon of cellular membrane permeability called "sonoporation" (Lindner, 2004, Newman & Bettinger, 2007).

Image fusion. Techniques for image fusion obtained by different imaging procedures allow the correlation of real-time ultrasound examination with CT or MRI images, enabling positioning of the needle in relation to the exact position of the tumor. The technique allows a better guidance both for biopsies and percutaneous ablative procedures, replacing CT guidance and thus avoiding irradiation. Combination with CEUS allows a better characterization of lesions as well as successful monitoring of percutaneous procedures or TACE effects (Sandulescu et al, 2011; Ewertsen et al, 2011).

Elastography. It was initially introduced in practice to assess the degree of fibrosis in chronic liver disease. In liver tumors it allows detection of liver nodules due to the difference of elasticity between the hepatic nodule and the parenchyma. There are few studies that try to assess the benign or malignant character of the lesion based only on elasticity. By combination with CEUS the method could be beneficial for early detection and characterization of HCC.

High Intensity Focused Ultrasound (HIFU). It is a new technique capable of destroying tumor tissue by hyperthermia, allowing percutaneous ablation without requiring tumor puncture. There are studies showing the efficacy of this technique in combination with TACE, with anti-tumor effect and better survival than using TACE alone (Wu, 2005). The method is expected to be an alternative to PEI and RFA because it avoids the puncture of the cirrhotic liver, but more studies are needed to prove its efficacy as a single therapy in the curative treatment of HCC (Maruyama et al, 2008).

Techniques for visualizing blood circulation independently from the angle of insonation based on transversal oscillation of red blood cells groups. This technique is now implemented on conventional transducers and can real time evidence different features of the blood flow visualized so far only on MRI angiography (Hansen et al, 2011).

6. Conclusions

Ultrasound exploration using current technologies has excellent possibilities for practical use. Several elements related to the lack of standardization and reproducibility of ultrasound procedures as well as operator-dependent nature of the method require structured approach to its use in liver tumors pathology (Bolondi et al, 2007). Structuring these applications and description of their actual performance are included in successive recommendations made by expert groups, known as "EFSUMB guidelines" (Albrecht et al, 2004; Claudon et al, 2008). In the current stage the following applications in liver pathology, especially in tumors are accepted as valid and represent indications for CEUS:

a. *characterization of nodular lesions found on non-cirrhotic liver.* Ultrasound examination is often the first imaging procedure performed in patients with abdominal pathology. Quite often lesions are detected and their nature has to be further on defined. Ultrasound procedures that allow achieving this purpose are multiple and complementary: 2D/3D ultrasound and elastography for morphometric informations; Doppler ultrasound (with its variants) and CEUS allow hemodynamic information. CEUS examination is the most specific of them as it is based on different behavior of contrast agent transiting liver masses depending on their nature. CEUS accuracy for characterization of focal lesions detected on noncirrhotic liver is similar to that of CT/MRI, being of 94.5% for metastases, 97% for hemangiomas, and of 90% for focal nodular hyperplasia. The method has a performance superior to 2D ultrasound and a high rate of diagnosis confidence regardless of the operator in what concerns tumor characterization and nodules count (Quaia et al, 2004).

b. *characterization of nodular lesions found on the cirrhotic liver.* Ultrasound examination is a "screening" procedure used to detect early HCC (Bolondi et al, 2001). The cirrhotic liver during the restructuring process develops nodules that often raise questions regarding their nature. The criteria used to determine the nature of these nodules involve size, circulation pattern (Doppler evaluated) and vascular bed behavior (CEUS evaluated). In over 90% of cases, HCC has a characteristic behavior. CEUS exploration has a sensitivity of 92-94% and a specificity of 87-96% in characterizing HCC (Tanaka et al, 2001, Nicolau et al, 2004).

In a linear study, covering 36 months, (January 2006 - December 2008), made on a cohort of 379 patients with liver tumors, (fig. 15), we had similar results concerning the performances of CEUS compared to other imaging procedures such as CT/MRI and histopathology as other groups (personal experience; unpublished results from the project Angiotumor nr. 138/2006 financed by the Ministry of Education and Research from Romania) (fig. 16) (Badea et al, 2008).

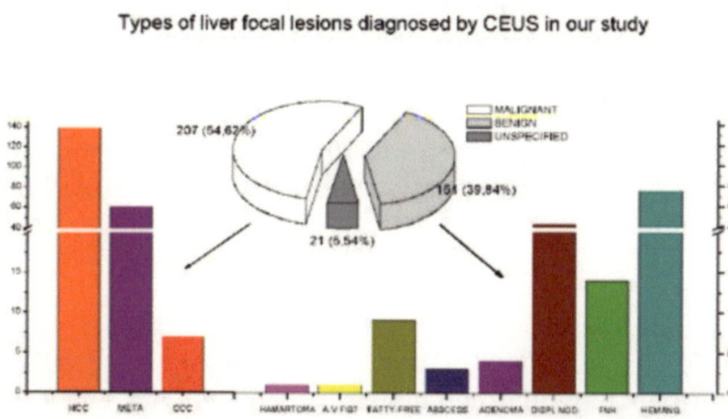

Fig. 15. Types of liver focal lesions diagnosed by CEUS in our study (HCC=hepatocellular carcinoma, META=liver metastasis, CCC=cholangiocarcinoma, A-V FIST=arterio-venous fistula, FATTY-FREE=fatyy-free area, DISPL NOD=cirrhotic displastic nodule, FNH=focal nodular hyperplasia, HEMANG=liver hemangioma)

c. *Detection and characterization of liver metastases.* Ultrasound is a method widely used in the early detection of liver metastases in patients with cancer pathology. Beyond the known limitations of the method, the examination is used because it is accessible, non-irradiant and it can detect metastases of quite small sizes and allows their characterization using vascular criteria. CEUS examination increases the performance of conventional ultrasound to values comparable with CT/MRI, becoming an alternative to these procedures in certain well defined situations (Dietrich et al, 2006).

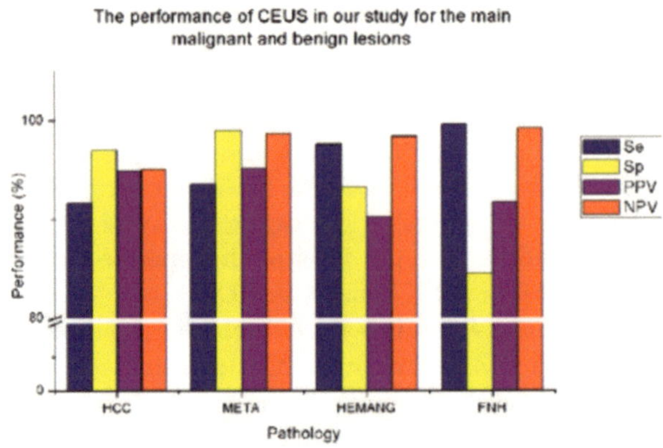

Fig. 16. The performance of CEUS in our study for the main malignant and benign lesions (HCC=hepatocellular carcinoma, META=liver metastasis, HEMANG=liver hemangioma, FNH=focal nodular hyperplasia, Se=sensitivity, Sp=specificity, PPV=positive predictive value, NPV=negative predictive value)

d. *Assessing therapeutic efficacy.* Using the vascular criteria allows the assessment of therapeutic efficacy under chemotherapy (Bolondi et al, 2007). Performing an interventional procedure (with diagnostic or therapeutic purpose) simultaneously with the administration of i.v. CAs increases the procedure's efficiency by a better visualization of the tumor and by correct guidance of the ablation needle in the active (vascularized) area of the tumor (Skjoldbye et al, 2002, Lencioni et al, 2004). After ablative procedures, or even better in one month after the procedure, the absence of the circulation bed in the tumor in arterial phase suggests an effective treatment (Solbiati et al, 2004; Vilana et al, 2006, Bartolotta et al, 2008). This principle is also true for chemotherapy with antiangiogenic agents. Even under these conditions combination of CEUS with i.v. contrast CT examination is required to detect small metastases between procedures (Bartolotta et al, 2008).

7. References

Andreana L, Isgrò G, Pleguezuelo M, Germani G, Burroughs A (2009). Surveillance and diagnosis of hepatocellular carcinoma in patients with cirrhosis. *World J Hepatol* October 31; 1(1):48-61. ISSN 1948-5182 (online)

Badea R, Badea Gh, Galatâr N, Crăciun C, Marin M, Bucher M (1991). Aspiration of fine needle biopsy - its relevance to higher accuracy of ultrasonic diagnosis of liver tumors - investigation of 165 patients. *Z Klin Med;* 46 (21): 1489 - 1493

Badea R, Badea Gh (1991). Sonographische Untersuchungen des Pfortadersystems bei Lebertumoren. *Ultraschall;* 12 (6): 272 - 276. ISSN 0172-4614

Badea R, Socaciu M, Lupsor M, Mosteanu O, Pop T (2007). Evaluating the liver tumors using three-dimensional ultrasonography. A pictorial essay. *J Gastrointestin Liv Dis;* 16 (1): 85-92. ISSN 1841-8724

Badea R, Socaciu M, Caraiani C, Mosteanu O, Pop T (2008). The use of second generation Ultrasound contrast agents (SonoVue) in the diagnosis and characterization of benign liver masses. *Romanian Journal of Hepatology.;* 4(1):11-9. ISSN 1841-6187

Bartolotta VT, Taibbi A, Midiri M, De Maria M 2008). Hepatocellular cancer response to radiofrequency tumor ablation: contrast-enhanced ultrasound. *Abdom Imaging* 33:501–511. ISSN 0942-8925 (print version) ISSN 1432-0509 (electronic version)

Bartolozzi C, Cioni D, Donati F, Granai G, Lencioni R (1999). Imaging evaluation of tumor response. In: Bartolozzi C, Lencioni R, editors. *Liver malignancies. Diagnostic and interventional radiology,* 1st ed. Berlin: Springer-Verlag,. pp. 467–487. ISBN-10: 3540647562 ISBN-13: 9783540647560

Bolondi L, S Sofia, S Siringo, S Gaiani, A Casali, G Zironi, F Piscaglia, L Gramantieri, M Zanetti, M Sherman (2001). Surveillance programme of cirrhotic patients for early diagnosis and treatment of hepatocellular carcinoma: a cost effectiveness analysis. *Gut*;48:251–259. Online ISSN 1468-3288

Bolondi L, Gaiani S, Celli N, Golfieri R, Grigioni WF, Leoni S, Venturi AM, Piscaglia F (2005). Characterization of small nodules in cirrhosis by assessment of vascularity: the problem of hypovascular hepatocellular carcinoma. *Hepatology*;42:27–34. Online ISSN: 1527-3350

Bolondi L, Correas JM, Lencioni R, Weskott HP, Piscaglia F (2007). New perspectives for the use of contrast-enhanced liver ultrasound in clinical practice. *Digestive and Liver Disease*; 39: 187–195. ISSN 1590-8658

Bruix J, Sherman M, Llovet JM, Beaugrand M, Lencioni R, Burroughs AK, Christensen E, Pagliaro L, Colombo M, Rodes J (2001). EASL Panel of Experts on HCC. Clinical management of hepatocellular carcinoma. Conclusions of the Barcelona-2000 EASL conference. European Association for the Study of the Liver. *J Hepatol*;35:421–430. ISSN 0168-8278

Bruix J, Sherman M (2005). Management of hepatocellular carcinoma. *Hepatology*;42:1208–1236. Online ISSN: 1527-3350

Bruix J, Sherman M (2011) AASLD Practice Guideline. Management of Hepatocellular Carcinoma: an Update. *Hepatology*; 53(3): 1020-1022. Online ISSN 1527-3350

Burns PN, Wilson SR, Hope Simpson D (2000). Pulse inversion imaging of liver blood flow: an improved method for characterization of focal masses with microbubble contrast. *Invest Radiol*; 35:58–71. ISSN 0020-9996.

Burns PN, Wilson SR (2006). Microbubble contrast for radiological imaging: 1. Principles. *Ultrasound Q*;22(1):5–13. PMID: 16641788

Cherrington JM, Strawn LM, Shawver LK (2000). New paradigms for the treatment of cancer: the role of anti-angiogenesis agents. *Adv Cancer Res*;79:1–38. ISSN 0065-230X

Choudhry S, Gorman B, Charboneau JW, Tradup JD, Beck RJ, Kofler JM, Groth DS (2000). Comparison of tissue harmonic imaging with conventional US in abdominal disease. *Radiographics*;20: 1127 – 1135. Print ISSN 0271-5333 Online ISSN 1527-1323

Claudon M, Cosgrove D, Albrecht T, Bolondi L, Bosio M, Calliada F, Correas JM, Darge K, Dietrich C, D'Onofrio M, Evans DH, Filice C, Greiner L, Jäger K, Jong N, Leen E, Lencioni R, Lindsell D, Martegani A, Meairs S, Nolsøe C, Piscaglia F, Ricci P, Seidel G, Skjoldbye B, Solbiati L, Thorelius L, Tranquart F, Weskott HP, Whittingham T (2008). Guidelines and good clinical practice recommendations for contrast enhanced ultrasound (CEUS)-update 2008. *Ultraschall Med*; 29: 28-44. ISSN 0172-4614.

Cosgrove D, Eckersley R (1997). Doppler indices in tumors - resolution of a dilemma? *Ultrasound in Obstetrics and Gynecology*, 10: 9 – 11. ISSN 1469-0705

Cosgrove D, Blomley M (2004). Liver tumors: evaluation with contrast-enhanced ultrasound. *Abdom Imaging*; 29: 446-454. ISSN: 0942-8925 (print version) ISSN 1432-0509 (electronic version)

Derchi LE, Claudon M (2009). Ultrasound: a strategic issue for radiology? *Eur Radiol*; 19: 1–6. Published online 15 August 2008. ISSN 0938-7994 (print version) ISSN 1432-1084 (electronic version)

Dietrich CF, Kratzer W, Strobe D, Danse E, Fessl R, Bunk A, Vossas U, Hauenstein K, Koch W, Blank W, Oudkerk M, Hahn D, Greis C. (2006). Assessment of metastatic liver disease in patients with primary extra-hepatic tumors by contrast-enhanced sonography versus CT and MRI. *World J Gastroenterol*;12:1699–1705. ISSN 1007-9327 (print) ISSN 2219-2840 (online)

Dromain C, de Baere T, Elias D, Kuoch V, Ducreux M, Boige V, Petrow P, Roche A, Sigal R (2002). Hepatic tumors treated with percutaneous radio-frequency ablation: CT and MR imaging follow up. *Radiology*; 223: 255-262. Print ISSN 0033-8419. Online ISSN 1527-1315

Ewertsen C, Henriksen B. M, Torp-Pedersen S,. Bachmann Nielsen M (2011). Characterization by Biopsy or CEUS of Liver Lesions Guided by Image Fusion between Ultrasonography and CT, PET/CT or MRI. Published online January 11, 2011 *Ultraschall in Med*; 32: 191–197. ISSN 0172-4614.

Frieser M, Kiesel J, Lindner A, Bernatik T, Haensler J. M., Janka R, Hahn E. G., Strobel D. (2011). Efficacy of Contrast-Enhanced US versus CT or MRI for the Therapeutic Control of Percutaneous Radiofrequency Ablation in the Case of Hepatic Malignancies. *Ultraschall in Med*. Published online 2011. ISSN 0172-4614.

Gaiani S, Volpe L, Piscaglia F, Bolondi L (2001). Vascularity of liver tumours and recent advances in Doppler ultrasound. *J Hepatol*;34:474–482. ISSN 0168-8278

Hansen PM, Pedersen MM., Kristoffer, Hansen KL., Bachmann Nielsen M, Jensen JA (2011). Demonstration of a Vector Velocity Technique. *Ultraschall in Med*; 32:213-215. ISSN 0172-4614.

Horigome H, Nomura T, Saso K, Itoh M, Joh T, Ohara H (1999). Limitations of imaging diagnosis for small hepatocellular carcinoma: comparison with histological findings. *J Gastroenterol Hepatol*; 14: 559 –565. Online ISSN 1440-1746

International Working Party (1995). Terminology of nodular hepatocellular lesions. *Hepatology*;22:983–993. Online ISSN 1527-3350

Jang HJ, Kim TK, Wilson SR (2009). Small nodules (1-2 cm) in liver cirrhosis: characterization with contrast-enhanced ultrasound. *Eur J Radiol*; 72: 418-424. ISSN 0720-048X

Kojiro M (2004). Focus on dysplastic nodules and early hepatocellular carcinoma: an Eastern point of view. *Liver Transpl*;10:S3–S8. Online ISSN 1527-6473

Konopke R, Kersting S, Saeger HD, Bunk A (2005). Detection of liver lesions by contrast-enhanced ultrasound -- comparison to intraoperative findings. *Ultraschall in Med*; 26: 107-113. ISSN 0172-4614.

Kreft B, Pauleit D, Bachmann R, Conrad R, Krämer A, Schild HH (2001). Incidence and significance of small focal liver lesions in MRI. *Rofo*; 173: 424-429. PubMed: 11414150. Available from www.ncbi.nlm.nih.gov

Larsen LPS (2010). Role of contrast enhanced ultrasonography in the assessment of hepatic metastases: A review. *World J Hepatol* January 27; 2(1): 8-15. ISSN 1948-5182 (online)

Lassau N, Chami L, Chebil M, Benatsou B, Bidault S, Girard E, Abboud G, Roche A (2011). Dynamic Contrast-Enhanced Ultrasonography (DCE-US) and Anti-angiogenic Treatments. *Discovery Medicine*. Published online. ISSN 1539-6509; eISSN 1944-7930

Lencioni R, Crocetti L, Cioni D, Della Pina C, Bartolozzi C (2004). Percutaneous radiofrequency ablation of hepatic colorectal metastases. Technique, indications, results, and new promises. *Invest Radiol*;39:689–697. ISSN 0020-9996

Lencioni R, Piscaglia F, Bolondi L (2008). Contrast-enhanced ultrasound in the diagnosis of hepatocellular carcinoma. *Journal of Hepatology* 48 848–857. ISSN 0168-8278

Lim HS, Jeong YY, Kang HK, Kim JK, Park JG (2006). Imaging features of hepatocellular carcinoma after transcatheter arterial chemoembolization and radiofrequency ablation. *Am J Roentgenol;* 187: W341-W349. Print ISSN: 0361-803X Online ISSN: 1546-3141

Lindner J (2004). Microbubbles in medical imaging: current applications and future directions. Nature;3:527-532. ISSN 0028-0836, eISSN: 1476-4687

Llovet JM, Bru ́C, Bruix J (1999). Prognosis of hepatocellular carcinoma: the BCLC staging classification. *Semin Liver Dis;*19:329–338. Print ISSN 0272-8087, e ISSN 1098-8971

Llovet JM, Burroughs A, Bruix J (2003). Hepatocellular carcinoma. *Lancet;*362:1907–1917. Print ISSN 0140-6736.

Llovet JM, Bruix J (2008). Novel advancements in the management of hepatocelular carcinoma in 2008. *Journal of Hepatology;* 48: S20 - S37. ISSN 0168-8278

Luo W, Numata K, Morimoto M, Kondo M, Takebayashi S, Okada M, Morita S, Tanaka K (2009). Focal liver tumors: characterization with 3D perflubutane microbubble contrast agent-enhanced US versus 3D contrast-enhanced multidetector CT. *Radiology;* 251(1):287–95. Print ISSN 0033-8419. Online ISSN 1527-1315

Maruyama H, Yoshikawa M, Yokosuka O (2008). Current role of ultrasound for the management of hepatocellular carcinoma. *World J Gastroenterol;* 14: 1710-1719. ISSN 1007-9327

Matsui O (2004). Imaging of multistep human hepatocarcinogenesis by CT during intra-arterial contrast injection. *Intervirology;* 47: 271-276. print ISSN 0300–5526, eISSN 1423–0100

Minami Y, Kudo M (2010). Hepatic malignancies: Correlation between sonographic findings and pathological features. *World J Radiol* 28;2(7):249-256. ISSN 1949-8470 (online)

Molins IG, Fernández Font JM, Álvaro JC, Navarro JLL, Gil MF, Rodríguez CMF (2010). Contrast-enhanced ultrasound in diagnosis and characterization of focal hepatic lesions. *World J Radiol* 2010 December 28; 2(12): 455-462. ISSN 1949-8470 (online)

Newman & T Bettinger (2007). Gene therapy progress and prospects: Ultrasound for gene transfer. *Gene Therapy* 14, 465–475. ISSN 0969-7128, eISSN 1476-5462

Nicolau C, Catala V, Vilana R (2004). Evaluation of hepatocellular carcinoma using Sonovue, a second generation ultrasound contrast agent: Correlation with cellular differentiation. *Eur Radiol;*14:1092–1099. print ISSN 0938-7994, eISSN 1432-1084

Nicolau C, Vilana R, Bianchi L, Brú C (2007). Early-stage hepatocellular carcinoma: the high accuracy of real-time contrast-enhanced ultrasonography in the assessment of response to percutaneous treatment. *Eur Radiol;* 17(Suppl 6): F80-88. print ISSN 0938-7994 , eISSN: 1432-1084

Parkin DM, Bray F, Ferlay J, Pisani P (2005). Global cancer statistics 2002. *CA Cancer J Clin;*55:74–108. Print ISSN: 0007-9235 eISSN: 1542-4863

Piscaglia F, Corradi F, Mancini M, Giangregorio F, Tamberi S, Ugolini G, Cola B, Bazzocchi A, Righini R, Pini P, Fornari F, Bolondi L (2007). Real time contrast enhanced ultrasonography in detection of liver metastases from gastrointestinal cancer. *BMC Cancer;* 7: 171. ISSN 1471-2407

Quaia E, Calliada F, Bertolotto M, Rossi S, Garioni L, Rosa L, Pozzi-Mucelli R. (2004) Characterization of focal liver lesions with contrast- specific US modes and a sulfur hexafluoride-filled microbubble contrast agent: diagnostic performance and confidence. *Radiology;*232(2): 420–30. Print ISSN 0033-8419. Online ISSN 1527-1315

Quaia E, Palumbo A, Rossi S, Degobbis F, Cernic S, Tona G, Cova M (2006). Comparison of Visual and Quantitative Analysis for Characterization of Insonated Liver Tumors After Microbubble Contrast Injection. *AJR;* 186:1560–1570. ISSN 1007-9327

Sandulescu DL, Dumitrescu D, Rogoveanu I, Saftoiu A (2011). Hybrid ultrasound imaging techniques (fusion imaging). *World J Gastroenterol;* 17(1):49-52. ISSN 1007-9327 (print) ISSN 2219-2840 (online)

Skjoldbye B, Pedersen MH, Struckmann J, Burcharth F, Larsen T (2002). Improved detection and biopsy of solid liver lesions using pulse-inversion ultrasound scanning and contrast agent infusion. *Ultrasound Med Biol;*28:439–444. ISSN 0301-5629

Solbiati L, Ierace T, Tonolini M, Cova L (2004). Guidance and monitoring of radiofrequency liver tumor ablation with contrast-enhanced ultrasound. *Eur J Radiol;* 51(Suppl): S19-23. print ISSN 0938-7994 eISSN 1432-1084

Solbiati L, Tonolini M, Cova L (2004). Monitoring RF ablation. *Eur Radiol;*14:34–42. print ISSN 0938-7994 eISSN 1432-1084

Spârchez Z, Radu P, Anton O, Socaciu M, Badea R (2009). Contrast-Enhanced Ultrasound in Assessing Therapeutic Response in Ablative Treatments of Hepatocellular Carcinoma. *J Gastrointestin Liver Dis* Vol.18 No 2, 243-248. ISSN 1841-8724

Strobel D, Kleinecke C, Hänsler J, Frieser M, Händl T, Hahn EG, Bernatik T (2005). Contrast-enhanced sonography for the characterisation of hepatocellular carcinomas-correlation with histological differentiation. *Ultraschall in Med;*26:270–276. ISSN 0172-4614.

Tanaka S, Ioka T, Oshikawa O, Hamada Y, Yoshioka F (2001). Dynamic sonog- raphy of hepatic tumors. *Am J Roentgenol;*177:799–805. Online ISSN 1546-3141

Vilana R, Bianchi L, Varela M, Nicolau C, Sánchez M, Ayuso C, García M, Sala M, Llovet JM, Bruix J, Bru C; BCLC Group (2006). Is microbubble-enhanced ultrasonography sufficient for assessment of response to percutaneous treatment in patients with early hepatocellular carcinoma? *Eur Radiol;*16:2454–2462. print ISSN 0938-7994 eISSN 1432-1084

von Herbay A, Vogt C, Westendorff J, Häussinger D, Gregor M (2009). Correlation between SonoVue Enhancement in CEUS, HCC Differentiation and HCC Diameter: Analysis of 130 Patients with Hepatocellular Carcinoma (HCC). *Ultraschall in Med;* 30: 544–550. ISSN 0172-4614.

Weidener N, Semple JP, Welch WR, Folkman J (1991). Tumor angiogenesis and metastasis – correlation in invasive breast carcinoma. *N. Engl. J. Med,* 324, 1 – 7. Available from: http://www.nejm.org/doi/full/10.1056/NEJM199101033240101

Wernecke K, Rummeny E, Bongartz G, Vassallo P, Kivelitz D, Wiesmann W, Peters PE, Reers B, Reiser M, Pircher W (1991). Detection of hepatic masses in patients with carcinoma: comparative sensitivities of sonography, CT, and MR imaging. *Am J Roentgenol;* 157: 731-739. Online ISSN 1546-3141

Wu F, Wang ZB, Chen WZ, Zou JZ, Bai J, Zhu H, Li KQ, Jin CB, Xie FL, Su HB (2005). Advanced hepatocellular carcinoma: treatment with high-intensity focused ultrasound ablation combined with transcatheter arterial embolization. *Radiology;* 235: 659-667. Print ISSN 0033-8419. Online ISSN 1527-1315

Zapata E, Zubiaurre L, Castiella A, Salvador P, García-Bengoechea M, Esandi P, Arriola A, Beguiristain A, Ruiz I, Garmendia G, Orcolaga R, Alustiza JM. (2010). Are hepatocellular carcinoma surveillance programs effective at improving the therapeutic options? *Rev Esp Enferm Dig;* 102: 484-488. ISSN 1130-0108

6

Liver Tumor Detection in CT Images by Adaptive Contrast Enhancement and the EM/MPM Algorithm

Yu Masuda et al.*
Department of Science and Engineering, Ritsumeikan Univesity, Shiga, Japan

1. Introduction

Liver cancer is considered one of the major causes of death in humans [1]. Early detection of tumors is essential for increasing the survival chances of patients. Recent advancements in medical imaging modalities have enabled the acquisition of high-resolution CT datasets, and thus, allowing physicians to identify both small and large tumors by manual visual inspection. Owing to the large number of images in medical datasets, it is difficult to manually analyze all images, and useful diagnostic information may be overlooked. Moreover, the diagnoses are mainly based on the physician's subjective evaluation and are dependent on the physician's experience. Therefore, computer assisted diagnosis (CAD) and computer assisted surgery have become one of the major research subjects.

Until now, many methods have been proposed for tumor detection and segmentation in liver CT images. These methods can be classified as semi-automatic [2][3] and automatic [4][5]. Smeets *et al.* have proposed a semi-automatic level set method, which combines a spiral scanning technique with supervised fuzzy pixel classification [2]. Mala *et al.* employed wavelet-based texture features in order to train a neural network for use in tumor detection [4]. In the method proposed by Park *et al.* [5], the voxels representing the liver vessels are removed from liver images and a bimodal histogram is assumed for the intensity distribution of the liver and tumors. The optimal threshold to segment tumors is determined by a "mixture probability density" algorithm. In our previous study [6], we proposed tumor detection [7], which is a technique combining the expectation maximization algorithm and a three-dimensional region of interest (ROI) detection method. However, if the image contrast is low, it is difficult to accurately remove vessels from the image. All the above-mentioned methods can locate tumors that are sufficiently large and have distinct boundaries. Semi-automatic approaches for handling a large number of tumors would need extensive user interactions, and therefore are error prone and tedious.

---

* Tomoko Tateyama[1], Wei Xiong[2], Jiayin Zhou[2], Makoto Wakamiya[3], Syuzo Kanasaki[3], Akira Furukawa[3] and Yen Wei Chen[1]
1 Department of Science and Engineering, Ritsumeikan Univesity, Shiga, Japan,
2 Institute for Infocomm Research, Singapore,
3 Shiga University of Medical Science, Shiga, Japan.

We propose a new method for detecting tumors in CT images. Our method is based on adaptive contrast enhancement and the expectation maximization / maximization of the posterior marginal (EM/MPM) algorithm. User interaction is not required and both large and small tumors can be accurately found. Compared with our previously reported method [6], the newly proposed method is also suitable for images with poor contrasts. We describe the method in Sections 2-6 and present the experimental results in Section 7, followed by our conclusions.

2. Overview of the proposed method

Our method is composed of seven steps: (1) read the CT images; (2) extract the liver region using a well-established liver region segmentation program [8]; (3) smooth out the noise from the CT images; (4) enhance the CT image contrast by using probability density functions (PDFs) estimated from the training data; (5) remove vessels by applying Maximum likelihood method; (6) detect tumor candidates by employing the EM/MPM algorithm; and (7) detect and segment the tumor regions by using a shape filter.

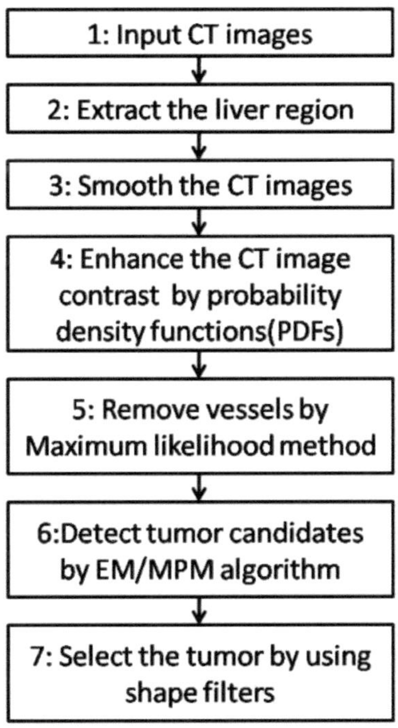

Fig. 1. The flowchart of our proposed method for tumor detections

3. Contrast enhancement

As tumor detection is mainly based on the intensity of CT images, the contrast of the images is very important. Two typical histograms of CT images having high and low contrasts are shown in Figs. 2(a) and 2(b), respectively. As shown in Fig.2(a), if the contrast of CT images is high, the tumor is in a different intensity range (left small peak) with the liver (right large peak) and the tumor can be easily detected by the intensity threshold, while if the contrast of

CT images is low, the tumor is in the same narrow intensity range as the liver as shown in Fig.2(b) and it is difficult to detect the tumor from the liver volume. Density value of all objects is in a narrow range as shown in Fig.2(b). So we have to enhance the contrast of CT images as a preprocessing.

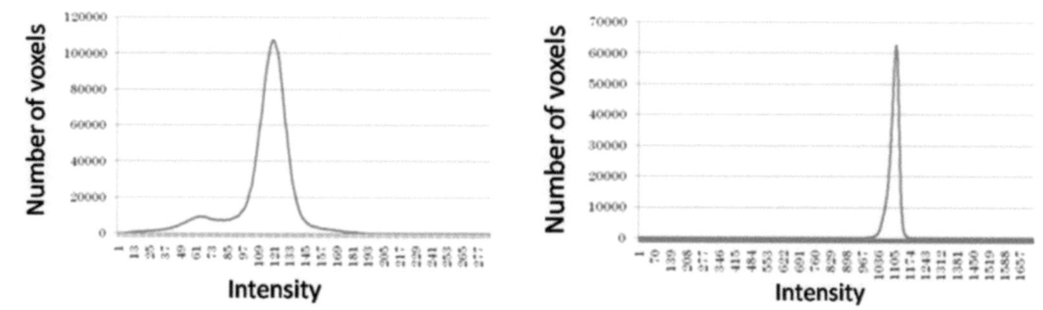

(a) (b)

Fig. 2. Histograms with (a) high (b) low contrasts

A piecewise linear histogram transformation is usually employed to enhance the intensity contrast. However, it is difficult to determine a fixed set of lower and upper limits of the transformation slope for all images because they are data dependent. In this study, we automatically and adaptively determine the parameters from each image. In liver CT images, there are three classes of tissues: tumor, healthy liver, and vessels. First, sample voxels of the three classes are manually selected from the training data. The intensity PDFs of each class is estimated.

We also compute their mean values (μ^A_{tumor}, μ^A_{liver}, μ^A_{vessel}), their standard derivations (σ_{tumor}, σ_{liver}, σ_{vessel}), and M^A. M^A is the intensity value which has the highest probability in the liver class. The mean values have the property of $\mu^A_{tumor} < \mu^A_{liver} < \mu^A_{vessel}$. In Fig. 3(a), the three curves, from left to right, represent the PDFs of the tumor, the (healthy) liver, and the vessel classes. The mean and standard deviation values may differ among images, but the mean value of the (healthy) liver is always larger than that of the tumor and smaller than that of the vessels. This can be used for the classification of the three classes. The pattern of these three curves is called Curve Pattern A.

Given a new image and its segmented liver volume, we first compute the intensity histogram of all voxels in the liver volume. We find the intensity value M^B, which has the most component in the liver class, and assume that M^B corresponds to the probability density peak of the class of healthy liver tissues in the new liver volume. Such an assumption is viable because the healthy tissues normally dominate the volume.

As a result, the mean values of the tumor and vessels are estimated as $\mu_{tumor} = M^B - M^A + \mu^A_{tumor}$ and $\mu_{vessel} = M^B - M^A + \mu^A_{vessel}$, respectively. Now, we set the lower limit as $T_{\min} = \mu_{tumor} - 3\sigma_{tumor}$ and the upper limit as $T_{\max} = \mu_{vessel} + 3\sigma_{vessel}$. The intensity transform formula for the range 0–255 is given in Eq. (1). Using the formula, the intensity histograms of the liver images are re-estimated [Fig. 3(c)] for later use.

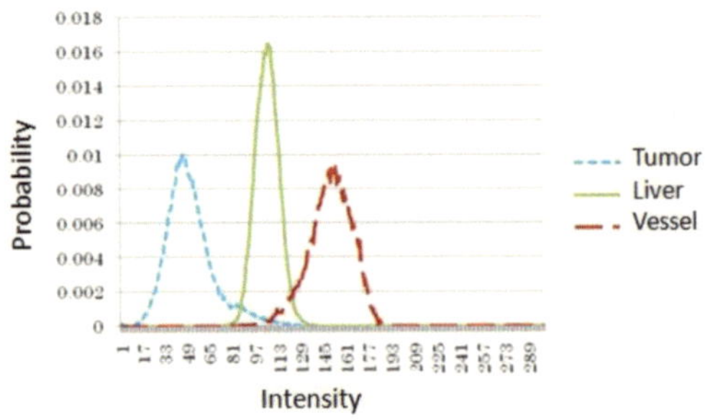

(a)

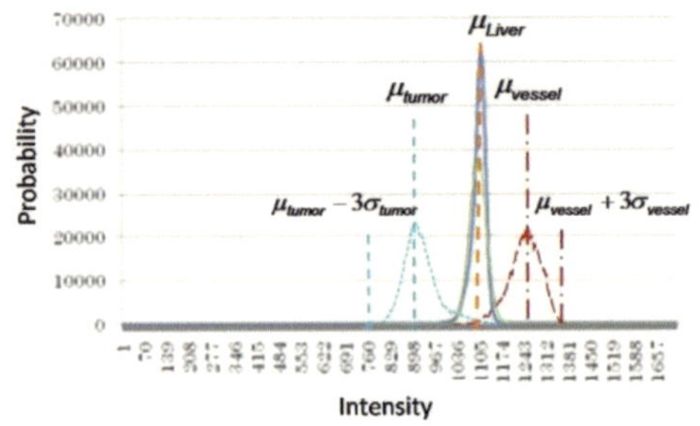

(b)

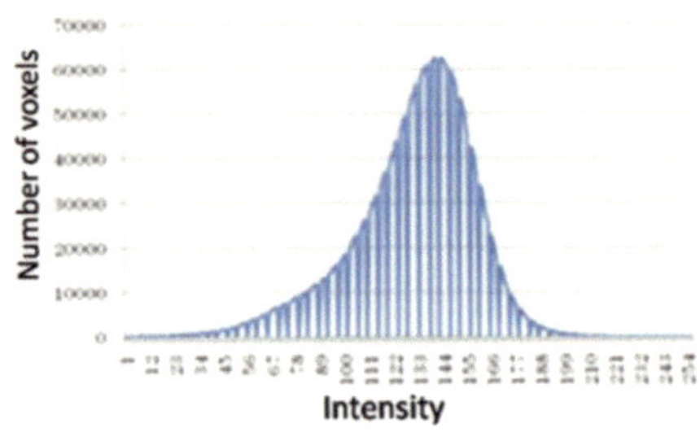

(c)

Fig. 3. (a) Estimated intensity PDFs for tumor (curve on the left), liver (curve in the center), and vessel (curve on the right); (b) Overlap the Curve Pattern A to the new image's liver volume histogram; (c) Histogram obtained after our histogram transformation

$$\begin{cases} \dfrac{(x_i - T_{\min})}{(T_{\max} - T_{\min})}(255-1)+1 & if\,(T_{\min} \le x_i \le T_{\max}) \\ 0 & if\,(x_i < T_{\min} \cup x_i > T_{\max}) \end{cases} \tag{1}$$
$$T_{\min} : \mu_{tumor} - 3\sigma, T_{\max} : \mu_{vessel} + 3\sigma$$

4. Removement of vessels by applying Maximum likelihood method

Before tumor detection step, we first remove vessels from CT images. In the conventional method [5], as the intensity of vessels is higher than those of health liver tissues and tumor tissues, intensity threshold method is used to remove vessels. We classify the CT volume into 3 classes by using Maximum likelihood method. And then, voxels of the class with the highest mean are removed as vessels. After this process, CT images only include tumor and healthy liver tissues. The tumor detection problem can be simplified as a 2-class classification problem. This process will also significantly reduce the detection time.

5. Tumor candidate detection by using EM/MPM algorithm

To extract tumor candidate, we used the EM/MPM algorithm [9]. It is based on a Bayesian framework that assumes a Gaussian mixture to model intensity distribution and concurrently estimates both the labels of the voxels and the model parameters. In MPM, the cost function is defined to minimize the total number of misclassified voxels. It can be proved that minimization of the cost function is equivalent to maximization of the posterior marginal probability of the label fields (Eq. 2) [10].

$$\hat{x}_{s_{MPM}} = \arg\max_{x} P_{X_s|Y}(x_s \mid y,\theta) = \arg\max_{x} \sum_{X\in\Omega_{k,s}} P_{X|Y}(x \mid y,\theta) \tag{2}$$

In Eq. (2), x, y, and θ are the label vector, feature vector, and model parameters, respectively, s is a pixel, k is the label of pixel s, and Ω refers to all possible labels of the image in which the label of pixel s equals k. The posterior probability is composed of two factors, namely the likelihood function and the prior probability. The likelihood function is a multiplication of the Gaussian distribution function and the prior probability is modeled by Markov random field (Eq. 3).

$$P_{X_s|Y}(x_s \mid y,\theta) = \sum_{X\in\Omega_{k,s}} P_{X|Y}(x \mid y,\theta) \propto \sum_{X\in\Omega_{k,s}} \left\{ \left[\prod_{i=1}^{N} \frac{1}{\sqrt{2\pi\sigma_{x_i}^2}} \right] \cdot \exp\left(-\sum_{i=1}^{N} \frac{(y_i - \mu_{x_i})^2}{2\sigma_{x_i}^2} - \sum_{\{r,s\}\in c} \frac{1}{T(n)} \delta(x_r, x_s) \right) \right\} \tag{3}$$

In Eq. (3), N is the total number of voxels, (μ_{xi}, σ_{xi}^2) are model parameters of class x_i, y_i is the intensity of a voxel, $T(n)$ is called temperature, and $\delta(x_r, x_s)$ is a function that contributes to the labels of the neighboring voxels (r) when determining the label of s. For all neighboring voxels whose labels (x_r) same as x_s, the output of the weighting function is zero. Otherwise, a value of 0.5 or 1 is assigned according to Fig. 3. In our method, we consider six neighboring voxels; four in the same slice and two in the upper and the lower slices (Fig. 4.)

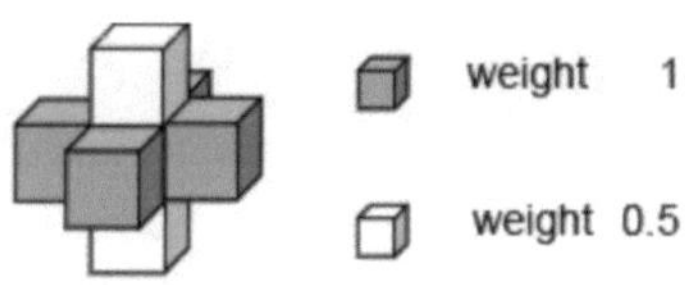

Fig. 4. Weight functions for 6-neighbours of a voxel.

Optimization of Eq. (2) is not simple. We use the simulated annealing method to iteratively determine an estimate [9], which is given by $T(n) = T_1 / \log(n + c)$. Here, T_1 is the initial temperature which is a large constant, c is a constant number and n is the iteration number. After determining the MPM estimate (the E-step), the model parameters are calculated (the M-step). We continue the iteration of the two steps until convergence is achieved. As a result, we obtain tumor candidates that may include both true and false positive regions. In our experiments, we assign the values of 1.4 to c, 50 to n, and 2.0 to T_1 through several testing runs. To remove false results, we use the shape information described below.

6. Candidate selection with shape filter

The tumor candidates, which were detected in the previous section, include many false positives because the detection used only intensity information. Therefore, in this step, we perform a selection process using a shape filter. We define the following five evaluation criteria: (1) size, (2) shape of each slice, (3) regional variation among the slices, (4) location in the image, and (5) numbers of connectivity among the slices.

In this study, we assume that the shape of a tumor is approximately spherical. Therefore, for the second criteria, we use a shape filter as shown in Fig. 5. For each tumor candidate, we first find a center of gravity, and then calculate distances from it to the 12 points which are on the edge of tumor candidate as shown in Fig.5. 4 points are cross points with the bounding box (line of a rectangle), which are shown in Fig.5 as diamond points. 8 points are boundary points sampled at intervals of 45 degree, which are shown in Fig.5 as small circle points. The ratio of maximum distance and minimum distance is used as a measure of shape. The ratio is a value larger than or equal to 1. If the candidate's shape is like a circle, the ratio will be 1. Since the tumor is considered having a spherical shape, the candidates are rejected if their ratio is larger than a pre-defined threshold (in our research, the threshold is set as 4).

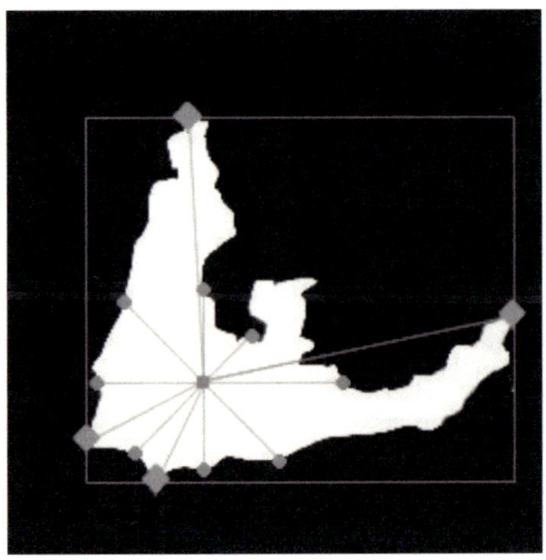

Fig. 5. Illustration of a shape filter

Though most false positive candidates can be rejected by the use of above 5 criterions, some tumor points will also be rejected. In order to recover the rejected true tumors, we use a new criterion, which is shown in Fig. 6 to check the rejected candidates. For each rejected tumor candidate, we first generate an edge image, and then superimpose it with two circles L_{in} and L_{out} having radius r_{in} and r_{out}, respectively, and centers corresponding to the center of the tumor candidate's 2D ROI. Their parameters are defined in Eq. 4.

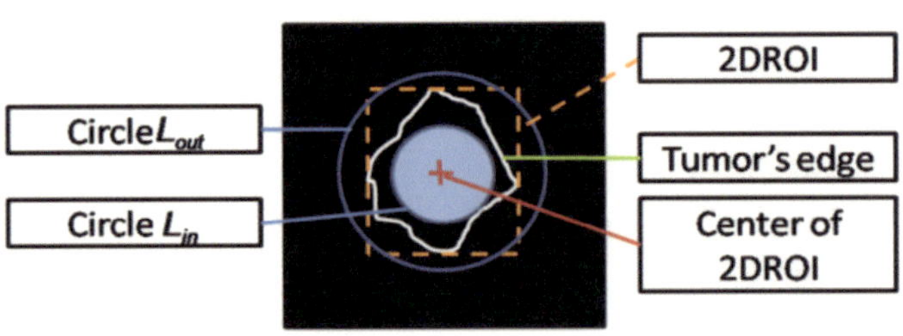

Fig. 6. Illustration of a shape filter for recheck

$$\begin{cases} r_{out} = 4 + L/2, & r_{in} = r_{out}/2, \quad if(L \geq 10) \\ r_{out} = 2 + L/2, & r_{in} = r_{out}/2 - 1, if(L < 10) \end{cases} \tag{4}$$

Here, L is the longer side length of 2D ROI. If the shape of a tumor candidate is approximately spherical, then a major portion of the tumor region is bounded by the circle L_{in} and the edge of the tumor is between the circles L_{in} and L_{out}.

7. Experimental results

We applied our proposed method to five sets of CT images. Information on each image is shown in Table 1. Data sets 1, 2, and 3 were used in the JAMIT CAD contest in July 2010, while Data sets 4 and 5 were used in the MICCA Liver Tumor Segmentation Challenge 2008 [11]. Table 2 shows the results of tumor detection. In this study, if a part of a tumor is detected in the correct region, we consider the result as a true positive. Because only the ground truth for Data sets 1, 2, and 3 were known, Table 2 shows comparisons between the detected results and the ground truth for Data sets 1–3. The proposed method provides accurate detection results for Data sets 1 and 2. For Data set 3, the detection rate is about 50% because the image includes numerous minute tumors.

Data set	Size			Spacing		
	x	y	z	x	y	z
1	512	512	156	0.625	0.625	1.00
2	512	512	191	0.732	0.732	1.00
3	512	512	200	0.72	0.72	1.00
4	512	512	173	0.59	0.59	1.50
5	512	512	172	0.77	0.77	1.50

Table 1. Information on each dataset

Data set	False negative	True Positive	Actual number
1	0	2	2
2	0	5	5
3	7	6	13

Table 2. Number of detected tumors

Fig. 7 shows the results of tumor detection using the EM/MPM algorithm and the method based on [6]. It removed high intensities without employing Maximum likelihood method and applied the EM algorithm. The results show that our proposed method is superior to the previous one. The reason is considered to be the use of histogram transformation with PDFs. In the previous method, the EM algorithm took more time to converge compared with that in our proposed method; this was because the proposed method employs Maximum likelihood method. Moreover, irregular shapes could be removed by using the shape filter [Fig. 7(d)].

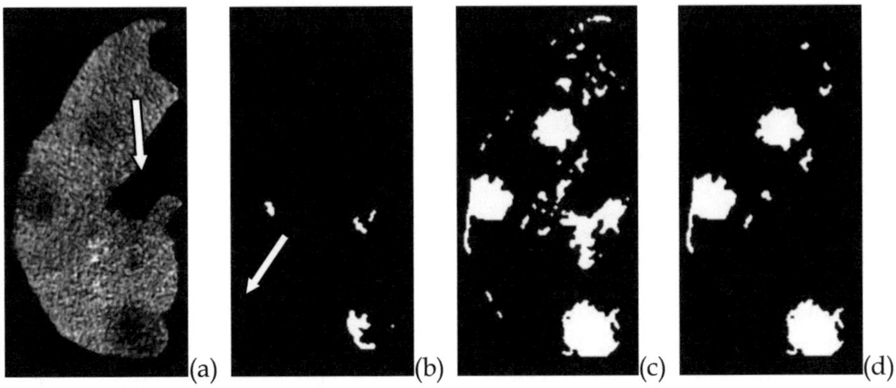

Fig. 7. (a) the original image (Data set 4). The tumor detection result obtained (b) using the method based on [6], (c) the proposed method, and (d) by the application of a shape filter to the image in (c). (In (b)–(d), the detected regions are white and the arrows indicate the locations of the detected tumors.)

Fig. 8 show the results of the experiments for Data set 3. We used four methods: EM with and without preprocessing (contrast enhancement) and EM/MPM with and without preprocessing. As we used different pre-processing for EM and EM/MPM, it may affect the result a little. However, Figures 8(c)–(f) are the images obtained after morphology operations. Figures 8(c), (d) demonstrate the effectiveness of our histogram transformation. Comparing Figs. 8(c), (e) with Figs. 8(d), (f), we find that using EM/MPM improves performance.

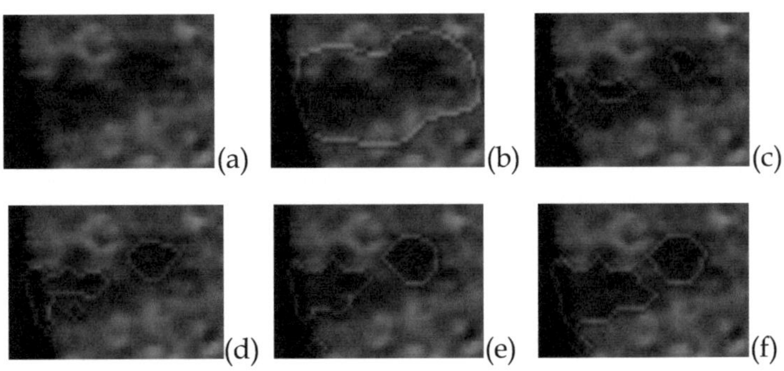

Fig. 8. Results after morphology (white lines) (a) Smoothed original image (b) answer (c) EM without preprocessing (d) EM with preprocessing (e) EM/MPM without preprocessing (f) EM/MPM with preprocessing

Next, we quantitatively evaluate the tumor segmentation performance in terms of the metrics proposed in the MICCAI Liver Tumor Segmentation Challenge 2008 [11]. The metrics are the volumetric overlap error (Overlap Error), absolute relative volume difference (Vol. dif.), average symmetric surface distance (Ave. Dist.), RMS symmetric surface distance (RMS Dist.), and maximum surface distance (Max. Dist.). For ideal segmentation, all metrics should be zero. Table 3 shows the results obtained for one slice of a segmented region in a tumor by the metrics given in [11]. For Data set 1, regions in which tumors are detected are not solely represented by dark regions but also by bright voxels around them. Our proposed method can detect dark tumor regions; however, it cannot detect the bright tumor regions. Therefore, we excluded the results for Data set 1 and included only the results for the other data sets. We compared the current method with the previous method on the basis of the abovementioned method [6]. It is obvious from the results that we have improved on all metrics.

Data	Method	Overlap Error [%]	Vol. dif. [%]	Ave Dist. [mm]	RMS Dist. [mm]	Max. Dist. [mm]
2	previous	74.27	68.09	1.28	1.84	5.00
	proposed	59.54	50.92	0.84	1.45	5.00
3	previous	75.63	72.08	2.76	4.20	13.45
	proposed	66.43	61.29	1.84	3.08	11.18
4	previous	84.29	84.29	4.84	6.57	16.27
	proposed	16.87	8.45	0.17	0.65	5.00
5	previous	6.71	4.53	0.04	0.28	4.24
	proposed	5.82	1.94	0.04	0.24	3.60

Table 3. Performance comparisons

8. Conclusions

We have proposed a new method to detect tumors automatically in CT image. By using contrast enhancement with PDFs of different tissue classes in a newly devised histogram transformation method, we can enhance the image contrast. Moreover, by using the EM/MPM algorithm, we can detect tumors more accurately. We plan to improve our work to handle the large morphology variation of tumors.

9. Acknowledgement

We thank associate professor Akinobu Shimizu of Tokyo University of Agriculture and Technology for providing liver region extract program. We also thank JAMIT and MICCAI for providing CT images. This work was supported in part by the Grant-in Aid for Scientific Research from the Japanese Ministry for Education, Science, Culture and Sports under the Grant No. 21300070 and 22103513, and in part by the Research fund from Ritsumeikan Global Innovation Research Organization (R-GIRO). Wei Xiong and Jiayin Zhou acknowledge supports from Singapore A*STAR project JCOAG03_FG05_2009.

10. References

[1] Center for Cancer Control and Information Services, National Cancer Center, Japan, http://ganjoho.jp/public/statistics/pub/statistics01.html

[2] D. Smeets, D. Loeckx, B. Stijnen, B. De Dobbelaer, D. Vandermeulen, P. Suetens, Semi-automatic level set segmentation of liver tumors combining a spiral scanning technique withsupervised fuzzy pixel classification, Medical image analysis, vol. 14, no. 1, pp. 13-20, February 2010.

[3] Häme, Y., Alhonnoro, T., Pollari, M.: Image Analysis for Liver Tumor Ablation Treatment Planning, Hands-on Image Processing 2009, Robotiker-Tecnalia.

[4] K. Mala, V. Sadasivam, S. Alagappan, "Neural Network Based Texture Analysis of Liver Tumor from Computed Tomography Images, " International Journal of Biomedical Sciences 2, 33–40, 2006.

[5] Seung-Jin Park, Kyung-Sik Seo, Jong-An Park: "Automatic Hepatic Tumor Segmentation Using Statical Optimal Threshold", Computational Science - ICCS 2005, Springer Berlin / Heidelberg, Volume 3514, pp 934-940, 2005.

[6] Y. Masuda, A. H. Foruzan, T. Tateyama, Y. W. Chen, "Automatic liver tumor detection using EM/MPM algorithm and shape information ", IEICE technical report 110(28), 25-30, 2010-05-13

[7] Y. Masuda, A. H. Foruzan, T. Tateyama, Y. W. Chen, "Automatic liver tumor detection using EM algorithm and 3DROI," Kamsao-section Joint Convention of Institutes of Electrical Engineerin, G310, 2009.

[8] A. Shimizu, http://www.tuat.ac.jp/~simizlab

[9] M.L. Comer and E. J. Delp. The EM/MPM Algorithm for Segmentation of Textured Images: Analysis and Further Experimental Results, IEEE Transactions on Image Processing. , 9 (10) 1731-1744 October 2000.

[10] J.L. Marrquin, S. Mitter and T. Poggie. Probabilistic Solution of Ill-Posed Problems in Computational Vision, Journal of American Statistical Association, 28 (397) 76-89 March 1987.

[11] X. Deng and G. Du:"Editorial: 3D Segmentation in the Clinic: A Grand Challenge II – Liver Tumor Segmentation", http://grand-challenge2008.bigr.nl/proceedings/liver/articles.html

7

Surgical Strategies for Locally Advanced Hepatocellular Carcinoma

Shugo Mizuno and Shuji Isaji
Department of Hepatobiliary-Pancreatic and Transplant Surgery, Mie University School of Medicine, Tsu, Mie, Japan

1. Introduction

Patients with advanced liver tumors extending into the portal vein or hepatic vein exhibit extremely poor prognosis after undergoing several nonsurgical therapeutic modalities, including transcatheter arterial chemoembolization (TACE) and radiofrequency ablation (RFA). Aggressive surgical treatments have been recommended in selected patients with advanced liver tumors accompanied with intravascular tumor thrombus (1). Complete surgical resection of the advanced liver tumors with tumor thrombus extending to the inferior vena cava (IVC) is beneficial for patients since it prevents the risk of pulmonary embolisms and prolongs long-term prognosis. However, IVC involvement increases the surgical risk and has been considered as a limiting factor for the curative resection of advanced tumors. The difficulty of surgery varies according to the tumor type and the region of the IVC involved; especially, the resection of tumors invading the junction of hepatic veins and the IVC is challenging. When the tumor thrombi extend above the diaphragm, cardiopulmonary bypass (CPB) is often suggested (2). Traditionally, it is necessary to perform sternotomy or thoracotomy for intrathoracic IVC isolation and to achieve adequate tumor-free margin and prevent emboli formation from the tumor thrombi (3). However, the set-up time for CPB exceeds 30 minutes (4) and the procedure of sternotomy needs additional 20 minutes or so, including the time required for closing the sternum wound. Furthermore, the complications and risks of CPB are similar to those observed in certain types of heart surgery (5). Moreover, the postoperative pain and wound adhesion caused by sternotomy and coagulopathy, and the central nervous complications inherent to the CPB and circulatory arrest have prompted the search for an alternative technique (6, 7).

Therefore, many surgeons continue to perform this aggressive surgery but try to avoid median sternotomy and CPB (8-11). This chapter introduces surgical approaches to loop the supradiaphragmatic IVC by avoiding sternotomy and thoracotomy (Figure 1).

Miyazaki et al. (8) first reported an approach to reach intrapericardial IVC through the abdominal cavity without sternotomy (Fig 1a). They suggested that after dissecting the coronary and triangular ligaments and mobilizing the bilateral hepatic lobes, the bilateral diaphragm just below the pericardial cavity can be transversely incised. The bottom of the pericardium is consecutively incised, and the intrapericardial cavity is reached. While the left lobe of the liver is retracted caudally, long-curved vascular forceps are inserted into the intrapericardial cavity, and the IVC is encircled just below the confluence into the atrium.

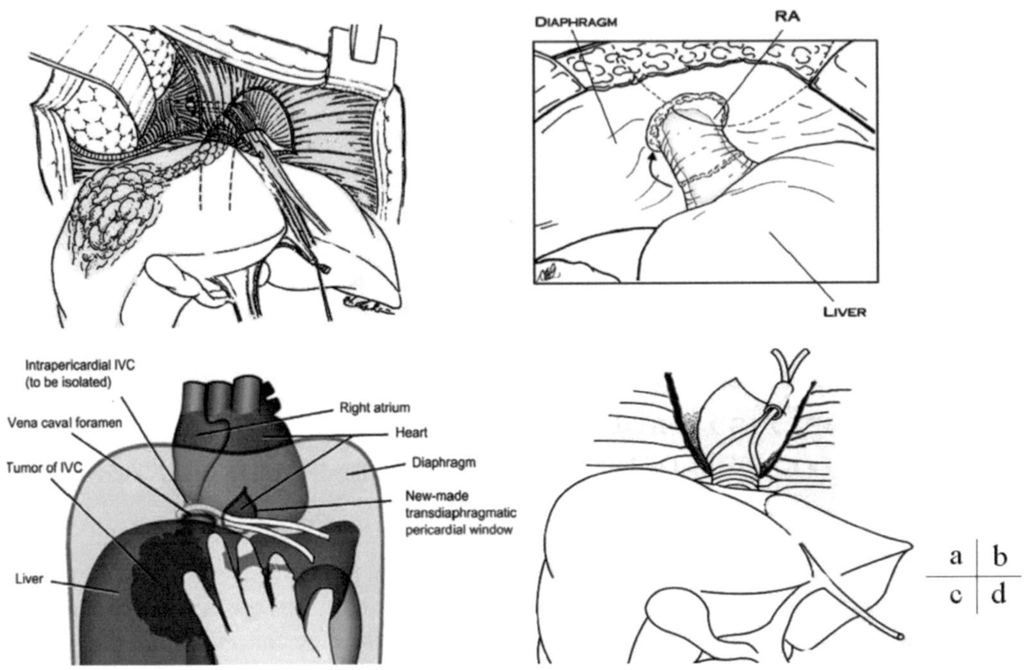

Fig. 1. Approach to the intra-thoracic IVC. (a) Miyazaki's technique: The figure was copied from the original paper (8), with permission from Thieme. (b) Ciancio's technique: The figure was copied from the original paper (9), with permission from Elsevier. (c) Chen's technique: The figure was copied from the original paper (10), with permission from Elsevier. (d) Our technique: The figure was copied from the original paper (11), with permission from Springer.

Ciancio et al. (9) showed the technique to gain access to the supradiaphragmatic IVC by circumferentially dissecting the central diaphragm tendon (Fig 1b, 2). The falciform ligament is divided using a cautery probe, and the incision is continued around each portion of the divided falciform ligament up to the right superior coronary ligament. The left triangular ligament and the central diaphragm tendon are dissected until the supradiaphragmatic, intrapericardial IVC is identified. The dissection should be circumferential so that the intrapericardial IVC can be encircled below or above the confluence into the right atrium.

Chen et al. (10) reported the method of IVC isolation through a transdiaphragmatic pericardial window (Fig 1c, 3). They suggested that the left lateral segment of the liver can be mobilized, and a plane between the liver and the diaphragm developed carefully to create a transdiaphragmatic pericardial window, about 5 × 5 cm. Through this window, the intrapericardial IVC is isolated with an umbilical tape by blunt and sharp dissection.

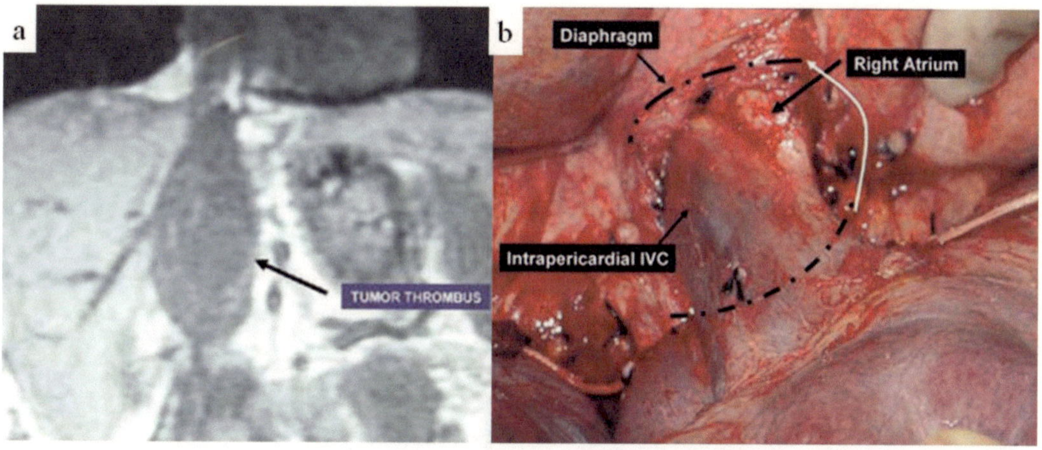

Fig. 2. Ciancio's technique (9). (a) Magnetic resonance imaging of RCC. Arrow indicates tumor thrombus in IVC extending above diaphragm into right atrium. (b) Diaphragm dissected off suprahepatic IVC. Intrapericardial IVC and right atrium exposed through abdominal cavity.

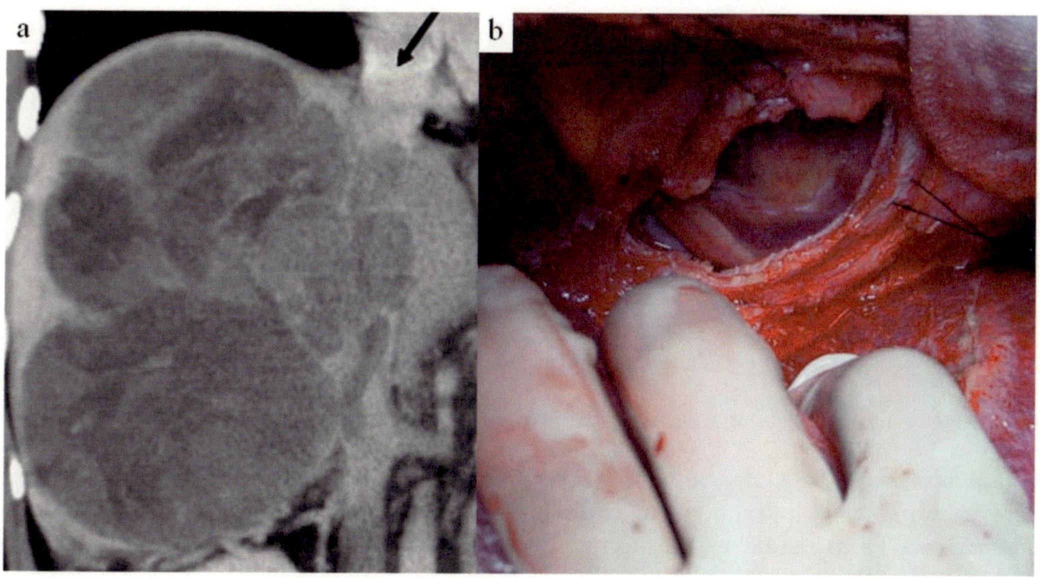

Fig. 3. Chen's technique (10). (a) Computed tomography image of an adrenocortical carcinoma. The arrow indicates the tumor thrombus extending to the junction of the hepatic vein and the inferior vena cava. (b) Transdiaphragmatic pericardial window approach for intrapericardial isolation of the inferior vena cava.

With regard to the adverse events of cutting the pericardium, there are intraoperative and postoperative problems. Intraoperatively, opening the pericardium increases the right ventricular end-diastolic and end-systolic volumes, resulting in diminished right ventricular ejection fraction (12). Postoperatively, there have been many case reports suggesting that pericardial effusion, constrictive and/or purulent pericarditis, and cardiac tamponade develop after cardiac or noncardiac surgery (13, 14).

Our technique is simpler, easier to perform, and less invasive, as compared to these approaches because it does not involve opening of the thoracic cavity and cutting of the pericardium (Fig 1d). We focused on the line of the fusion of pericardium to diaphragm (LFPD) (8), which is connected between the pericardium and diaphragm but can be easily disconnected (Fig. 4).

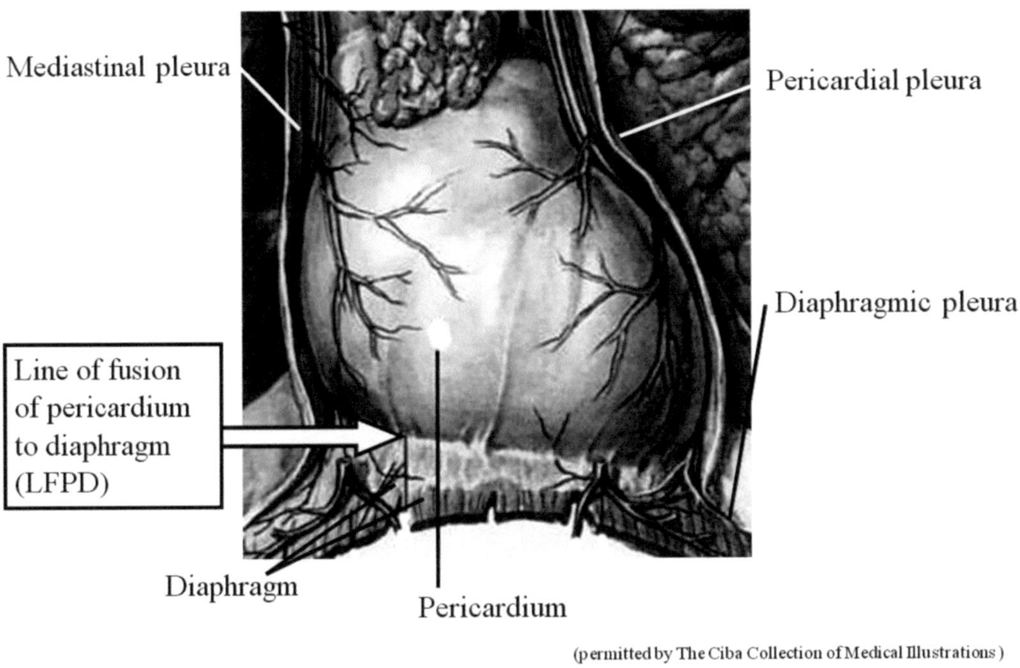

Fig. 4. The anatomy of the line of fusion of pericardium to diaphragm (LFPD)

For advanced hepatocellular carcinoma (HCC) patients (Fig. 5), LFPD was dissected, and the pericardium and diaphragm were completely separated without causing injury to the pericardium. From just below the xiphoid process to the IVC, the diaphragm was vertically dissected using LigaSure® without median sternotomy. Then, the intrathoracic IVC was exposed easily and was encircled with an umbilical tape to prevent emboli formation from the tumor thrombi (Fig. 6). After liver parenchyma transection, total hepatic vascular exclusion (THVE) was achieved by clamping the intrathoracic IVC, the infrahepatic IVC, right hepatic vein, right hepatic artery, and right portal vein. During the THVE, IVC wall was cut at the root of the left hepatic vein, and then the intracaval tumor thrombus and the left lobe of the liver were removed *en bloc* (Figure 7). The IVC defect was closed by a continuous suture with 5-0 monofilament.

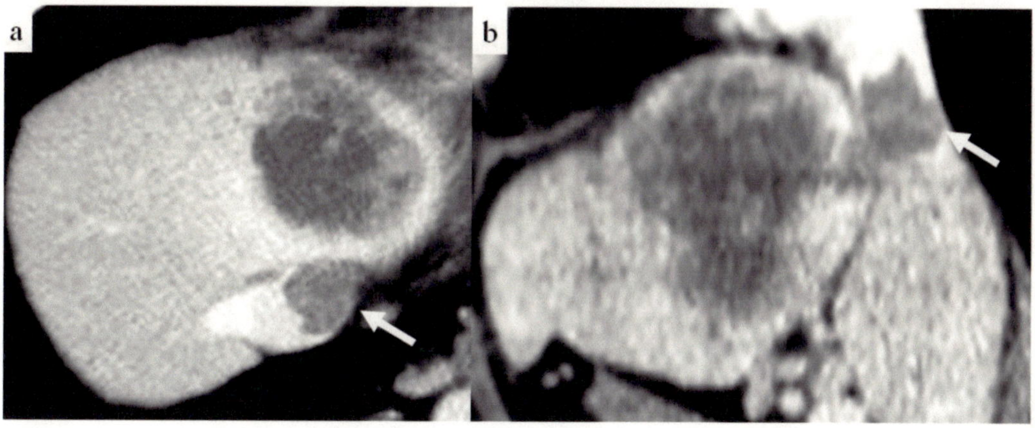

Fig. 5. Computed tomography image of hepatocellular carcinoma. The arrow indicates the tumor thrombus extending to the intra-pericardial inferior vena cava. (a) transverse sections, (b) sagittal section.

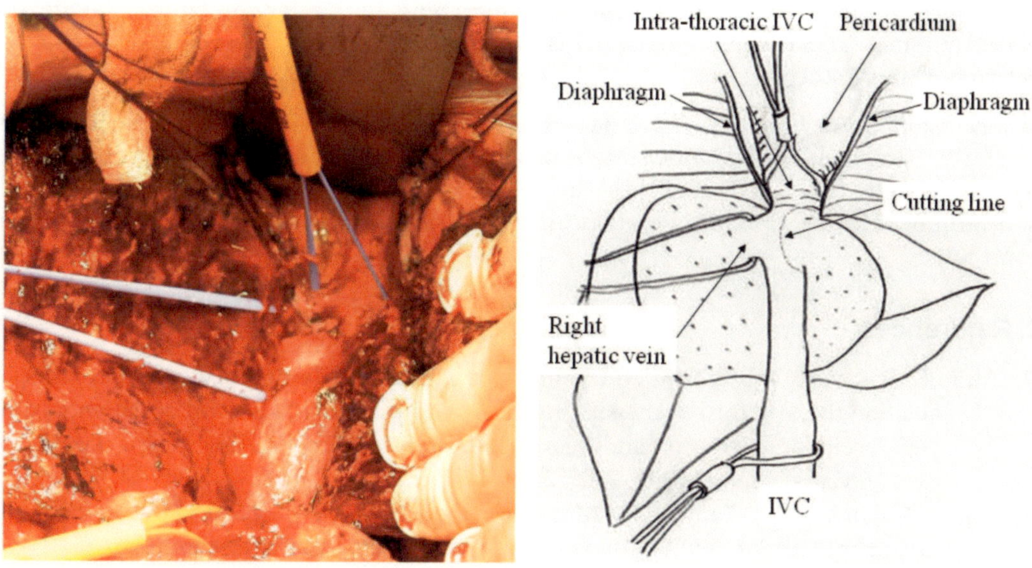

Fig. 6. After detachment of the line of fusion of pericardium to diaphragm (LFPD) and transection of the liver parenchyma, the infrahepatic IVC, right hepatic vein, right hepatic artery and right portal vein were taped.

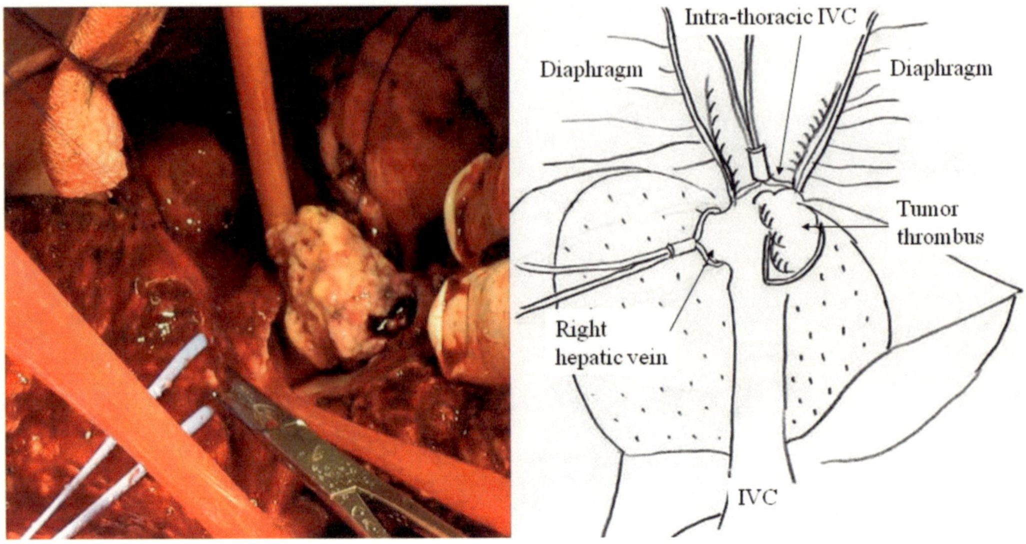

Fig. 7. During the THVE, the wall of the IVC was cut at the root of the left hepatic vein, and tumor thrombus was exposed.

Before applying THVE, we have to assess the preoperative hepatic functional reserve and carefully monitor intraoperative hemodynamic changes (16). Our selection criteria for liver resection are the same as Makuuchi criteria (17): the resection volume of the liver is determined based on total bilirubin and the Indocyanine green retention rate at 15 minutes. However, since THVE runs the risk of ischemic liver damage, these criteria should be determined more strictly.

In conclusion, the technique we have described here appears to be easy and beneficial in the surgical treatment of IVC tumors, since it provides a longer tumor-free margin of the IVC; short operative time; and abolishes the need for sternotomy, CPB, and cutting the pericardium. However, more experience is necessary to validate the benefits of this approach.

2. References

[1] Taura K, Ikai I, Hatano E, Fujii H, Uyama N, Shimahara Y. Implication of frequent local ablation therapy for intrahepatic recurrence in prolonged survival of patients with hepatocellular carcinoma undergoing hepatic resection: an analysis of 610 patients over 16 years old. *Ann Surg*. 2006; 244: 265-73.

[2] Togo S, Shimada H, Tanaka K, Masui H, Fujii S, Endo I, et al. Management of malignant tumor with intracaval extension by selective clamping of IVC. *Hepatogastroenterology*. 1996; 43: 1165-71.

[3] Nesbitt JC, Soltero ER, Dinney CP, Walsh GL, Schrump DS, Swanson DA, et al. Surgical management of renal cell carcinoma with inferior vena cava tumor thrombus. *Ann Thorac Surg.* 1997; 63: 1592-600.
[4] Hiroura M, Furusawa T, Amino M, Moriya T, Goto H, Fukaya Y, et al. Clinical experience of a vacuum- assisted non-roller extra-corporeal circulation system. J Extra Corpor Technol 2000; 32: 148–51.
[5] Salis S, Mazzanti VV, Merli G, Salvi L, Tedesco CC, Veglia F, et al. Cardiopulmonary bypass duration is an independent predictor of morbidity and mortality after cardiac surgery. *J Cardiothorac Vasc Anesth.* 2008; 22: 814-22.
[6] Novick AC, Kaye MC, Cosgrove DM, Angermeier K, Pontes JE, Montie JE, et al. Experience with cardiopulmonary bypass and deep hypothermic circulatory arrest in the management of retroperitoneal tumors with large vena cava thrombi. Ann Surg 1990; 212: 472–6.
[7] Taylor KM. Central nervous system effects of cardiopulmonary bypass. Ann Thorac Surg 1998; 66: S20–4.
[8] Miyazaki M, Ito H, Nakagawa K, Shimizu H, Yoshidome H, Shimizu Y, et al.. An approach to intrapericardial inferior vena cava through the abdominal cavity, without median sternotomy, for total hepatic vascular exclusion. *Hepatogastroenterology.* 2001; 48: 1443-6.
[9] Ciancio G, Soloway M. Renal cell carcinoma with tumor thrombus extending above diaphragm: avoiding cardiopulmonary bypass. Urology 2005; 66: 266–70.
[10] Chen TW, Tsai CH, Chou SJ, Yu CY, Shih ML, Yu JC, et al.. Intrapericardial isolation of the inferior vena cava through a transdiaphragmatic pericardial window for tumor resection without sternotomy or thoracotomy. *Eur J Surg Oncol.* 2007; 33: 239-42.
[11] Mizuno S, Kato H, Azumi Y, Kishiwada M, Hamada T, Usui M, et al. Total vascular hepatic exclusion for tumor resection: a new approach to the intrathoracic inferior vena cava through the abdominal cavity by cutting the diaphragm vertically without cutting the pericardium. *J Hepatobiliary Pancreat Sci.* 2010 Mar;17(2):197-202
[12] Mathru M, Kleinman B, Dries DJ, Rao T, Calandra D. Effect of opening the pericardium on right ventricular hemodynamics during cardiac surgery. *Chest.* 1990; 98: 120-3.
[13] Sihvo EI, Räsänen JV, Hynninen M, Rantanen TK, Salo JA. Gastropericardial fistula, purulent pericarditis, and cardiac tamponade after laparoscopic Nissen fundoplication. *Ann Thorac Surg.* 2006 Jan;81(1):356-8.
[14] Sangalli F, Colagrande L, Manetti B, Avalli L, Celotti S, Maniglia P, et al. Hemodynamic instability after cardiac surgery: transesophageal echocardiographic diagnosis of a localized pericardial tamponade. *J Cardiothorac Vasc Anesth.* 2005; 19: 775-6.
[15] Netter FH. A compilation of paintings on the normal and pathologic anatomy and physiology, embryologic, and diseases of the Heart. In: Yonkman FF, editors. The Ciba Collection of Medical Illustrations. New Jersey: CIBA; 1974, p. 2-5.

[16] Jamieson GG, Corbel L, Campion JP, Launois B. Major liver resection without a blood transfusion: is it a realistic objective? *Surgery*. 1992; 112: 32-6.
[17] Makuuchi M, Kosuge T, Takayama T, et al. Surgery for small liver cancers. *Semin Surg Oncol*. 1993;9:298–304.

8

Treatment Strategy for Recurrent Hepatocellular Carcinoma

Charing Ching Ning Chong and Paul Bo San Lai
Division of Hepato-Biliary and Pancreatic Surgery, Department of Surgery
Prince of Wales Hospital, the Chinese University of Hong Kong
Hong Kong, SAR

1. Introduction

Hepatocellular carcinoma is an important malignancy of global significance. It is the seventh commonest cancer and the fourth leading cause of cancer deaths worldwide (GLOBOCAN, 2008). While hepatectomy remains to be the gold standard for treating HCC, long-term prognosis after curative resection remains unsatisfactory with high incidence of recurrence. The reported cumulative 5-year recurrence rate after curative partial hepatectomy averages above 70% in both Eastern and Western centers and the remnant liver is the commonest site of recurrence (Chong et al., 2011; Ercolani et al., 2003; Poon et al., 2001; Yeh et al., 2002).

Intra-hepatic metastasis from the primary resected tumor and multicentric occurrence of a new tumor in the liver remnant are the two major patterns of intra-hepatic recurrence of HCC. In general, intrahepatic metastasis represented early recurrence (within 1 year after hepatectomy) and is associated with the vascular invasion and the subsequent intrahepatic venous spread while multicentric occurrence is associated with the underlying liver status and represented late recurrence (Jwo et al., 1992; Matsumata et al., 1989; Yamamoto et al., 1998). Although the exact mechanism has not been clarified, many studies had shown that late recurrence was associated with a better survival than early recurrence (Poon et al., 1999; Poon et al., 2000; Shimada et al., 1996).

Appropriate treatment for intrahepatic recurrence is crucial in improving long-term outcome after initial hepatectomy. Increased survival rates after aggressive treatment of post-resection HCC recurrence have been reported (Itamoto et al., 2007; Matsuda et al., 2001; Sugimachi et al., 2001; Tralhao et al., 2007; Wu et al., 2009; Zhou et al., 2010). Currently, various therapeutic modalities such as repeat hepatectomy, local ablation therapy and transcatheter arterial chemoembolization (TACE) have been used to treat recurrent HCC. However, there is no standard strategy for selection among different modalities so far.

2. Treatment options for recurrent HCC

2.1 Liver transplantation

Theoretically, liver transplantation would be the optimal treatment for HCC within Milan criteria as it allows radical resection of the tumor together correction of the underlying liver cirrhosis. However, due to the shortage in organ supply and long waiting time, recommending liver transplantation as the standard treatment for recurrent HCC deems logistically impractical.

2.2 Re-hepatectomy

Repeat hepatic resection has been widely recognised as one of the most effective treatments for intra-hepatic recurrent HCC compared to other therapeutic modalities (Chen et al., 2004; Itamoto et al., 2007; Minagawa et al., 2003; Sugimachi et al., 2001; Tralhao et al., 2007; Wu et al., 2009; Zhou et al., 2010). It should be the treatment of choice in suitable patients with preserved liver function and functional status. The safety and long-term results of repeated resection has been well-established, with operative mortality rates ranging from 0% to 8.5% and the reported cumulative 5-year survival rate after a second hepatectomy was comparable to the survival after initial hepatectomy for primary HCC (Aeii et al., 1998; Farges et al., 1998; Hu et al., 1996; Itamota et al., 2000; Kakazu et al., 1993; Matsuda Y et al., 1993; Minagawa et al., 2003; Nagano et al., 2009; Nagasue et al., 1996; Poon et al., 1999; Shimada et al., 1996, 1998; Suenaga M et al., 1994; Sugimachi et al., 2001; Zhou et al., 2010).

In a recent systemic review where studies reporting in at least 10 patients are included, Zhou et al analysed 29 studies of repeat hepatectomy for recurrent HCC with a curative intent (Zhou et al., 2010). A total of 1149 patients underwent repeat hepatectomy for recurrent HCC and the rate of repeat hepatectomy ranged from 8.7% to 44%. The median or mean operating time ranged from 136 to 365 minutes and the median or mean estimated blood loss ranged from 211 to 1980 ml. Majority of patients received minor resection at the time of repeat resection. The reported ranges of the 1-, 3- and 5-year survival were 69% to 100%, 21% to 87% and 25% to 87% respectively.

These results may support the use of repeat resection for recurrent HCC. Moreover, it is noteworthy that the rate of extra-hepatic spread after hepatic resection is low. The reported incidence of extra-hepatic metastases after primary liver resection was 5% to 20% while that after second resection was almost the same (Belghiti et al., 1991; Bismuth et al., 1995; Kosuge et al., 1993; Makuuchi et al., 1998). Nevertheless, repeat resection is technically demanding and difficult due to possible adhesions between the raw liver surface and the surrounding organs, distortion and anatomical disorientation caused by the rotation of liver remnant as a result of regeneration and limited liver reserve after previous resection (Figure. 1).

So far, no consensus has been reached for the standard selection criteria for re-hepatectomy. In general, patients with good performance status and adequate liver functional reserve could be selected for re-hepatectomy if oncological clearance can be achieved (Zhou et al., 2010). The main consideration remains the probability of patients developing post-hepatectomy liver failure.

An important finding reported by the Japanese groups is that the overall survival after second hepatectomy was significantly poorer in patients who recurred within 1 year after first hepatectomy than those who recurred more than 1 year after initial operation (Minagawa et al., 2003; Nagano et al., 2009). The authors postulated that many of these cases of early recurrence might be a result of intrahepatic metastasis from primary HCC and hence, associated with a poorer outcome. As a result, Minagawa et al, after reviewed 67 patients received repeated hepatectomy for recurrent HCC, concluded that a disease-free interval of more than 1 year after primary hepatectomy, single HCC at primary resection, and negative portal vein invasion at repeated resection were favourable prognostic factors after repeated resection with excellent 3- and 5-year survival rates of 100% and 86% respectively. They, therefore, recommended these patients should be indicated for repeat resection even if they have undergone major hepatic resection as the primary hepatectomy as long as the liver function can be preserved (Minagawa et al., 2003).

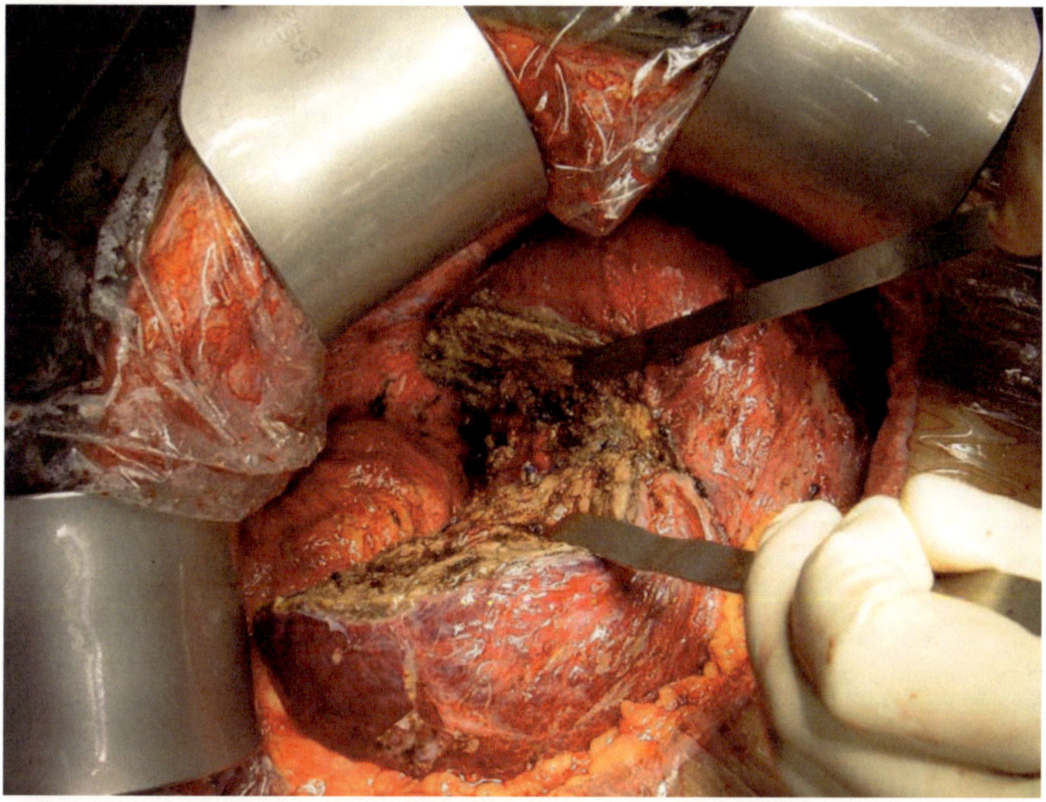

Fig. 1. Intra-operative picture of a patient who underwent right posterior sectionectomy for a recurrent HCC at segment VIII. Multiple adhesions over liver surface were also showed.

The good results from repeat hepatectomy should be interpreted with caution as patients selected for repeat hepatectomy were usually patients with better prognosis, e.g. better liver reserve and smaller tumours.

Recently, laparoscopic hepatectomy is well accepted as a safe and feasible treatment for primary HCC in selected patients with similar result to the open approach (Lee et al., 2007; Vignano et al., 2009). It is recommended for peripheral lesion requiring limited hepatectomy or left lateral sectionectomy (Lee et al., 2011; Vignano et al., 2009). Feasibility of repeat laparoscopic liver resection in recurrent HCC had been reported (Belli et al., 2009; Cheung et al., 2010; Hu et al., 2011; Liang et al., 2009). However, all these reports only focused on the technical aspects and the short-term outcomes. The importance of careful patient selection should be emphasized when considering laparoscopic re-resection and it should only be done by surgeons who are highly experienced in both laparoscopic and open hepatic surgeries.

2.3 Local ablation therapies

Tumor ablation is defined as the direct application of chemical or thermal therapies to a tumor to achieve eradication or substantial tumor destruction. Although repeat hepatectomy is the most effective treatment for recurrent HCC, impaired liver function and the presence of multicentric tumours often precludes repeat hepatectomy in more than 80% of patients with recurrent HCC (Arii, et al. 1998; Kakazu et al., 1993; Lu et al., 2005; Minagawa et al., 2003; Poon et al., 1999; Shimada et al., 1996; Suenaga et al., 1993). Local ablative therapies have been increasingly used to treat recurrent HCC. They are particularly suitable for treatment of recurrent HCC as recurrence can usually be detected at an early stage on the surveillance imaging after hepatectomy while the nodules are still small.

Radiofrequency ablation (RFA), microwave coagulation therapy (MCT) and percutaneous ethanol injection (PEI) are the three most commonly used local ablative treatment modalities for treatment of small primary HCC. Reports on the use of PEI in treating HCC recurrence are scarce. Both RFA and MCT can be applied percutaneously, laparoscopically, or at open surgery. From the experience in treating primary HCC, RFA and MCT are able to destroy bigger tumor up to 6cm or 7cm in diameter and require fewer treatment sessions than PEI and are therefore gaining attention as a valuable treatment options for ablating recurrent HCC (Goldberg & Gazelle, 2001; Ikeda et al., 2001; Livraghi et al., 1999; Lu et al., 2001; Seki et al., 1999). Currently, most of the currently available results on local ablative therapy for recurrent HCC were using RFA.

2.3.1 Radiofrequency ablation (RFA)

RFA is a thermo-ablative technique, which works by using a high-frequency alternating current applied via electrodes placed within the tissue to induce temperatures changes and generate areas of coagulative necrosis and tissue desiccation. RFA has been increasingly used to treat small primary or recurrent HCC (<5cm) in patients with poor liver reserve (Lau & Lai, 2009). High complete ablation rate (over 90%) and long-term survival comparable to those achieved by hepatectomy have been reported by cohort studies on RFA to treat recurrent HCC after partial hepatectomy. The reported 3-year survival rate averaged above 60% and the 5-year overall survival rate ranged from 18%-51.6% (Camma et al., 2005; Chen et al., 2006; Choi et al., 2007; Lu et al., 2005; Poon et al., 2002; Tateishi et al., 2005; Taura K et al., 2006; Yang et al., 2006).

Besides the good results it achieves, RFA also has a few advantages over the repeat hepatectomy. First of all, it can be used in patients with poor liver function who might not be able to tolerate a repeat hepatectomy. Being a minimally invasive technique, RFA can be applied percutaneously in suitable patients and avoid the risk associated with general anesthesia and laparotomy (Figure. 2). Furthermore, RFA can be applied repeatedly for repeated treatment of recurrence. It is particularly important since in the background of liver cirrhosis, HCC tends to recur repeatedly and repeated treatment may be necessary. Hence, treatment with minimal damage to the non-tumoral hepatic parenchyma may be more preferable.

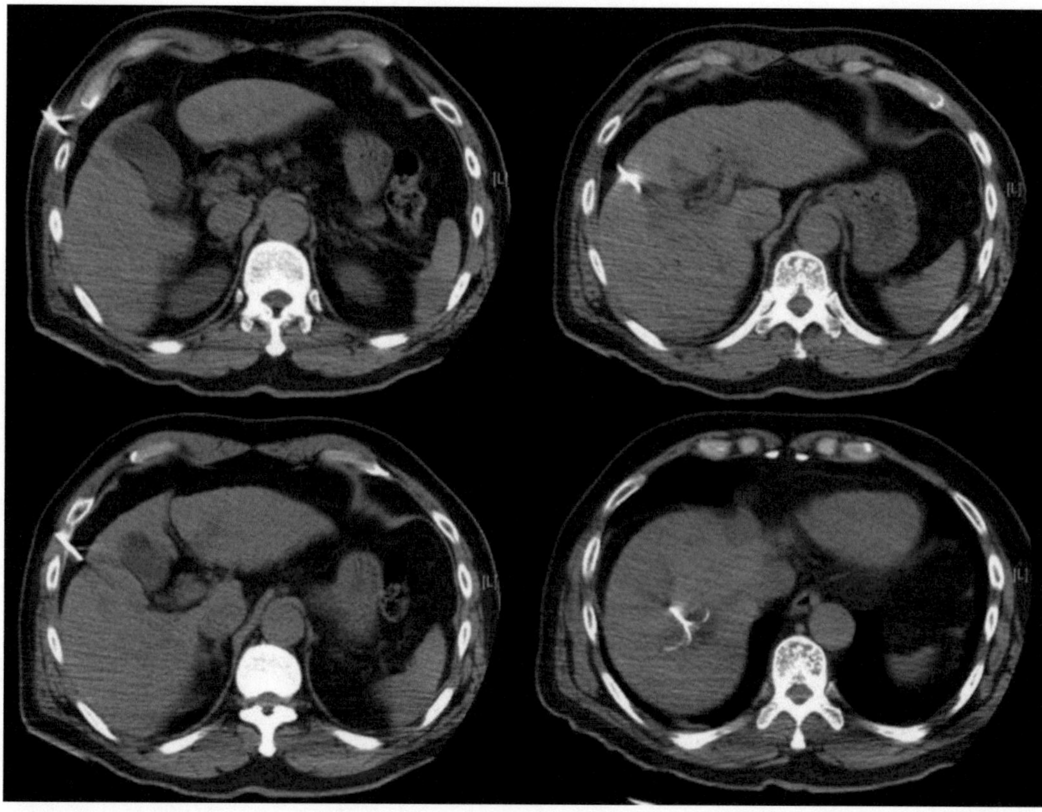

Fig. 2. CT image of a CT-guided percutaneous RFA of a segment VIII recurrent HCC which was performed under local anaesthesia.

Liang et al compared the long-term survival outcomes of percutaneous RFA and repeat partial hepatectomy for recurrent HCC (Liang et al., 2009). They found that there was no significant difference in the overall survival of patients with recurrent HCC treated by repeat hepatectomy or RFA while RFA had the advantage over hepatectomy in being less invasive and causing fewer treatment-related morbidities. The authors attempted to make the baseline demographics in two arms comparable by using the same selection criteria to identify patients received repeat hepatectomy and percutaneous RFA in order to minimize the selection bias. The criteria included fewer than three recurrent tumours with the largest one less than 5cm, no radiological evidence of venous invasion, no extrahepatic metastases, no severe liver dysfunction (Child-Pugh class C), no significant coagulopathy, and no history of encephalopathy, refractory ascites or variceal bleeding.

Of note, as in repeat hepatectomy, the benefit of RFA was more promising for patients with a longer disease-free interval from hepatectomy (Liang et al., 2009; Yang et al., 2006). Yang et al studied 41 patients with 76 recurrent HCC who received percutaneous RFA after hepatectomy. Early and late recurrences were defined as recurrence that occurred within 1 year and after 1 year respectively (Yang et al., 2006). The late-recurrence group had a significantly longer overall survival than the early-recurrence group (mean overall survival 42.9 months *versus* 16.4 months).

Needle tract dissemination is one of the major complications of great concern in percutaneous ablations. (Figure. 3) In a phase II study assessing the treatment-related complications and response rate of RFA in 32 patients by Llovet et al reported that the incidence of needle tract dissemination after radiofrequency ablation was as high as 12.5% (Llovet et al., 2001).

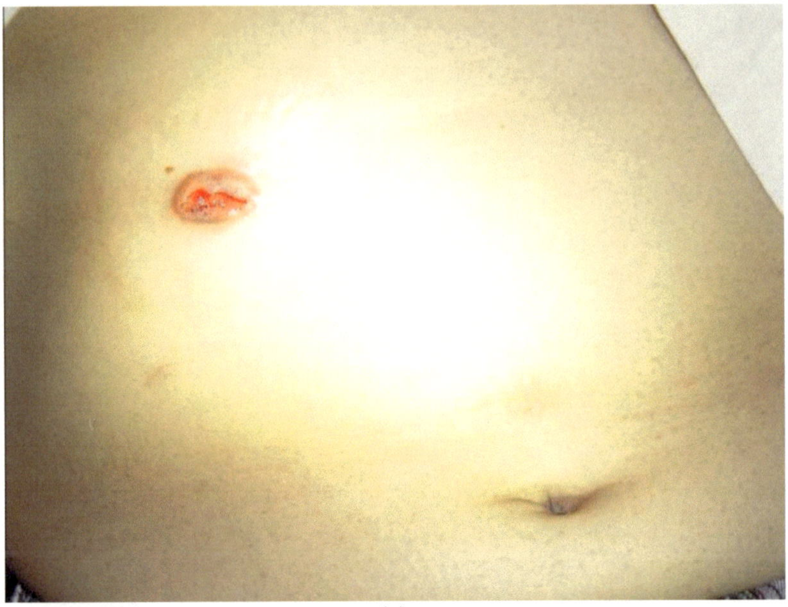

(a)

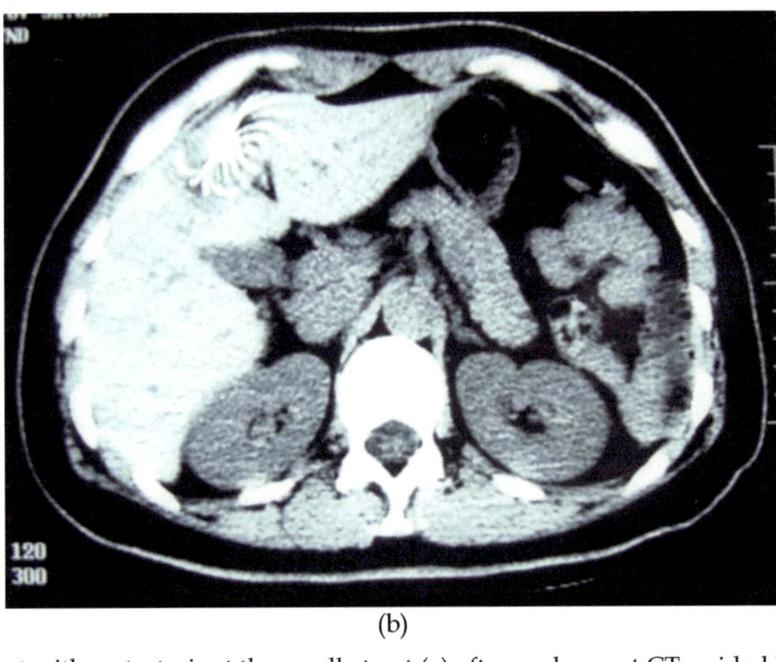

(b)

Fig. 3. Patient with metastasis at the needle tract (a) after underwent CT-guided RFA for HCC (b).

2.3.2 Microwave Coagulation Therapy (MCT)

Initially developed for intra-operative haemostasis during hepatectomy, MCT has now developed as a new ablative therapy for treatment of HCC with high ablation rate, even for tumor with wider diameters, rapid ablation time and low morbidity and mortality rates and minimal heat sink effect (Itoch et al., 2011; Lloyd et al., 2011) (Figure. 4 & 5).

MCT works by agitating water molecules in the surrounding tissue and producing friction and heat, hence inducing cellular death via coagulative necrosis (Simon et al., 2005) (Figure. 5). Although reports on the efficacy of MCT in primary HCC are numerous, results of MCT on recurrent HCC are limited. Boutros et al reported their experience with MCT in 60 patients with unresectable HCC (Boutros et al., 2010). Complete ablations were achieved in 57 of the 60 patients (95%) judged by contrast-enhanced CT carried out 1-2 weeks after procedure and 1-2 months after discharge. However, 39 of the 60 patients (65%) had recurrence and 7 (11.6%) had local recurrence resulting in a low recurrence-free survival. Among these 60 patients, 45 had recurrent HCC. The reported 1- and 3-year recurrence-free survival rates of the patients who underwent MCT for recurrent HCC were 41.6% and 8.8% respectively.

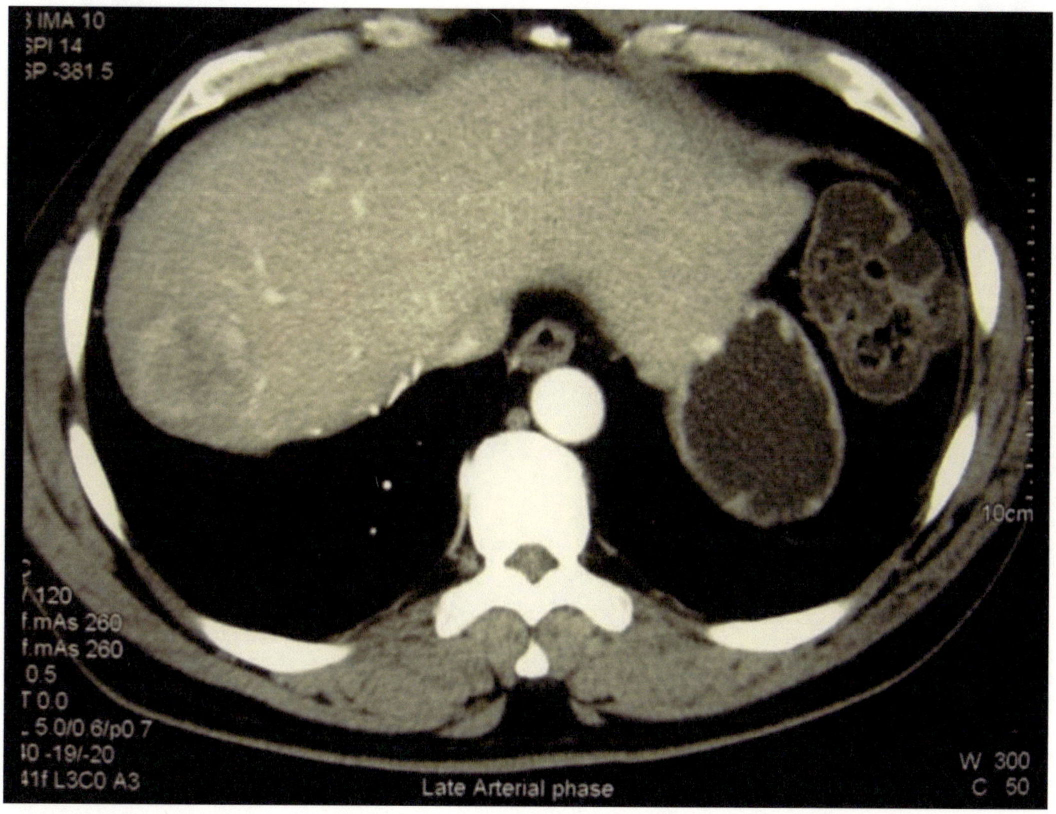

Fig. 4a. Pre-operative CT image of a recurrent HCC at segment VIII of liver.

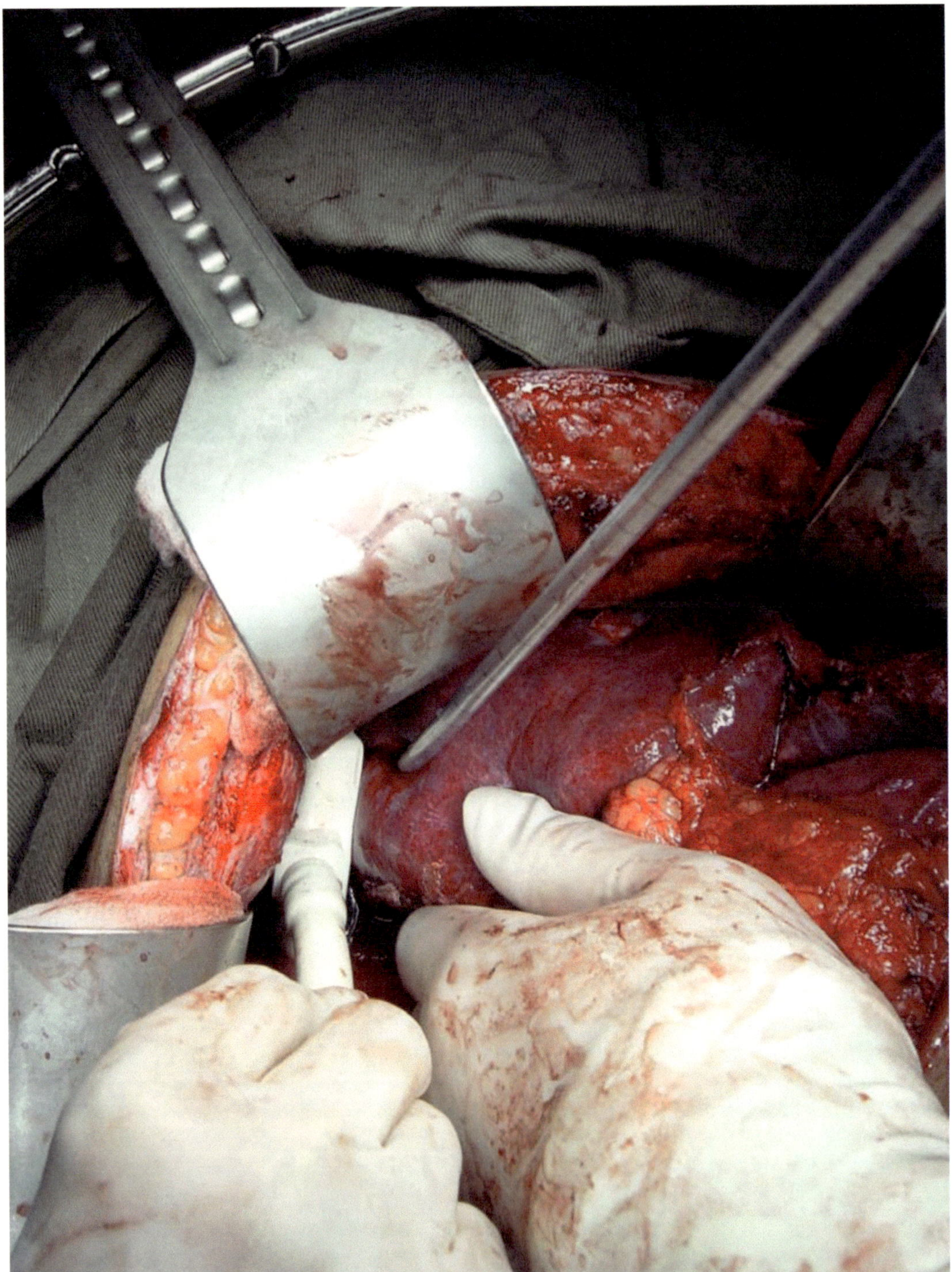

Fig. 4b. Open MCT for segment VIII recurrence guided by operative USG.

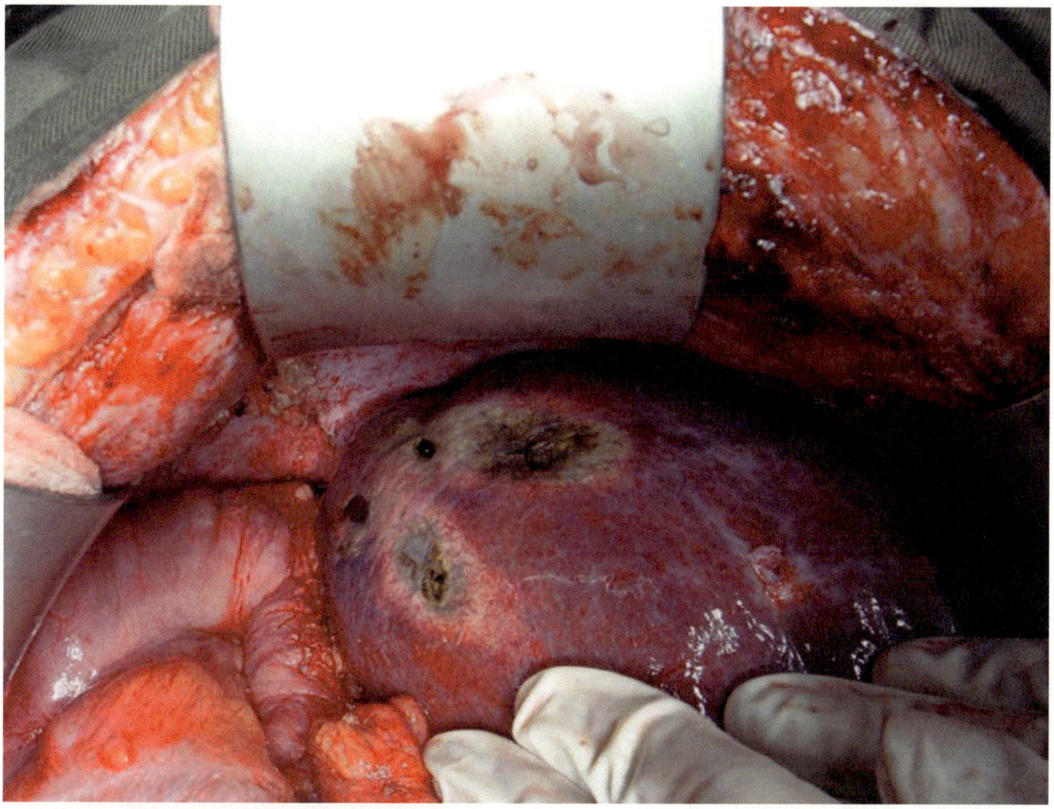

Fig. 4c. Segment VIII tumor after open MCT ablation.

Several studies compared RFA to MCT in treating hepatic tumour (Lu et al., 2005; Ogata et al., 2008; Ohmoto & Yamamoto, 2006; Shibata et al., 2002; Xu et al., 2005). Most of them failed to detect a superiority of one over another. With the currently available evidence, MCT is a safe and effective treatment for HCC. However, further prospective studies with long-term results are needed in order to confirm its role in treatment of recurrent HCC and its performance compared to RFA or liver resection.

2.4 Transarterial therapies

Hepatic flow to the hepatocellular carcinoma and liver parenchyma has a very unique pattern. Typical hepatocarcinoma nodules are highly vascularized with arterial afferents originating from the hepatic artery, whereas the hepatic parenchymal flow is largely derived from the portal vein. This forms the basis of the transarterial therapies.

2.4.1 Transarterial Chemoembolization (TACE)

Despite the results from repeat hepatic resection for intra-hepatic recurrence was well recognised, the re-resection rate is low because of the impairment of functional reserve in the liver remnant and multiplicity of nodules (Eguchi et al., 2006; Kanematsu et al., 1984; Poon et al., 2002). Local ablation should be best performed in patients with recurrences featuring three or fewer small nodules (Shimada et al., 2007). In contrast, transarterial chemoembolization (TACE) can be applied in any type of HCC, irrespective of tumor size, location, or number of lesions provided that patients have reasonable liver function. In addition, the benefit of TACE on survival in patients with unresectable HCC had already been demonstrated (Llovet & Bruix, 2003; Shim et al., 2009). Therefore, TACE is widely applicable and practical in patients with intra-hepatic HCC recurrence (Choi et al., 2009; Eguchi et al., 2008; Shim et al., 2010).

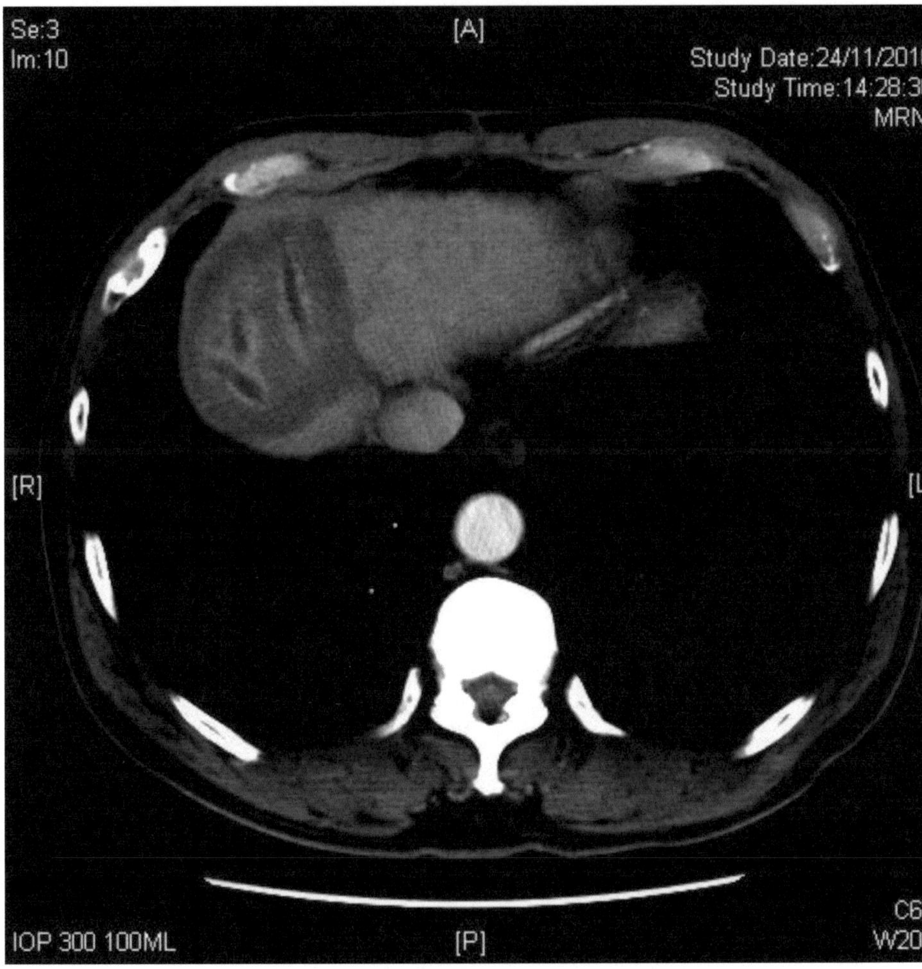

Fig. 5. CT image of a patient with a 5cm segment VIII recurrent HCC at 6 months after microwave ablation. Three passes were performed for a bigger ablative zone and the needle tracts were showed on the follow up scan.

TACE is the intra-arterial administration of chemotherapy combined with arterial embolization and is commonly used as an alternate treatment for recurrent HCC (Figure. 6). There is no standardized protocol in the optimal time interval between treatments and also the choice, dosage, concentration, rate of injection of the chemotherapeutic and the embolizing agents.

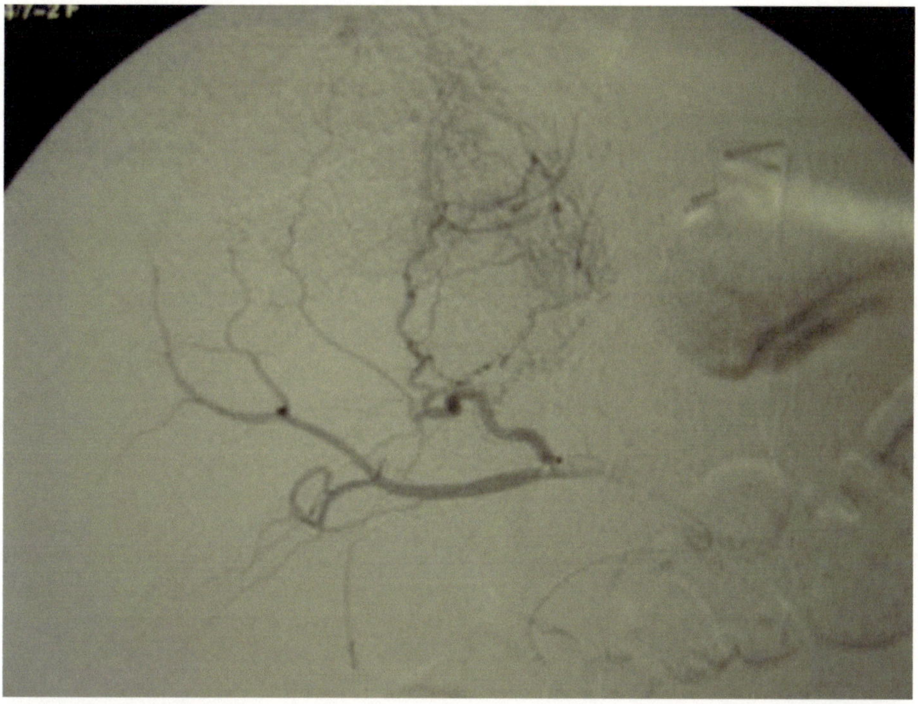

Fig. 6a. Hepatic angiogram showing a hypervascular tumor supplied by left hepatic artery.

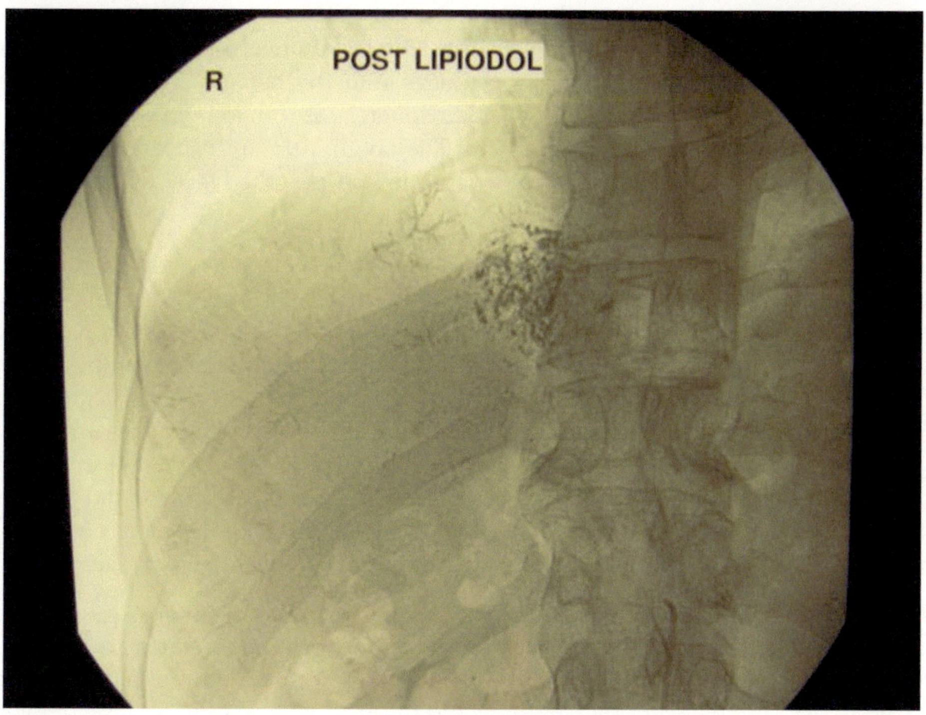

Fig. 6b. The tumor was stained by lipiodol after TACE.

Shim et al analysed data from 199 consecutive HCC patients who underwent curative liver resection and later received repeat TACE for intra-hepatic HCC recurrence. They found that complete tumor necrosis after repeated TACE offered favorable long-term survival outcomes to HCC-recurrent patients, with a median survival time after first TACE of 48.9 months. Despite this, unlike repeat hepatectomy and RFA, TACE cannot be regarded as a curative treatment for recurrent HCC yet.

Although it is not a surgical procedure, the problems of decreased liver reserves and anatomic changes due to previous operation still exist. Moreover, neovascularisation or collaterals that feed the recurrent tumour, damage to the non-tumorous liver tissue, and accumulation of drug toxicity from repeated TACE sessions are the main concern for the use of TACE. Post-embolization syndrome, which is a combination of fever, abdominal pain, nausea and vomiting, elevated liver enzymes and white cell counts for a few hours to a few days, is the most common complication of TACE. Although this syndrome is experienced after 80-90% of TACE procedures, it is mostly self-limited and the treatment is mainly symptomatic. Occasionally, more severe complications like acute cholecystitis, biliary tract necrosis, pancreatitis, gastric erosion or even ulcers can occur as a result of inadvertent injection of the chemotherapeutic and embolizing agents into these organs. Liver failure can develop after TACE and may result in mortality after TACE especially in patients with borderline liver function before treatment. Therefore, patients with portal vein thrombosis or poor liver function are contraindication to TACE.

2.4.2 Selective Internal Radiation Treatment (SIRT)

Selective internal radiation treatment (SIRT) is the delivery of radiation treatment via intrahepatic arterial administration of yttrium 90 (Y-90) microspheres. This technique involved the administration of Y-90 microspheres into the hepatic arterial via the trans-femoral route. The administered Y-90 microspheres are then entrapped within the microvasculature and release irradiation. The high tumor concentration of Y-90 microspheres results in an effective tumoricidal radiation-absorbed level while the radiation injury to the normal liver parenchyma is limited.

Its role as a safe and effective therapeutic option for patients with unresectable hepatocellular carcinoma is increasingly recognized. Recently, Lau et al (Lau et al, 2011) reviewed the role of SIRT with Y-90 microspheres for hepatocellular carcinoma, including recurrent unresectable HCC. SIRT is a recommended option of palliative therapy for large or multifocal HCC without major portal vein invasion or extrahepatic spread. It can be used as a bridging therapy before liver transplantation or as a tumor downstaging treatment, or as a curative treatment for patients who are not fit for surgery. However, the evidence was limited to cohort studies and comparative studies with historical control and was mainly targeted on primary HCC. Future research may yield more information on its role on recurrent HCC and the efficacy when compared to chemoembolization or target therapy.

In contrary to chemoembolization, optimal perfusion is required to enhance the free radical-dependent cell death in SIRT. In order to minimize the treatment-related toxicity, hepatic scintigraphy with technetium Tc 99m (^{99m}Tc) macro-aggregate albumin (MAA) should be performed to determine the arterial anatomy and to calculate the shunt fraction delivered to the lungs before subjecting the patient to SIRT. Pulmonary shunt fraction greater than 15%

on ^{99m}Tc-MAA scan predisposes to radiation pneumonitis and is therefore a contraindication for SIRT. In addition to radiation pneumonitis, other serious complication associated with SIRT include gastric or duodenal ulcers or perforation as a result of reflux of Y-90 microspheres into the gastrointestinal vascular bed and radiation hepatitis resulting from a radiation dose higher than the tolerable level. Nevertheless, most patients only reported mild symptoms like abdominal pain, lethargy or nausea, which may require symptomatic treatment. (Rossi et al, 2010) In most cases, it is a well-tolerated minimally invasive therapy.

3. Extrahepatic recurrence

Extra-hepatic recurrence or extra-hepatic metastasis occurs as a result of tumor extension from the liver or direct spreading to adjacent structures such as the diaphragm, the bowel and the adrenal gland; haematogenous spread via the systemic circulation to the lung; lymphatic spread from the liver to the portal and abdominal lymph nodes; or peritoneal dissemination from tumor rupture. Lung and abdominal lymph nodes are the commonest sites of metastasis, followed by musculoskeletal system, adrenal gland and peritoneum (Katyal et al., 2000; Yang et al., 2007).

There were very few studies addressing the aggressive management of extra-hepatic recurrence after liver resection. This is probably related to the extremely poor prognosis in these patients before the introduction of sorafenib.

3.1 Systemic treatment

In general, extra-hepatic metastasis is regarded as an advanced systemic disease and therefore, only systemic chemotherapy or supportive treatment will be offered only. Unfortunately, the response rate of HCC to systemic chemotherapy such as adriamycin is very low and the results were mostly disappointing (Simonetti et al., 1997).

With better understanding of the mechanism of hepatocarcinogenesis, effective molecularly targeted agents, such as sorafenib, have been emerged and improved survival benefits have been demonstrated in large, placebo-controlled phase III trials in Europe and Asia for patients with advanced HCC (Cheng et al., 2009; Llovet et al., 2008). While some may criticize that the benefit gained from sorafenib over placebo in patients with extra-hepatic metastasis from HCC was marginal only, the extra months gain may well be extremely valuable to patients.

3.2 Surgical resection

Recently, the role of resection of extra-hepatic metastasis from hepatocellular carcinoma has been reviewed (Chua & Morris, 2011). From the results reported in the literatures, prolonged survival after surgical resection may be achieved in selected patients with solitary extra-hepatic recurrence at the sites of the abdominal lymph node, adrenal gland, lung, and peritoneum. Surgical resection might be an effective option in patients with one or two isolated extrahepatic metastases if the patient has otherwise good performance status, good hepatic functional reserve, and well-controlled intrahepatic HCC recurrence. However, it might just reflect a group of patients with a more favourable natural course of disease (Chan et al., 2009; Lam et al., 1998; Nakayama et al., 1999; Sakamoto et al., 1999).

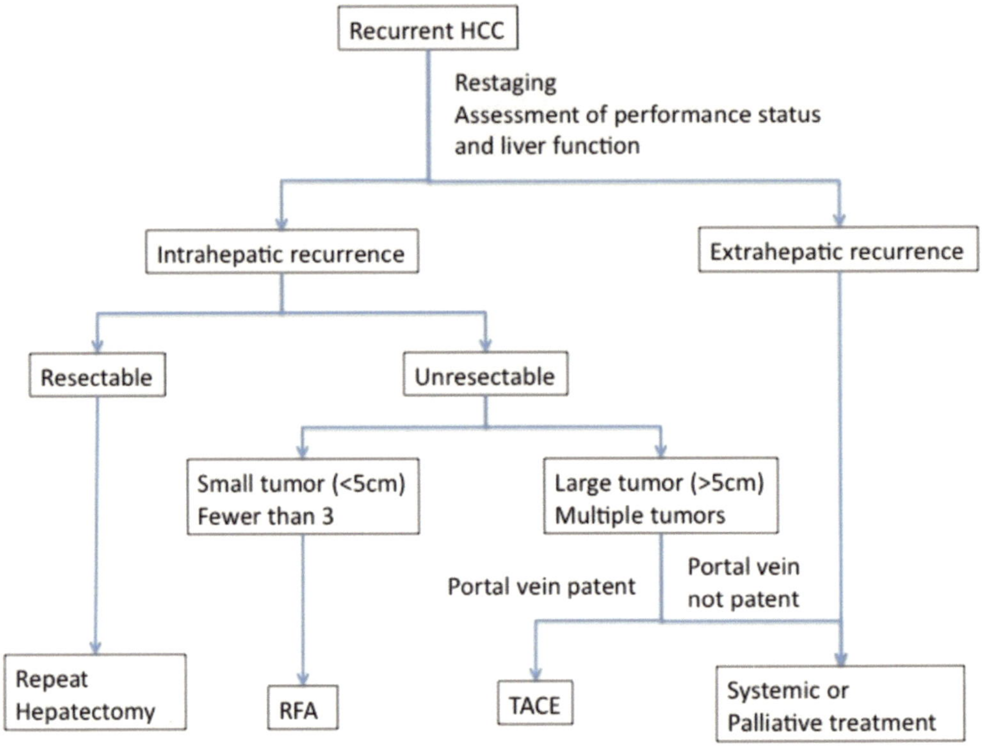

Fig. 7. Algorithm protocol for treatment of recurrent HCC

4. Prevention

Unfortunately, there is still no universally accepted form of adjuvant therapy for preventing recurrence after hepatic resection (Lau et al., 2009). Adjuvant regional therapy and anti-viral therapy are the two main directions that researches on this field are working on.

4.1 Role of adjuvant regional therapy

The preventive effect of TACE on recurrence after operation had been studied by prospective (Peng et al., 2009; Zhong et al., 2009) and retrospective series (Ren et al., 2004; Xi et al., 2007) mostly in eastern centers. The survival benefit of adjuvant TACE after hepatic resection was demonstrated in patients with high risk factors for recurrence while the effect in low risk for recurrence remains questionable. However, the quoted high risk factors for recurrence varied between studies, namely large tumor, multiple nodules, vascular invasion and presence of portal vein tumor thrombus. With the currently available evidence, the adjuvant regional chemotherapy with or without embolization or combination of systemic chemotherapy does not provide any additional benefit (Chan et al., 2000; Lau et al., 2009; Schwartz et al., 2002). Adjuvant transarterial treatments with ^{131}I-lipiodol and adjuvant immunotherapy with interferon had demonstrated early promising results, which may have a role in preventing early intra-hepatic recurrence (Boucher et al., 2003; Ikeda et al., 2000;

Kudo et al., 2002; Lau et al., 2008; Partensky et al., 2000; Sun et al., 2006; Takjayama et al., 2000). However, its role remains to be confirmed by further studies.

4.2 Antiviral therapy

In Asia, chronic hepatitis B virus (HBV) infection is the major cause of HCC. The risk for HCC development is closely associated with hepatitis B e antigen (HBeAg) status and the serum HBV-DNA level. Recent studies showed that tumour recurrence after curative treatment of HCC was increased with the level of HBV-DNA and alanine aminotransferase (ALT) (Cheung et al., 2008; Huang et al., 2008). This implies that HBV viral replication may play a role in HCC development and tumour recurrence. Scattered results from perspective and retrospective studies have shown that continuous treatment with nucleotide analogue in patients with chronic hepatitis B or cirrhosis could reduce the risk of HCC development (Liaw et al., 2004; Matsumoto et al., 2005). Wong et al reviewed the results of nine cohort studies including more than 500 patients in a recent meta-analysis concluded that anti-viral therapy could significantly reduce the risk of HCC recurrence after curative treatment of HBV-related HCC (Wong et al., 2011). Furthermore, anti-viral therapy might also allow salvage therapy in case of HCC recurrence by better-preserved liver function as supported by the result of two other studies (Kuzuya et al., 2007; Piao et al., 2005). Hence, anti-viral therapy with nucleotide analogues should be considered after curative treatment of HBV-related HCC for the potential benefit in tumor recurrence and overall survival.

5. Conclusion

The principles of therapy for recurrent HCC should be, in fact, the same as those for primary HCC. Patients should have proper pre-operative assessment for their general functional status and evaluation of the functional liver reserve. Active hepatitis seems to be an important factor for patients considered for repeated liver resection, and therefore viral status, viral activity and finally liver function have to be evaluated thoroughly before resection. Depending on the local availability of various imaging modality, detail workup for restaging the disease and to rule out extra-hepatic metastasis is an important part in the decision of the best treatment for patient with recurrent HCC. Re-hepatectomy should be the treatment of choice if the tumour is resectable in terms of patient's performance status, tumour staging and functional reserve of the liver remnant. For patients with small recurrence and borderline liver functional, local ablation therapy is a safe and effective treatment option. In case of multiple intra-hepatic recurrences, TACE can be considered in patients with good liver function as long as the portal veins remain patent.

6. References

Arii, S.; Monden, K.; Niwano, M.; Furutani, M.; Mori, A.; Mizumoto, M. & Imamura, M. (1998). Results of surgical treatment for recurrent hepatocellular carcinoma: comparison of outcome among patients with multicentric carcinogenesis, intrahepatic metastasis, and extrahepatic recurrence. *Journal of Hepato-biliary-pancreatic Surgery*, Vol.5, No.1, (1998), pp. 86–92, ISSN 0944-1166

Belghiti, J.; Panis, Y.; Farges, O.; Benhamou, JP. & Fekete, F. (1991). Intrahepatic recurrence after resection of hepatocellular carcinoma complicating cirrhosis. *Annals of Surgery,* Vol.214, No.2, (August 1998), pp. 114–117, ISSN 0003-4932

Belli, G.; Cioffi, L.; Fantini, C.; D'Agostino, A.; Russo, G.; Limongelli, P. & Belli, A. (2009). Laparoscopic redo surgery for recurrent hepatocellular carcinoma in cirrhotic patients: feasibility, safety, and results. *Surgical Endoscopy,* Vol.23, No.8, (August 2009), pp. 1807–1811, ISSN 0930-2794

Bismuth, H.; Chiche, L. & Castaing, D. (1995). Surgical treatment of hepatocellular carcinomas in non-cirrhotic liver: experience with 68 liver resections. *World Journal of Surgery,* Vol.19, No.1, (January-February 1995), pp. 35–41, ISSN 0364-2313

Boucher, E.; Corbinais, S.; Rolland,Y.; Bourguet, P.; Guyader, D.; Boudjema, K.; Meunier, B. & Raoul, JL. (2003). Adjuvant intra-arterial injection of iodine-131-labeled lipiodol after resection of hepatocellular carcinoma. *Hepatology,* Vol.38, No.5, (November 2003), pp. 1237-1241, ISSN 1457-8862

Boutros, C.; Somasundar, P.; Garrean, S.; Saied, A. & Espat, NJ. (2010). Microwave coagulation therapy for hepatic tumors: review of the literature and critical analysis. *Surgical Oncology,* Vol.19, No.1, (March 2010), pp: 22-32, ISSN 0960-7404

Camma, C.; Marco, VD.; Orlando, A.; Sandonato, L.; Casaril, A.; Parisi, P.; Alizzi, S.; Sciarrino, E.; Virdone, R.; Pardo, S.; Di Bona, D.; Licata, A.; Latteri, F.; Cabibbo, G.; Montalto, G.; Latteri, MA.; Nicoli, N. & Craxì, A. (2005). Treatment of hepatocellular carcinoma in compensated cirrhosis with radiofrequency thermal ablation (RFTA): a prospective study. *Journal of Hepatology,* Vol.42, No.4, (April 2005), pp: 535–540, ISSN 0168-8278

Chan, KM.; Yu, MC.; Wu, TJ.; Lee, CF.; Chen, TC.; Lee, WC. & Chen, MF. (2009). Efficacy of surgical resection in management of isolated extrahepatic metastases of hepatocellular carcinoma. *World Journal of Gastroenterology,* Vol.15, No.43, (November 2009), pp: 5481-5488, ISSN 1007-9327

Chen, MS.; Li, JQ.; Zheng, Y.; Cuo, RP.; Liang, HH.; Zhang, YQ.; Lin, XJ. & Lau, WY. (2006). A prospective randomized trial comparing percutaneous local ablative therapy and partial hepatectomy for small hepatocellular carcinoma. *Annals of Surgery,* Vol.243, No.3, (March 2006), pp: 321–328, ISSN 0003-4932

Chen, WT.; Chau, GY.; Lui, WY.; Tsay, SH.; King, KL.; Loong, CC. & Wu, CW. (2004). Recurrent hepatocellular carcinoma after hepatic resection: prognostic factors and long-term outcome. *European Journal of Surgical Oncology,* Vol.30, No.4, (May 2004), pp: 414–420, ISSN 0748-7983

Cheng, AL.; Kang, YK.; Chen, Z.; Tsao, CJ.; Qin, S.; Kim, JS.; Luo, R.; Feng, J.; Ye, S.; Yang, TS.; Xu, J.; Sun, Y.; Liang, H.; Liu, J.; Wang, J.; Tak, WY.; Pan, H.; Burock, K.; Zou, J.; Voliotis, D. & Guan, Z. (2008). Efficacy and safety of sorafenib in patients in the Asia-Pacific region with advanced hepatocellular carcinoma: a phase III randomised, double-blind, placebo-controlled trial. *Lancet Oncology,* Vol.10, No.1, (January 2008), pp: 25-34, ISSN 1470-2045

Cheung, TT.; Ng, KK.; Poon, RT.; Chan, SC.; Lo, CM. & Fan, ST. (2010). A case of laparoscopic hepatectomy for recurrent hepatocellular carcinoma. *World Journal of Gastroenterology,* Vol.16, No.4, (January 2010), pp: 526–530, ISSN 1007-9327

Cheung, YS.; Chan, HL.; Wong, J.; Lee, KF.; Poon, TC.; Wong, N. & Lai, PB. (2008). Elevated perioperative transaminase level predicts intrahepatic recurrence in hepatitis B-related hepatocellular carcinoma after curative hepatectomy. *Asian Journal of Surgery*, Vol.31, No.2, (April 2008), pp: 41–49, ISSN 1015-9584

Choi, D.; Lim, HK.; Rhim, H.; Kim, YS.; Yoo, BC.; Pail, SW.; Joh, JW. & Park, CK. (2007). Percutaneous radiofrequency ablation for recurrent hepatocellular carcinoma after hepatectomy: long-term results and prognostic factors. *Annals of Surgical Oncology*, Vol.14, No.8, (August 2007), pp: 2319-2329, ISSN 1068-9265

Choi, JW.; Park, JY.; Ahn, SH.; Yoon, KT.; Ko, HK.; Lee, do Y.; Lee, JT.; Kim, KS.; Choi, JS.; Han, KH.; Chon, CY. & Kim, do Y. (2009). Efficacy and safety of transarterial chemoembolization in recurrent hepatocellular carcinoma after curative surgical resection. *American Journal of Clinical Oncology*, Vol.32, No.6, (December 2009), pp: 564-569, ISSN 0277-3732

Chong, CC.; Lee, KF.; Ip, PC.; Wong, JS.; Cheung, SY.; Wong, J.; Ho, SC. & Lai, PB. (2011). Pre-operative predictors of post-hepatectomy recurrence of hepatocellular carcinoma: Can we predict earlier?, *The Surgeon (2011)*, doi:10.1016/j.surge.2011.07.004. In press.

Chua, TC. & Morris, DL. (2011). Exploring the role of resection of extrahepatic metastases from hepatocellular carcinoma. *Surgical Oncology*, (Mar 2011), ISSN 0960-7404. [Epub ahead of print]

Eguchi, S.; Ijtsma, AJ.; Slooff, MJ.; Porte, RJ.; de Jong, KP.; Peeters, PM.; Gouw, AS. & Kanematsu, T. (2006). Outcome and pattern of recurrence after curative resection for hepatocellular carcinoma in patients with a normal liver compared to patients with a diseased liver. *Hepatogastroenterology*, Vol.53, No.70, (July-August 2006), pp: 592–596, ISSN 0172-6390

Eguchi, S.; Matsumoto, S.; Hamasaki, K.; Takatsuki, M.; Hidaka, M.; Tajima, Y.; Sakamoto, I. & Kanematsu, T. (2008). Re-evaluation of lipiodolized transarterial chemoembolization therapy for intrahepatic recurrence of hepatocellular carcinoma after curative liver resection. *Journal of Hepato-biliary-pancreatic Surgery*, Vol.15, No.6, (November 2008), pp: 627-633, ISSN 0944-1166

Ercolani, G.; Grazi, GL.; Ravaioli, M.; Del Gaudio, M.; Gardini, A.; Cescon, M.; Varotti, G.; Cetta, F. & Cavallari, A. (2003). Liver resection for hepatocellular carcinoma on cirrhosis: univariate and multivariate analysis of risk factors for intrahepatic recurrence. *Annals of Surgery*, Vol.237, No.4, (April 2003), pp: 536-543, ISSN 0003-4932

Farges, O.; Regimbeau, JM. & Belghiti, J. (1998). Aggressive management of recurrence following surgical resection of hepatocellular carcinoma. *Hepatogastroenterology*, Vol.45, No.3, (August 1998), pp: 1275–1280, ISSN 0172-6390

Globocan 2008, Cancer Incidence and Mortality Worldwide in 2008, In: *World Health Organisation*, 1st August 2011, Available from: < http://globocan.iarc.fr/ >

Goldberg, SN. & Gazelle, GS. (2001). Radiofrequency tissue ablation: physical principles and techniques for increasing coagulation necrosis. *Hepatogastroenterology*, Vol.48, No.38, (March-April 2001), pp: 359–367, ISSN 0172-6390

Hu, M.; Zhao, G.; Xu, D. & Liu, R. (2011). Laparoscopic repeat resection of recurrent hepatocellular carcinoma. *World Journal of Surgery*, Vol.35, No.3, (March 2011), pp: 648-655, ISSN 0364-2313

Hu, RH.; Lee, PH.; Yu, SC.; Dai, HC.; Sheu, JC.; Lai, MY. & Chen, DS. (1996). Surgical resection for recurrent hepatocellular carcinoma: prognosis and analysis of risk factors. *Surgery*, Vol.120, No.1, (July 1996), pp: 23–29, ISSN 0039-6060

Huang, Y.; Wang, Z.; An, S.; Zhou, Y.; Chan, HL. & Hou, J. (2008). Role of hepatitis B virus genotypes and quantitative HBV DNA in metastasis and recurrence of hepatocellular carcinoma. *Journal of Medical Virology*, Vol.80, No.4, (April 2008), pp: 591–597, ISSN 0146-6615

Ikeda K, Arase Y, Saitoh S, Kobayashi M, Suzuki Y, Suzuki F, Tsubota A, Chayama K, Murashima N & Kumada H. (2000). Interferon beta prevents recurrence of hepatocellular carcinoma after complete resection or ablation of the primary tumor-A prospective randomized study of hepatitis C virus-related liver cancer. *Hepatology*, Vol.32, No.2, (August 2000), pp: 228-232, ISSN 0270-9139

Ikeda, M.; Okada, S.; Ueno, H.; Okusaka, T. & Kuriyama, H. (2001). Radiofrequency ablation and percutaneous ethanol injection in patients with small hepatocellular carcinoma: a comparative study. *Japanese Journal of Clinical Oncology*, Vol.31, No.7, (July 2001), pp: 322-326, ISSN 0368-2811

Itamoto, T.; Nakahara, H.; Amano, H.; Kohashi, T.; Ohdan, H.; Tashiro, H. & Ashara, T. (2007). Repeat hepatectomy for recurrent hepatocellular carcinoma. *Surgery*, Vol.141, No.5, (May 2007), pp: 589–597, ISSN 0039-6060

Itoh, S.; Ikeda, Y.; Kawanaka, H.; Okuyama, T.; Kawasaki, K.; Eguchi, D.; Korenaga, D. & Takenaka, K. (2011). Efficacy of Surgical Microwave Therapy in Patients with Unresectable Hepatocellular Carcinoma. *Annals of Surgical Oncology*, (June 2011), ISSN 1068-9265, [Epub ahead of print]

Jwo, SC.; Chiu, JH.; Chau, GY.; Loong, CC. & Lui, WY. (1992). Risk factors linked to tumor recurrence of human hepatocellular carcinoma after hepatic resection. *Hepatology*, Vol.16, No.6, (December 1992), pp: 1367–1371, ISSN 0270-9139

Kakazu, T.; Makuuchi, M.; Kawasaki, S.; Miyagawa, S.; Hashikura, Y.; Kosuge, T.; Takayama, T. & Yamamoto, J. (1993). Repeat hepatic resection for recurrent hepatocellular carcinoma. *Hepatogastroenterology*, Vol.40, No.4, (August 1993), pp: 337–341, ISSN 0172-6390

Kanematsu, T.; Takenaka, K.; Matsumata, T.; Furtuta, T.; Sugimachi, K. & Inokuchi, K. (1984). Limited hepatic resection effective for selected cirrhotic patients with primary liver cancer. *Annals of Surgery*, Vol.199, No.1, (January 1984), pp: 51–56, ISSN 0003-4932

Katyal, S.; Oliver, III JH.; Peterson, MS.; Carr, BS. & Baron, RL. (2000). Extrahepatic Metastases of Hepatocellular Carcinoma. *Radiology*, Vol.216, No.3, (September 2000), pp: 698-703, ISSN 0033-8419

Kosuge, T.; Makuuchi, M.; Takayama, T.; Yamamoto, J.; Shimada, K. & Yamasaki, S. (1993). Long-term results after resection of hepatocellular carcinoma: experience of 480 cases. *Hepatogastroenterology*. Vol.40, No.4, (August 1993), pp: 328–332, ISSN 0172-6390

Kubo, S.; Nishiguchi, S.; Hirohashi, K.; Tanaka, H.; Shuto, T. & Kinoshita, H. (2002). Randomized clinical trial of long-term outcome after resection of hepatitis C virus-related hepatocellular carcinoma by postoperative interferon therapy. *British Journal of Surgery*, Vol.89, No.4, (April 2002), pp: 418-422, ISSN 0007-1323

Kuzuya, T.; Katano, Y.; Kumada, T.; Toyoda, H.; Nakano, I.; Hirooka, Y.; Itoh, A.; Ishigami, M.; Hayashi, K.; Honda, T. & Goto, H. (2007). Efficacy of antiviral therapy with lamivudine after initial treatment for hepatitis B virus-related hepatocellular carcinoma. *Journal of Gastroenterology and Hepatology*, Vol.22, No.11, (Novvember 2007), pp: 1929– 1935, ISSN 0815-9319

Lam, CM.; Lo, CM.; Yuen, WK.; Liu, CL. & Fan, ST. (1998). Prolonged survival in selected patients following surgical resection for pulmonary metastasis from hepatocellular carcinoma. *British Journal of Surgery*, Vol.85, No.9, (September 1998), pp: 1198-200, ISSN 0007-1323

Lau, WY.; Lai, EC.; Leung, TW. & Yu, SC. (2008). Adjuvant intra-arterial iodine-131-labeled lipiodol for resectable hepatocellular carcinoma: a prospective randomized trial-update on 5-year and 10-year survival. *Annals of Surgery*, Vol.247, No.1, (January 2008), pp: 43-48, ISSN 0003-4932

Lau, WY. & Lai, EC. (2009). The current role of radiofrequency ablation in the management of hepatocellular carcinoma: a systematic review. *Annals of Surgery*, Vol.249, No.1, (January 2009), pp: 20-25, ISSN 0003-4932

Lau, WY.; Lai, EC. & Lau, SH. (2009). The current role of neoadjuvant/adjuvant/chemoprevention therapy in partial hepatectomy for hepatocellular carcinoma: a systemic review. *Hepatobiliary and Pancreatic Disease International*, Vol.8, No.2, (April 2009), pp: 124-133, ISSN 1499-3872

Lau, WY.; Lai, EC.; Leung TW. (2011) Current role of selective internal irradiation with yttrium-90 microspheres in the management of hepatocellular carcinoma: a systematic review. *International Journal of Radiation Oncology, Biology, Physics*, Vol.81, No. 2, (Oct 2011), pp: 460-467, ISSN 0360-3016

Lee, KF.; Cheung, YS.; Chong, CN.; Tsang, YY.; Ng, WW.; Ling, E.; Wong, J. & Lai, PB. (2007). Laparoscopic versus open hepatectomy for liver tumours: a case control study. *Hong Kong Medical Journal*, Vol.13, No.6, (December 2007), pp: 442–448, ISSN 1024-2708

Lee, KF.; Chong, CN.; Wong, J.; Cheung, YS.; Wong, J.; Lai, P. (2011). Long-Term Results of Laparoscopic Hepatectomy Versus Open Hepatectomy for Hepatocellular Carcinoma: A Case-Matched Analysis. *World Journal of Surgery*, (August 2011), ISSN 0361-2313, [Epub ahead of print]

Liang, X.; Cai, XJ.; Yu, H.; Wang, YF. & Laing, YL. (2009). Second laparoscopic resection for recurrent hepatocellular carcinoma after initial laparoscopic hepatectomy: case report. *Chinese Medical Journal*, Vol.122, No.11, (June 2009), pp: 1359–1360, ISSN 0366-6999

Livraghi, T.; Goldberg, SN.; Lazzaroni, S.; Meloni, F.; Solbiati, L. & Gazelle, GS. (1999). Small hepatocellular carcinoma: treatment with radio-frequency ablation versus ethanol injection. *Radiology*, Vol.210, No.3, (March 1999), pp: 655–661, ISSN 0033-8419

Llovet, JM. & Bruix, J. (2003). Systematic review of randomized trials for unresectable hepatocellular carcinoma: Chemoembolization improves survival. *Hepatology*, Vol.37, No.2, (Febuary 2003), pp: 429–442, ISSN 0815-9319

Llovet, JM.; Ricci, S.; Mazzaferro, V.; Hilgard, P.; Gane, E.; Blanc, JF.; de Oliveira, AC.; Santoro, A.; Raoul, JL.; Forner, A.; Schwartz, M.; Porta, C.; Zeuzem, S.; Bolondi, L.; Greten, TF.; Galle, PR.; Seitz, JF.; Borbath, I.; Häussinger, D.; Giannaris, T.; Shan, M.; Moscovici, M.; Voliotis, D. & Bruix, J. (2008). Sorafenib in advanced

Hepatocellular Carcinoma. The *New England Journal of Medicine*, Vol.359, No.4, (July 2008), pp: 378-390, ISSN 0028-4793

Llovet, JM.; Vilana, R.; Brú, C.; Bianchi, L.; Salmeron, JM.; Boix, L.; Ganau, S.; Sala, M.; Pagès, M.; Ayuso, C.; Solé, M.; Rodés, J. & Bruix, J. (2001). Increased risk of tumor seeding after percutaneous radiofrequency ablation for single hepatocellular carcinoma. *Hepatology*, Vol.33, No.3, (May 2001), pp: 1124–1129, ISSN 0815-9319

Lu, MD.; Chen, JW.; Xie, XY.; Liu, L.; Huang, XQ.; Liang, LJ. & Huang, JF. (2001). Hepatocellular carcinoma: US-guided percutaneous microwave coagulation therapy. *Radiology*, Vol.221, No.1, (October 2001), pp: 167- 172, ISSN 0033-8419

Lu, MD.; Xu, HX.; Xie, XY.; Yin, XY.; Chen, JW.; Kuang, M.; Xu, ZF.; Liu, GJ. & Zheng, YL. (2005). Percutaneous microwave and radiofrequency ablation for hepatocellular carcinoma: a retrospective comparative study. *Journal of Gastroenterology*, Vol.40, No.11, (November 2005), pp: 1054-1060, ISSN 0944-1174

Lu, MD.; Yin, XY.; Xie, XY.; Xu, HX.; Xu, ZF.; Liu, GJ.; Kuang, M. & Zheng, YL. (2005). Percutaneous thermal ablation for recurrent hepatocellular carcinoma after hepatectomy. *British Journal of Surgery*, Vol.92, No.11, (November 2005), pp: 1393-1398, ISSN 0007-1323

Makuuchi, M.; Takayama, T.; Kubota, K.; Kimura, W.; Midorikawa, Y.; Miyagawa, S. & Kawasaki, S. (1998). Hepatic resection for hepatocellular carcinoma: Japanese experience. *Hepatogastroenterology.* Vol.45, No.3, (August 1998), pp: 1267–1274, ISSN 0172-6390

Matsuda, M.; Fujii, H.; Kono, H. & Matsumoto, Y. (2001). Surgical treatment of recurrent hepatocellular carcinoma based on the mode of recurrence: repeat hepatic resection or ablation are good choices for patients with recurrent multicentric cancer. *Journal of Hepato-biliary-pancreatic Surgery,* Vol.8, No.4, (2001), pp: 353–359, ISSN 0944-1166

Matsuda, Y.; Ito, T.; Oguchi, Y.; Nakajima, K. & Izukura, T. (1993). Rationale of surgical management for recurrent hepatocellular carcinoma. *Annals of Surgery*; Vol.217, No.1, (January 1993), pp: 28-34, ISSN 0003-4932

Matsumata, T.; Kanematsu, T.; Takenaka, K.; Yoshida, Y.; Nishizaki, T. & Sugimachi, K. (1989). Patterns of intrahepatic recurrence after curative resection of hepatocellular carcinoma. *Hepatology,* Vol.9, No.3, (March 1989), pp: 457–460, ISSN 0270-9139

Minagawa, M.; Makuuchi, M.; Takayama, T. & Kokudo, N. (2003). Selection criteria for repeat hepatectomy in patients with recurrent hepatocellular carcinoma. *Annals of Surgery,* Vol.228, No.5, (November 2003), pp: 703-710, ISSN 0003-4932

Nakayama, H.; Takayama, T.; Makuuchi, M.; Yamasaki, S.; Kosuge, T.; Shimada, K. & Yamamoto, J. (1999). Resection of peritoneal metastases from hepatocellular carcinoma. *Hepatogastroenterology,* Vol.46, No.26, (March - April 1999), pp: 1049–1052, ISSN 0172-6390

Ohmoto, K. & Yamamoto, S. (2006). Comparison between radiofrequency ablation and percutaneous microwave coagulation therapy for small hepatocellular carcinomas. *Clinical Radiology,* Vol.61, No.9, (September 2006), pp: 800-801, ISSN 009-9260

Ogata, Y.; Uchida, S.; Hisaka, T.; Horiuchi, H.; Mori, S.; Ishibashi, N.; Akagi, Y. & Shirouzu, K. (2008). Intraoperative thermal ablation therapy for small colorectal metastases to the liver. *Hepatogastroenterology.* Vol.55, No.82-83, (March - April 2008), pp: 550-556, ISSN 0172-6390

Partensky, C.; Sassolas, G.; Henry, L.; Pallard, P. & Maddern, GJ. (2000). Intra-arterial iodine 131-labeled lipiodol as adjuvant therapy after curative liver resection for hepatocellular carcinoma: a phase 2 clinical study. *Archives of Surgery*, Vol.135, No.11, (November 2000), pp: 1298-1300, ISSN 0004-0010

Peng, BG.; He, Q.; Li, JP. & Zhou, F. (2009). Adjuvant transcatheter arterial chemoembolization improves efficacy of hepatectomy for patients with hepatocellular carcinoma and portal vein tumor thrombus. *American Journal of Surgery*, Vol.198, No.3, (September 2009), pp: 313-318, ISSN 0002-9610

Piao, CY.; Fujioka, S.; Iwasaki, Y.; Fujio, K.; Kaneyoshi, T.; Araki, Y.; Hashimoto, K.; Senoh, T.; Terada, R.; Nishida, T.; Kobashi, H.; Sakaguchi, K. & Shiratori, Y. (2005). Lamivudine treatment in patients with HBV-related hepatocellular carcinoma - using an untreated, matched control cohort. *Acta Medica Okayama*, Vol.59, No.5, (October 2005), pp: 217–224, ISSN 0386-300X

Poon, RTP.; Fan, ST.; Lo, CM.; Liu, CL. & Wong, J. (1999). Intrahepatic recurrence after curative resection for hepatocellular carcinoma: long-term results of treatment and prognostic factors. *Annals of Surgery*, Vol.229, No.2, (Febuary 1999), pp: 216-222, ISSN 0003-4932

Poon, RT.; Fan, ST.; Ng, IO.; Lo, CM.; Liu, CL. & Wong, J. (2000). Different risk factors and prognosis for early and late intrahepatic recurrence after resection of hepatocellular carcinoma. *Cancer, Vol.89, No.3.* (August 2000), pp: 500-507, ISSN 0008-543X

Poon, RT.; Fan, ST.; Lo, CM.; Ng, IO.; Liu, CL.; Lam, CM. & Wong, J. (2001). Improving survival results after resection of hepatocellular carcinoma: a prospective study of 377 patients over 10 years. *Annals of Surgery*, Vol.234, No.1, (Jul 2001), pp: 63-70, ISSN 0003-4932

Poon, RT.; Fan, ST.; O'Suilleabhain, CB. & Wong, J. (2002). Aggressive management of patients with extrahepatic and intrahepatic recurrences of hepatocellular carcinoma by combined resection and locoregional therapy. *Journal of the American College of Surgeons*, Vol.195, No.3, (September 2002), pp: 311–318, ISSN 1072-7515

Poon, RT.; Fan, ST.; Tsang, FH. & Wong, J. (2002). Locoregional therapies for hepatocellular carcinoma: a critical review from the surgeon's perspective. *Annals of Surgery*, Vol.235, No.4, (April 2002), pp: 466-486, ISSN 0003-4932

Ren, ZG.; Lin, ZY.; Xia, JL.; Ye, SL.; Ma, ZC.; Ye, QH.; Qin, LX.; Wu, ZQ.; Fan, J. & Tang, ZY. (2004). Postoperative adjuvant arterial chemoembolization improves survival of hepatocellular carcinoma patients with risk factors for residual tumor: a retrospective control study. *World Journal of Gastroenterology*, Vol.10, No.19, (October 2004), pp: 2791-2794, ISSN 1007-9327

Rossi, L.; Zoratto, F.; Papa, A.; Iodice, F.; Minozzi, M.; Frati, L. & Tomao, S. (2010). Current approach in the treatment of hepatocellular carcinoma. *World Journal of Gastrointestinal Oncology*, Vol.2, No. 9, (September 2010), pp: 348-359, ISSN 1948-5204

Sakamoto, Y.; Kubota, K.; Mori, M.; Inoue, K.; Abe, H.; Harihara, Y.; Bandai, Y. & Makuuchi, M. (1999). Surgical management for adrenal gland metastasis of hepatocellular carcinoma. *Hepatogastroenterology*. Vol.46, No.26, (March - April 1999), pp: 1036-1041, ISSN 0172-6390

Seki, T.; Wakabayashi, M.; Nakagawa, T.; Imamura, M.; Tamai, T.; Nishimura, A.; Yamashiki, N.; Okamura, A. & Inoue, K. (1999). Percutaneous microwave coagulation therapy for patients with small hepatocellular carcinoma: comparison with percutaneous ethanol injection therapy. *Cancer,* Vol.85, No.8, (April 1999), pp: 1694-1702, ISSN 0008-543X

Shibata, T.; Iimuro, Y.; Yamamoto, Y.; Maetani, Y.; Ametani, F.; Itoh, K. & Konishi, J. (2002). Small hepatocellular carcinoma: comparison of radio-frequency ablation and percutaneous microwave coagulation therapy. *Radiology,* Vol.223, No.2, (May 2002), pp: 331-337, ISSN 0033-8419

Shim, JH.; Park, JW.; Choi, JI.; Kim, HN.; Lee, Wj. & Kim, CM. (2009). Does postembolization fever after chemoembolization have prognostic significance for survival in patients with unresectable hepatocellular carcinoma? *Journal of Vascular and Interventional Radiology,* Vol.20, No.2, (Febuary 2009), pp: 209–216, ISSN 1051-0443.

Shim, JH.; Kim, KM.; Lee, YJ.; Ko, GY.; Yoon, HK.; Sung, KB.; Park, KM.; Lee, SG.; Lim, YS.; Lee, HC.; Chung, YH.; Lee, YS, & Suh, DJ. (2010). Complete necrosis after transarterial chemoembolization could predict prolonged survival in patients with recurrent intrahepatic hepatocellular carcinoma after curative resection. *Annals of Surgical Oncology,* Vol.17, No.3, (Machr 2010), pp: 869-877, ISSN 1068-9265

Shimada, K.; Sakamoto, Y.; Esaki, M.; Kosuge, T.; Morizane, C.; Ikeda, M.; Ueno, H.; Okusaka, T.; Arai, Y. & Takayasu, K. (2007). Analysis of prognostic factors affecting survival after initial recurrence and treatment efficacy for recurrence in patients undergoing potentially curative hepatectomy for hepatocellular carcinoma. *Annals of Surgical Oncology,* Vol.14, No.8, (August 2007), pp: 2337-2347, ISSN 1068-9265

Shimada, M, Takenaka K, Gion T, Fujiwara Y, Kajiyama K, Maeda T, Shirabe K, Nishizaki T, Yanaga K & Sugimachi K. (1996). Prognosis of recurrent hepatocellular carcinoma: a 10-year surgical experience in Japan. *Gastroenterology,* Vol.111, No.3, (September 1996), pp: 720–726, ISSN 0016-5085

Shimada, M.; Takenaka, K.; Taguchi, K.; Fujiwara, Y.; Gion, T.; Kajiyama, K.; Maeda, T.; Shirabe, K.; Yanaga, K. & Sugimachi, K. (1998). Prognostic factors after repeat hepatectomy for recurrent hepatocellular carcinoma. *Annals of Surgery,* Vol.227, No.1, (January 1998), pp: 80-85, ISSN 0003-4932

Simon, CJ.; Dupuy, DE. & Mayo-Smith, WW. (2005). Microwave ablation: principles and applications. *Radiographics,* Vol.25, Suppl 1, (October 2005), S69-83, ISSN 0271-5333

Simonetti, RG.; Liberati, A.; Angiolini, C. & Pagliaro, L. (1997). Treatment of hepatocellular carcinoma: a systematic review of randomized controlled trials. *Annals of Oncology,* Vol.8, No.2, (February 1997), pp: 117-136, ISSN 0923-7534

Suenaga, M.; Sugiura, H.; Kokuba, Y.; Uehara, S. & Kurumiya, T. (1994). Repeated hepatic resection for recurrent hepatocellular carcinoma in eighteen cases. *Surgery,* Vol.115, No.4, (April 1994), pp: 452– 457, ISSN 0039-6060.

Sugimachi, K.; Maehara, S.; Tanaka, S.; Shimada, M. & Sugimachi, K. (2001). Repeat hepatectomy is the most useful treatment for recurrent hepatocellular carcinoma. *Journal of Hepato-biliary-pancreatic Surgery,* Vol.8, No.5, (2001), pp: 410-416, ISSN 0944-1166

Sun, HC.; Tang, ZY.; Wang, L.; Qin, LX.; Ma, ZC.; Ye, QH.; Zhang, BH.; Qian, YB.; Wu, ZQ.; Fan, J.; Zhou, XD.; Zhou, J.; Qiu, SJ. & Shen, YF. (2006). Postoperative interferon alpha treatment postponed recurrence and improved overall survival in patients after curative resection of HBV-related hepatocellular carcinoma: a randomized clinical trial. *Journal of Cancer Research and Clinical Oncology*, Vol.132, No.7, (July 2006), pp: 458-465, ISSN 0171-5216

Takayama T, Sekine T, Makuuchi M, Yamasaki S, Kosuge T, Yamamoto J, Shimada K, Sakamoto M, Hirohashi S, Ohashi Y & Kakizoe T. (2000). Adoptive immunotherapy to lower postsurgical recurrence rates of hepatocellular carcinoma: a randomized trial. *Lancet*, Vol.356, No.9232, (September 2000), pp: 802-807, ISSN 0140-6736

Tateishi R, Shiina S, Teratani T, Obi S, Sato S, Koike Y, Fujishima T, Yoshida H, Kawabe T & Omata M. (2005). Percutaneous radiofrequency ablation for hepatocellular carcinoma: an analysis of 1000 cases. *Cancer*, Vol.103, No.6, (March 2005), pp: 1201-1209, ISSN 0008-543X

Taura, K.; Ikai, I.; Hatano, E.; Fukii, H.; Uyama, N. & Shimahara, Y. (2006). Implication of frequent local ablation therapy for intrahepatic recurrence in prolonged survival of patients with hepatocellular carcinoma undergoing hepatic resection: an analysis of 610 patients over 16 years old. *Annals of Surgery*, Vol.244, No.2, (August 2006), pp: 265-273, ISSN 0003-4932

Tralhão, JG.; Dagher, I.; Lino, T.; Roudié, J. & Franco, D. (2007). Treatment of tumour recurrence after resection of hepatocellular carcinoma. Analysis of 97 consecutive patients. *European Journal of Surgery Oncology*, Vol.33, No.6, (August 2007), pp: 746–751, ISSN 0748-7983

Viganò, L.; Tayar, C.; Laurent, A. & Cherqui, D. (2009). Laparoscopic liver resection: a systematic review. *Journal of Hepato-biliary-pancreatic Surgery*, Vol.16, No. 4, (June 2009), pp: 410–421, ISSN 0944-1166

Wong, JS.; Wong, GL.; Tsoi, KK.; Wong, VW.; Cheung, SY.; Chong, CN.; Wong, J.; Lee, KF.; Lai, PB. & Chan, HL. (2011). Meta-analysis: the efficacy of anti-viral therapy in prevention of recurrence after curative treatment of chronic hepatitis B-related hepatocellular carcinoma. *Alimentary Pharmacology and Therapeutics*, Vol.33, No.10, (May 2011), pp: 1104-1112, ISSN0269-2813

Wu, CC.; Cheng, SB.; Yeh, DC.; Wang, J. & Peng, FK. (2009). Second and third hepatectomies for recurrent hepatocellular carcinoma are justified. *British Journal of Surgery*, Vol.96, No.9, (September 2009), pp: 1049-1057, ISSN 0007-1323

Xi, T.; Yan, ZL.; Wang, K.; Li, J.; Xia, Y.; Shen, F. & Wu, MC. (2007). Role of post-operative transcatheter arterial chemoembolization in hepatocellular carcinoma with different pathological characteristics. *Zhonghua Wai Ke Za Zhi*, Vol.45, No.9, (May 2007), pp: 1587-1590, ISSN 0529-5815

Xu, HX.; Lu, MD.; Xie, XY.; Yin, XY.; Kuang, M.; Chen, JW.; Xu, Zf. & Liu, GJ. (2005). Prognostic factors for long-term outcome after percutaneous thermal ablation for hepatocellular carcinoma: a survival analysis of 137 consecutive patients. *Clinical Radiology*, Vol.60, No.9, (September 2005), pp: 1018-1025, ISSN 0009-9260

Yamamoto, J.; Kosuge, T.; Takayama, T.; Shimada, K.; Yamasaki, S.; Ozaki, H.; Yamaguchi, N. & Makuuchi, M. (1996). Recurrence of hepatocellular carcinoma after surgery. *British Journal of Surgery*, Vol.83, No.9, (Septemerb 1996), pp: 1219–1222, ISSN 0007-1323

Yang, W.; Chen, MH.; Yin, SS.; Yan, K.; Gao, W.; Wang, YB.; Huo, L.; Zhang, XP. & Xing, BC. (2006). Radiofrequency ablation of recurrent hepatocellular carcinoma after hepatectomy: therapeutic efficacy on early- and late-phase recurrence. *American Journal of Roentgenology*, Vol.186, 5 Supp, (May 2006), S275–S283, ISSN 0361-803X

Yang, Y.; Nagano, H.; Ota, H.; Morimoto, O.; Nakamura, M.; Wada, H.; Noda, T.; Damdinsuren, B.; Marubashi, S.; Miyamoto, A.; Takeda, Y.; Dono, K.; Umeshita, K.; Nakamori, S.; Wakasa, K.; Sakon, M. & Monden, M. (2007). Patterns and clinicopathologic features of extrahepatic recurrence of hepatocellular carcinoma after curative resection. *Surgery*, Vol.141, No.2, (February 2007), pp: 196-202, ISSN 0039-6060

Yeh, CN.; Chen, MF.; Lee, WC. & Jeng, LB. (2002). Prognostic factors of hepatic resection for hepatocellular carcinoma with cirrhosis: univariate and multivariate analysis. *Journal of Surgical Oncology*, Vol.81, No.4, (December 2002), pp: 195–202, ISSN 0022-4790

Zhong, C.; Guo, RP.; Li, JQ.; Shi, M.; Wei, W.; Chen, MS. & Zhang, YQ. (2009). A randomized controlled trial of hepatectomy with adjuvant transcatheter arterial chemoembolization versus hepatectomy alone for Stage III A hepatocellular carcinoma. *Journal of Cancer Research and Clinical Oncology*, Vol.135, No.10, (October 2009), pp: 1437-1445, ISSN 0171-5216

Zhou, Y.; Sui, C.; Li, B.; Yin, Z.; Tan, Y.; Yang, J. & Liu, Z. (2010). Repeat hepatectomy for recurrent hepatocellular carcinoma: a local experience and a systematic review. *World Journal of Surgical Oncology*, Vol.8, No.55, (July 2010), ISSN 1477-7819

9

Colorectal Liver Metastasis: Current Management

Alejandro Serrablo, Luis Tejedor, Vicente Borrego and Jesus Esarte
Miguel Servet University Hospital
Spain

1. Introduction

Colorectal cancer (CRC) is the third most frequent in men in developed countries (after lung and prostate tumours) and second among women (after breast cancer), with approximately one million new cases per year throughout the world (550,000 men and 470,000 women), representing 14.6% and 15.2% respectively of all malignant tumours diagnosed. The role of colonoscopy in the screening of this pathology is crucial. CRC affecting the intestine has a high rate of cure (45-50%) with radical surgery. The most frequent metastatic involvement in CRC, after lymph nodes invasion, is seen in the liver.

Several studies have analyzed the pre-operative prognostic factors in patients undergoing liver resection for liver metastases of CRC in order to select patients for surgical treatment. However, intraoperative and post-operative factors have been poorly studied and that could report on the aggressiveness of the tumour and the curative efficacy of the surgery performed. The purpose of surgery is resection of all liver lesions with a tumour-free margin, provided R0 resection (complete resection with no microscopic residual tumour) may be achieved with low morbidity and mortality (Choti et al. 2002; Marin et al. 2009; Lordan & Karanjia 2007) without endangering the life of the patient due to either liver insufficiency or post-operative complications. According to most authors, it should be noted that surgery, however extensive it is, does not prolong survival if residual microscopic or gross tumour is left (Harmantas et al. 1996; Kronawitter et al. 1999).

Since Woodington and Waugh reported the first favourable results of surgical treatment for CRC liver metastases (Woodington & Waugh, 1964), a disease previously considered incurable, to date, a 5- and 10-year survival rates of 35-58% and 20-25% respectively have been achieved, while survival without treatment is less than 2% (Ohlsson et al. 1998; Fong et al. 1999).

The key for indicating the most adequate treatment is the study conducted by a multidisciplinary team (Söreide et al. 2008; Artigas et al. 2007). The difficulty for assessing the indication stems from the fact that the presence of extrahepatic tumour, the possibility of achieving a tumour-free margin and the actual number of liver metastases are frequently known during the laparotomy. Different studies have analyzed the traditional pre-operative factors predicting survival in order to select patients in whom unnecessary surgery could be avoided. These were factors related to the patient, the primary tumour and the liver metastases (Fong et al. 1999; Nordlinger et al. 1996). However, some authors do not contraindicate surgery in patients with poor prognostic criteria provided a R0 resection may be obtained, as a number of prognostic factors are known only after resection (Marín et al. 2009). These factors include the histological study (number, resection margin size, microsatellites, type of growth, presence of tumour pseudocapsule, tumour differentiation grade, histological type, nuclear grade and number of mitoses/mm^2) and the immunohistochemical study of the resected specimen. The latter may combine the markers of cell proliferation and cell cycle control, p53 and Ki67. There is increasing evidence supporting the concept that in human cancer, a minority of cells (tumour stem cells) has acquired characteristics of uncontrolled growth and the ability to form metastases (Reya et al. 2001; Dalerba et al. 2007; Jordan et al. 2006). This hypothesis is supported by different experimental observations made initially in acute myeloid leukaemia (Bonnet D & Dick J 1997) and subsequently in human solid tumours, such as breast (Al-Hajj 2003), brain (Singh et al. 2004; Galli et al. 2004), colorectal (O' Brien et al. 2004; Ricci-Vitiani et al. 2007), head and neck (Prince et al. 2007) and pancreatic cancer (Li et al. 2007). However, this concept continues to be highly controversial and data reported on colorectal cancer are not yet conclusive (Ricci-Vitiani et al. 2007; Hill 2006).

It is therefore interesting to know both the qualitative and quantitative stem cell population in the tumour using markers, such as CD44, CD133, and CD166. The tissue microarray (TMA) technique allows for monitoring and simultaneous evaluation of a great number of samples or tumour series in a single experiment, ensuring homogeneity of the techniques between specimens and validation of the results obtained with various histological, immunohistochemical and in-situ hybridization (FISH) techniques (Battifora 1986; Kononen et al 1998; Milanes-Yearsley et al 2002).

In addition, over the last decade, a revolution in the approach to CRC liver metastases has occurred. Firstly, there was the advent of new chemotherapy drugs that have allowed better control of the disease, higher response rates and longer survival rates. Secondly, this has opened up a greater possibility of surgical rescue in more patients. Aggressive surgical management is called extreme liver surgery: ante-situ, in-situ and ex-situ liver resections are included (Mehrabi et al. 2011; Hoti et al. 2011; Oldhafer et al. 2001).

2. Current diagnostic tools

Imaging of the liver of CRC patients requires high sensitivity and reliable characterization of the lesions, allowing differentiation of malignant from benign tumours. Accurate and timely detection of hepatic metastases has long-range therapeutic and prognostic implications, since untreated liver metastases have a poor prognosis (5-year survival rate of 0–3%) while the resection with curative intent offers a much better one (5-year survival rate from 35% to 58%) (El Khodary et al. 2011). An understanding of the segmental anatomy of the liver is imperative for localization and appropriate management of hepatic neoplasms. The classification proposed by Couinaud (Couinaud 1957) and later modified by Bismuth (Bismuth 1982) provides the surgically relevant information and is easily applicable to cross-sectional imaging techniques, such as computed tomography (CT), magnetic resonance imaging (MRI) and ultrasonography (US).

The imaging assessment of potentially resectable CRC liver metastases, needed for a careful pre-operative selection of patients, should address the following five critical issues:

1. Evaluation of possible liver metastases. Number, size and segmental location of tumours must be determined, as well as their differential diagnosis with benign lesions.
2. Possible hilar lymph node involvement. As they represent metastases from the liver metastases, this lymphatic involvement carries a poor prognosis (survival rates after resection are 3-12%), although the pre-operative diagnosis is difficult.
3. Vascular invasion. Obviously, assessment of vascular invasion is critical when deciding the appropriate surgical strategy.
4. Liver volumetry. Measuring the volume of the future remnant liver when considering extended resections is recommended, since insufficient residual volume of liver parenchyma is a contraindication to surgery.
5. Presence of extrahepatic disease. Although peritoneal carcinomatosis may be very difficult to detect, other extrahepatic involvement is usually diagnosed pre-operatively (Valls et al. 2009).

Imaging techniques used nowadays for diagnosis of these lesions include US, multi-detector CT (MDCT), MRI and fluorine-18-fluorodeoxyglucose positron emission tomography (FDG PET). FDG PET and CT can be combined in order to provide fused images, allowing high spatial resolution and functional information in the same examination (FDG PET/CT). In studies with specificity higher than 85%, the sensitivity for detection of liver metastases is progressively increasing from US to CT, MRI and FDG PET (Kinkel et al. 2002). The extensive literature regarding the benefits and constraints of each of these modalities for detecting liver metastases shows several limitations: inadequate definition of inclusion and exclusion criteria, incomplete reporting of methods, lack of uniform references, etc. The best standard of reference is laparotomy with bimanual palpation and intraoperative ultrasonography (IOUS), but this was used in only a few studies (Valls et al 2001). When a suboptimal standard is used, underreporting of lesions and overestimation of detection rate are the results (van Erkel et al 2002). Another confounding factor is the different methods for reporting sensitivity: per patient (detection of at least one lesion per patient) and per lesion (detection of all lesions per patient). Therefore, it is important to inquire into the results of the current studies, also because improving technology can make results of prior studies superfluous (Lucey et al. 2006).

2.1 Ultrasonography

US is a rapid and non-invasive method for screening patients with suspected liver metastases but, although it is highly efficient in distinguishing patients with diffuse hepatic metastases that involve all the liver, it is more operator dependent than other imaging methods, fails to show parts of the liver in certain patients and its sensitivity (50-70%) and specificity are surpassed by other imaging studies.

The detection of hepatic metastases is substantially improved by contrast-enhanced US (CEUS) compared to conventional B-mode sonography, increasing the sensitivity per lesion from 71% to 87% (Oldenburg & Albrecht 2008). US contrast agents consist of microbubbles of gas that flood the blood pool after intravenous injection and are confined to the vascular compartment. These agents are safe, well tolerated and have very few contraindications.

Metastases behave characteristically in three phases: arterial, portal venous and delayed (El Khodary et al. 2011). CEUS sensitivity and specificity in staging liver metastases (80–95% and 84–98%, respectively) approach those of CT and MRI. In addition, CEUS is useful to improve the detection rate of metastases smaller than 1 cm or of those lesions that are isoechoic with respect to adjacent liver parenchyma, thus improving the performance of sonography in around 13.7% of the cases (Chami et al. 2008).

In general, if an examination of the liver by US is insufficient, then examination by CEUS will also be insufficient. CEUS has limited ability to observe certain parts of the liver, especially in obese patients and/or in cases of steatosis and it is not possible to simultaneously examine multiple lesions in the arterial and early portal phases. Hypervascular metastases and haemangiomas on one hand and metastases and small cysts on the other can be difficult to differentiate (Larsen 2010).

Intraoperative diagnosis is based on IOUS and on diagnostic laparoscopy. IOUS has higher sensitivity than transabdominal US, MDCT and MRI, and allows identification of metastases 0.5 cm in size and defining the relationship between lesion, vessels and biliary structures. With a sensitivity of 98% and a specificity of 95%, IOUS is generally considered the gold standard for detecting liver lesions and is regarded as a routine investigation, modifying the planned surgical intervention in 18-30% of the patients. In addition, Doppler and spectral Doppler facilitate the technique of surgical resection. Laparoscopy, which is not routinely used in the pre-operative evaluation of the advanced disease, allows an assessment of the peritoneal and pelvic spread of the primitive cancer and, with the combined use of laparoscopic ultrasound (LIOUS), enables detection of small metastases, varying the initial surgical plan in 20–30% of the cases (Guglielmi et al. 2005). Contrast enhanced IOUS (CE-IOUS) shows some benefit over pre-operative imaging and IOUS since it seems to improve the ability to characterize already detected lesions and facilitate the detection of new metastatic lesions (Fioole et al. 2008; Leen et al. 2006; Nakano et al. 2008; Torzilli et al. 2005).

2.2 Computed Tomography

MDCT has a sensitivity of 70–85% and a specificity of 90%, especially for lesions bigger than 1.5–2 cm. Sensitivity is lower for small subglissonian metastases, even though multi-slice CT allows identification of hepatic lesions of 0.5 cm in size (Guglielmi et al. 2005). Fast data acquisition and breath-hold scanning allows imaging of the liver twice. This bi-phasic contrast-enhanced scan during the arterial-dominant phase and the portal-venous perfusion phase after bolus-like contrast administration, prior to the equilibrium phase, is accepted as standard for the optimised display of the complex vascularization of the liver and potential hepatic lesions. Slice thicknesses of 2 or 4 mm are the most effective for detection of focal liver lesions, with an identical detection rate of 96% for both. 3-D data sets can be produced improving multiplanar imaging, which allows evaluation of subcapsular lesions, demonstration of vascular anatomy and better characterisation of the lesions. Together with improvements in bolus-tracking, MDCT scanning during the various vascular contrast and equilibrium phases allows performing CT-angiography of the liver and mesenteric vessels, which can be important in patients undergoing hepatic resection or transarterial chemo or radio-embolisation. MDCT portal venogram is useful in evaluation of the portal system. Additionally, quantitative perfusion studies can also be done. Thus, MDCT can be used for evaluating the liver lesion, liver parenchyma and hepatic vessels in the same sitting.

It is important to take account of the time elapsed between the radiological study and the operation. One recent study showed that the utility of MDCT as a pre-operative tool to evaluate CRC liver metastases is inversely proportional to the time interval between imaging and surgery, which may explain conflicting reports of the accuracy of MDCT in the literature (Yang et al. 2010).

Hepatic volumetry, necessary to evaluate the feasibility of major hepatectomies, especially in the case of atypical resections, is provided by MDCT software able to highlight different liver segments and to create vascular maps for arterial and portal afferences, and for hepatic vein drainage. The volume of each single segment can be calculated and a simulation of surgical resection can be performed. Information can be displayed using coloured maps or three-dimensional movies (Laghi et al. 2005).

2.3 Magnetic Resonance Imaging

MDCT is usually preferred because it is more widely available and because it is a well-established technique for surveying the extrahepatic abdominal organs and tissues. However, MRI has an advantage in the characterization of focal lesions and is also preferred for patients who cannot receive intravenous iodinated contrast material or when concerns about the risk of radiation from repeated exposure to CT, as in children or young adults, exists. In general, MRI sensitivity varies from 85-90% and its specificity is up to 95%, although a comparison of the performance of MDCT vs. MRI needs to be reassessed periodically, considering the rapid evolution of both technologies and the increase in therapeutic options available.

Contrast media are of two types: the extracellular agents (gadolinium chelates) and the liver specific agents. Gadolinium is used for lesion detection and characterisation while liver specific agents are used as functional agents. The most commonly used substance in contrast-enhanced dynamic MRI is extracellular gadolinium-chelate complex, which provides the greatest diagnostic sensitivity and specificity rates among cross-sectional techniques currently in use. The current standard MRI liver protocol includes a T2-weighted sequence, a T1-weighted sequence and a three-phase technique after administration of gadolinium (arterial-dominant, portal venous and hepatic venous or interstitial). Like CT, the detection of CRC liver metastases using MRI is maximized during the portal venous phase.

The administration of organ-specific contrast agents with hepatocyte specificity (mangafodipir trisodium [MnDPDP], gadobenate dimeglumine [Gd-BOPTA]) or reticuloendothelial system specificity (superparamagnetic iron oxide [SPIO] particles, captured by Kupffer cells) allows an increase in the sensitivity and specificity of the method (Bluemke et al. 2000; Vidiri et al. 2004), but data about their benefits are controversial. Furthermore, these agents are generally costly and not widely available.

Diffusion-weighted MR imaging (DWI) is a recently introduced technique to depict differences in molecular diffusion caused by the random motion of molecules. It provides excellent tissue contrast based on molecular diffusion, which is different from ordinary T1- and T2-weighted images, without the need for a contrast agent (El Khodary et al. 2011). An additional benefit of DWI is the ability to derive quantitative indices, which may be important in the assessment of disease response to novel therapeutics, including anti-vascular and anti-angiogenic therapy, since conventional assessment based on measuring lesion size is insensitive to early, treatment-related changes (Koh et al. 2006). In summary, DWI is a simple and sensitive method for screening focal hepatic lesions and is useful for differential diagnosis (Koike et al. 2009).

2.4 Positron Emission Tomography

FDG PET is a highly sensitive and specific imaging study detecting hepatic metastases from CRC (92–100% and 85–100% respectively), although for some authors the strength of these data is moderate (Lucey et al. 2006). Several studies have also shown the utility of FDG PET in identifying additional metastatic lesions when initial CT showed single hepatic metastases and, thus, changed the management strategy. Nevertheless, false negative and false positive findings in FDG PET for hepatic metastases are not negligible (Udayasankar et al. 2008) and its positive predictive value (PPV) is not high, leading to some authors to confirm histologically the FDG PET findings suggesting non-resectability (Valls et al. 2009).

Two meta-analyses have demonstrated high diagnostic values of PET in the evaluation of hepatic metastases (Bipat et al. 2005; Wiering et al. 2005), as well as a recent review (Patel et al. 2011) confirming the superior sensitivity of FDG PET for detecting liver metastases on a per patient basis, but not on a per lesion basis. Other papers have shown FDG PET/CT to be slightly less sensitive than MRI with liver-specific contrast agents or dedicated sequences for small lesions (Coenegrachts et al. 2009), but more sensitive than MDCT alone (Kong et al. 2008; Selzner et al. 2004), although its role is not yet clear owing to the small number of studies (Niekel et al. 2010). In the context of CRC metastases, the role of FDG PET/CT is to avoid unnecessary surgery, based on its ability to detect extrahepatic foci of disease (nodal metastases, lung nodules) that are not depicted or characterized as malignant by other imaging methods (Sørensen et al. 2007). In addition, this technology is not suitable for liver resection planning. In patients evaluated with FDG PET prior to surgery, a lower risk of "non-therapeutic laparotomy" (Pawlik et al. 2009) and improved survival (Fernandez et al. 2004) has been observed, reflecting better patient selection.

A recent meta-analysis reviewing more than 3,000 patients found that sensitivity of CT, MR imaging and FDG PET on a per lesion basis were 74.4%, 80.3% and 81.4%, respectively, while on a per patient basis, the sensitivities were 83.6%, 88.2% and 94.1%, respectively. Specificity estimates were comparable. No differences were seen for lesions measuring at least 10 mm. Data about FDG PET/CT were too limited for comparisons with other modalities (Niekel et al. 2010).

In brief, although every modality has benefited from advances in technology, MDCT scanning remains a dominant imaging modality not only for lesion detection and pre-operative planning, but also for treatment monitoring and post-treatment surveillance. High-resolution CT with contrast combined with FDG PET/CT may obviate the need for additional studies and may improve patient management (Bipat et al. 2007; Doan et al. 2010; Vauthey 2006). Dynamic gadolinium-based contrast-enhanced MRI should be reserved for problem solving. MRI has the highest sensitivity for lesion detection, but because of its low sensitivity in detecting extrahepatic disease in the peritoneum and chest, it is not a desirable primary imaging modality (Vauthey 2006) except for evaluating patients who have not previously undergone therapy (Lucey et al. 2006; Niekel et al. 2010). Ultimately, the modality used must be tailored not only to the patient and the clinical situation, but also to the imaging expertise within the institution.

3. Current criteria for resectability

Improvements in pre-operative imaging techniques, patient selection and surgical techniques, as well as the introduction of new cytotoxic and biologic agents for pre-operative and post-operative chemotherapy have improved the resectability rate and almost doubled the 5-year survival rate for patients with CRC liver metastases, from about 30% two decades ago to nearly 60%. In this setting, with the care of these patients rapidly evolving, the standards of care needed to be redefined. The criteria for resectability of these metastases have changed dramatically. Features such as the number of lesions (1 to 3 unilobar metastases), the size of the lesion (less than 5 cm), preferably presenting at least 12 months after resection of the primary tumour, resectable with a minimum margin of 1 cm in width and without hilar adenopathy or extrahepatic disease, are no longer considered as determinant factors regarding resectability and, thereby, are invalid to deny a patient the opportunity of lengthy survival.

Regarding the number of metastasis, Altendorf-Hofmann did not find long-term differences in the survival rates between patients with 1 to 3 metastasis and those with 4 or more, if a R0 resection had been obtained (Altendorf-Hofmann et al. 2003). Moreover, some studies have shown that the degree of response to chemotherapy is a stronger predictor factor for long-term survival than the number of metastasis. Regarding tumour size and prognosis, reports have been conflicting. Evidence shows that size is not a resectability factor, but a factor related to tumour aggressiveness.

It has been shown that the actual width of the surgical margin has no effect on survival as long as the margin is microscopically negative (Figueras et al. 2007; Lordan 2007; Pawlik et al. 2005). A margin greater than 10mm is considered to be optimum, although this has changed too (Casanova et al. 2004). Although surgeons should continue to plan hepatic resection to preserve a "safety zone" and should avoid routine use of "minimum margin" surgery, a predicted margin of less than 1 cm should no longer be considered an exclusion criterion for resection.

Historically, extrahepatic disease has been almost universally accepted as a contraindication to liver resection. Recently, however, some series have shown a 5-year survival rate of 12% to 37% after liver resection in selected patients with extrahepatic disease, independent of the location of that disease (lung, primary colorectal recurrence, retroperitoneal or hepatic pedicle lymph nodes, peritoneal carcinomatosis, miscellaneous) (Elias et al. 2003, 2005). In most cases, incidental peritoneal disease found at laparotomy would contraindicate hepatic resection. In general, resection in such patients should only be considered after documentation of stable/responsive disease with systemic chemotherapy and when an R0 resection of both intrahepatic and extrahepatic disease is feasible. From an anatomic and prognostic perspective, it seems appropriate to recommend that patients with combined liver and extrahepatic disease be reported separately from those meeting the traditional resectable criteria, and be designated as borderline resectable (Vauthey 2007).

Positive hilar lymph nodes are associated with a poor outcome and have been traditionally considered as a contraindication to hepatic resection of CRC liver disease. Recent papers have reported long-term survival in some patients with hilar nodal metastases and have concluded that this patient population may still benefit from hepatic resection and lymphadenectomy, provided that involved nodes are in the hepatoduodenal-retropancreatic area and not in the common hepatic artery/celiac-axis region (Adam et al. 2008; Jaeck 2003). Although patients with microscopic involvement may derive a benefit from hepatic resection, gross involvement of the hilar nodes should be considered a relative contraindication to resection.

At present, the criteria for resectability include any patient in whom all disease can be removed with a negative margin and who has adequate hepatic reserve. That is to say, instead of resectability being defined by what is removed, now it is sustained by what will remain after resection, including patients with extrahepatic disease (Pawlik et al. 2008). Interestingly, none of the traditional adverse prognostic indicators of recurrence, such as carcinoembryonic antigen more than 200 ng/mL, short disease-free interval, node-positive primary, tumour size more than 5 cm, multiple tumours, or synchronous presentation, precluded long-term survival, except for a positive resection margin (Vauthey 2007).

In 2006, the Consensus Conference on Colorectal Liver Metastases of the American Hepato-Pancreato-Biliary Association (AHPBA) established that CRC liver metastases should be defined as resectable when the disease can be completely resected, two adjacent liver segments can be spared with an adequate vascular inflow and outflow and biliary drainage, and the volume of the liver remaining after resection (future liver remnant [FLR]) will be adequate (at least 20% of the total estimated liver volume for normal parenchyma, 30–60% if the liver is injured by chemotherapy, steatosis or hepatitis, or 40–70% in the presence of cirrhosis, depending on the degree of underlying hepatic dysfunction) (Vauthey 2006). When hepatic metastatic disease is not optimally resectable based on insufficient remnant liver volume, pre-operative chemotherapy, portal vein embolization or staged liver resection can be considered. Also, ablative techniques may be considered alone or in conjunction with resection. All original sites of disease need to be amenable to ablation or resection (Abdalla et al. 2006; Adam et al. 2006; Donadon et al. 2007; Garden et al. 2006).

Resection should be offered to all patients who are suitable candidates and neoadjuvant chemotherapy should be considered in patients who are deemed unresectable at initial evaluation (Doan et al. 2010). Novel chemotherapeutic regimens combining 5-FU, folinic acid and oxaliplatin and/or irinotecan have been associated with improved response rates (approximately 50%), allowing 10-30% of the patients with initially unresectable disease to be successfully treated with liver surgery (Adam et al. 2004). In addition, combination with biologic agents that target angiogenesis and the epidermal growth factor receptor (EGFR), bevacizumab and cetuximab, achieves response rates of up to 70%, increasing these figures (Vauthey 2006). Re-evaluation for resection should be done after 2 or 3 months of pre-operative chemotherapy and every 2 months thereafter. Tumour progression before surgery is associated with a poor outcome, even after potentially curative hepatectomy. Tumour control before surgery is crucial to offer a chance of prolonged remission in patients with multiple metastases (Adam et al. 2004). Patients should be referred early for evaluation for resection. The peri-operative complication rate, including hepatobiliary complications, is higher with lengthy pre-operative chemotherapy and is likely related to the prolonged and sequential use of multiple regimens (de Haas et al. 2011).

Once patients have been diagnosed and a decision made in a multidisciplinary setting that resection is appropriate, it is essential to ensure that patients undergo repeat high quality abdominopelvic CT (or MRI) within a month of the date of surgery. Chest CT should also be performed at this time.

4. Chemotherapy and surgery

The high recurrence rate and the overall poor "true" survival after surgical resection of CRC liver metastases led to the incorporation of the use of chemotherapy. This treatment can be administered in different strategies: neoadjuvant, peri-operative, adjuvant and conversion or downstaging. The latter is administrated to patients with unresectable disease with the goal of downsizing the tumour, re-staging it and re-considering its resection.

Chemotherapy seems to improve outcomes compared with surgery alone. Current chemotherapeutic regimens lead to improved survival in patients with unresectable liver metastases. Resection of the primary tumour and the liver lesions is the optimal management of stage IV CRC with liver metastases. For patients with extensive liver metastases, FOLFOX (folinic acid, 5-fluorouracil and oxaliplatin) and FOLFIRI (irinotecan instead of oxaliplatin) have improved resection rates and survival. Upfront chemotherapy in the asymptomatic patient compared with resection of the primary tumour does not appear to affect survival significantly. However, given that 60% of the patients were alive after 2 years, resection of the primary lesion for palliative reasons and local control must be considered in rectal cancer (Cellini et al. 2010).

Optimal regimens and sequencing of chemotherapies when liver resection is an option are unclear. Some suggest that treatment of resectable liver metastases, in the absence of high-risk features (Fong score) should begin with surgery and consider adjuvant chemotherapy after surgery (Fong et al. 1999). If high-risk features are present, most physicians prefer a short course of systemic pre-operative chemotherapy. Peri-operative therapy and regional therapy with hepatic arterial infusion (HAI) increase disease-free survival (DFS) when compared with surgery alone. In unresectable disease, systemic chemotherapy with or without a biologic agent or HAI with systemic therapy must be considered. If the disease becomes resectable, adjuvant treatment should follow surgery. Adjuvant chemotherapy is usually FOLFOX, but HAI combined with systemic chemotherapy is also an option. The role of adjuvant treatment after liver resection should not be viewed in isolation, but rather in the context of prior treatment, surgical preference and individual patient characteristics. Conducting randomized trials examining the role of adjuvant chemotherapy has been difficult because of the rapidly changing chemotherapy regimens and drugs (Power & Kemeny 2010).

Operated patients with a perforated tumour or a considerable lymphatic burden are considered candidates for neoadjuvant chemotherapy before liver surgery, followed by a re-evaluation after 3 months (Garden et al. 2009). The algorithm of the treatment may be that shown in Figure 1 (Kopetz & Vauthey 2008).

During the treatment with 5-fluorouracil/folinic acid plus oxaliplatin or 5-fluorouracil/folinic acid plus irinotecan, the patients deemed to be resectable should be considered as surgical candidates regardless of the associated adverse predictive factors. The emergence of EGFR antibody agents, which act effectively in patients with K-ras wild-type tumour, fosters treatment individualization (Shimada et al. 2009).

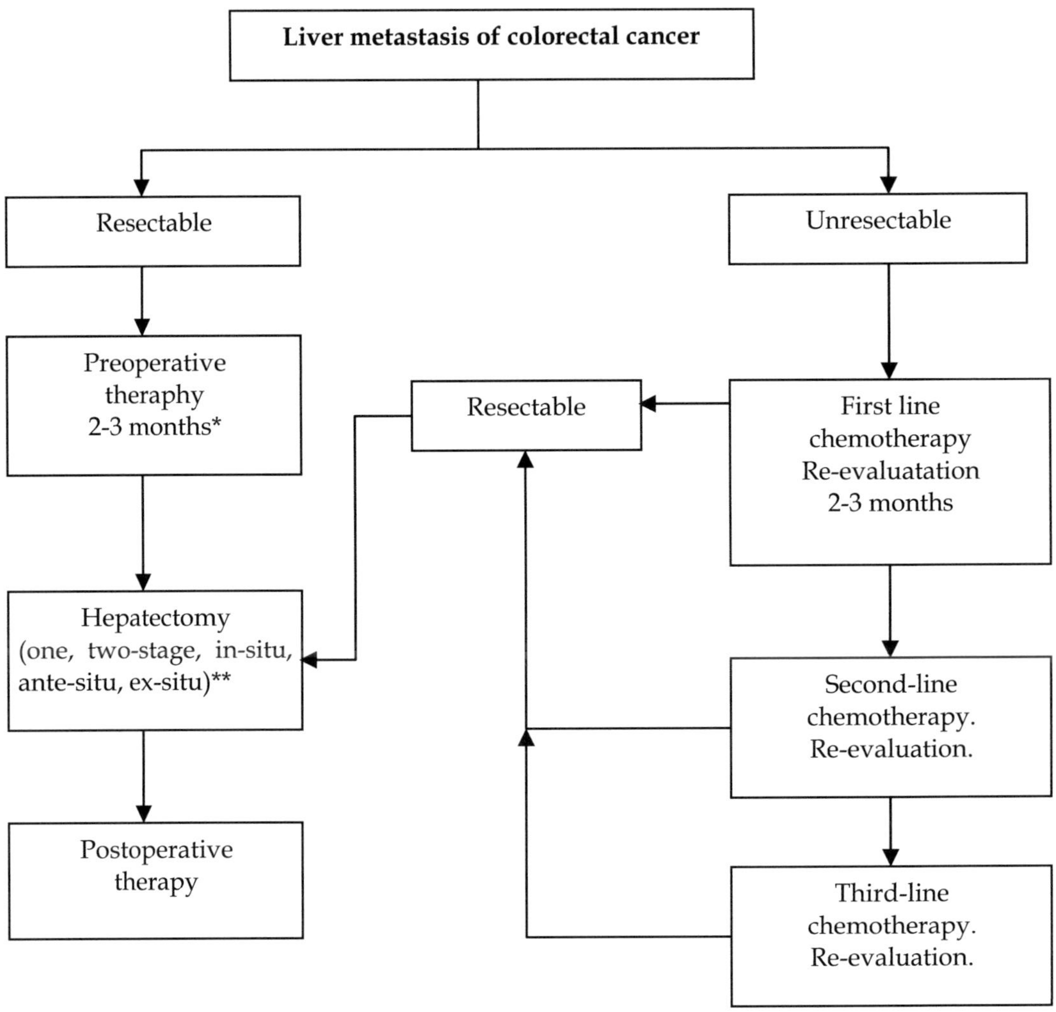

Fig. 1. *Pre-operative therapy depends on the multidisciplinary team and the analyses of the individual case. In some cases, the first option can be resection without pre-operative chemotherapy. **Portal vein embolization (PVE) can be associated to these approaches according to future liver remnants (FLR) volume and the status of the liver (normal, postchemotherapy and cirrhotic).

The efficacy of the peri-operative chemotherapy on survival benefit for resectable liver metastases has not been justified. However, the timing and the indication of the surgery are dramatically changing with the development of chemotherapeutic agents. The overwhelming majority of patients with resectable metastases receive some sort of chemotherapy, although it is not known if the adjuvant regimen is better than the neoadjuvant. The EORTC 40983 study did not demonstrate a clear advantage of pre-operative chemotherapy in patients with initially resectable metastasis, but it could not answer either if neoadjuvant, adjuvant or peri-operative chemotherapy is superior. Detractors claim that chemotherapy delays surgery while supporters point out that surgery is facilitated and that the treatment provides information on tumour biology (Nordlinger et al. 2008). The surgeon's main concern is to operate on patients with livers affected by chemotherapy, which are usually more rigid, more difficult to manage and tend to bleed more easily. The same study demonstrated that no patient progressed from a resectable disease to an unresectable one, that short cycles of treatment provided minimal liver toxicity, that morbidity was similar in both groups and that survival improved in the chemotherapy sub-group. However, the problem persists over the timing of administering chemotherapy and the management of "ghost lesions" after complete response that cannot be detected with IOUS.

5. Rescuing more patients

In 1986, Ekberg provided several contraindications for the surgery of liver metastases of colorectal origin (4 or more nodules, a size greater than 5 cm, presence of extrahepatic disease and the inability to resect with a margin greater than 1 cm). Others studies corroborated these findings. A thorough analysis of these papers could have reduced their influence realising that they had short series or that their statistical analysis was univariate. As previously stated, these criteria are deemed obsolete. So the question is: can all disease be resected while leaving a functional liver remnant? (Charnsangavej et al. 2006). There exist some innovative strategies that increase the volume of the hepatic remnant. Portal vein embolization (PVE) or ligation causes atrophy of the ipsilateral hemiliver and hypertrophy of the contralateral side. PVE appears to be particularly valuable in patients who present with underlying liver disease. The concomitant administration of chemotherapy may decrease both the tumour load and post-operative recurrences. Furthermore, aggressive approaches in selected cases can provide the only possible cure.

5.1 Downstaging chemotherapy

Downstaging chemotherapy is indicated for metastatic disease and for syncronicity in nonresectable disease. Intravenous or HAI downstaging chemotherapy showed a resectability of 20% (Fusai & Dadvison 2003). The advent of oxaliplatin and irinotecan reached response rates of up to 50% increased over 65% with the addition of bevazucimab and cetuximab. Although there are no reports of outcomes of liver resection after HAI, its complication rates are so high (57%) that it is dismissed as a first option.

When treating these patients, the question arises as to whether to continue treatment until reaching the maximal effect or stopping once the disease becomes resectable. In general, pre-operative chemotherapy should be stopped once the intrahepatic disease has been downsized to the point where hepatic resection is feasible. Surgery should be considered after 3 or 4 cycles in order to reduce liver toxicity, and therefore surgical morbidity, and to avoid a complete clinical response, difficult to trace intraoperatively. In most patients receiving chemotherapy, a complete response on CT scan does not mean cure (Benoist et al. 2006) due to the fact that in over 80% of the cases there are viable cancer cells in the initial site of the metastasis. Current management of these ghost lesions is to remove all of them if possible, considering the future liver remnant. In general, all the original sites of disease noted on the pre-therapy imaging need to be resected or ablated.

Since post-operative morbidity affects long-term survival (Laurent et al. 2003), length of chemotherapy treatment must be taken into account. In recent years more and more patients with stable long-term disease (more than 20 months) are considered for surgical treatment. Irinotecan and oxaliplatin have been associated with the development of steatohepatitis. Among patients receiving these drugs, the rates of complications and death after major liver resection are likely to be higher compared to patients not receiving chemotherapy, although this is not completely clear. Albeit systemic treatment is very effective in reducing tumour burden and facilitates the surgical therapy in previously unresectable patients, the recurrence rate is high because of the presence of residual microscopic disease.

5.2 Portal vein embolization

Based on objective date, consensus has been reached on what is an adequate liver remnant and what are the "safe" resection percentages depending on the quality and health of the liver (Zorzi et al. 2007). Figure 2.

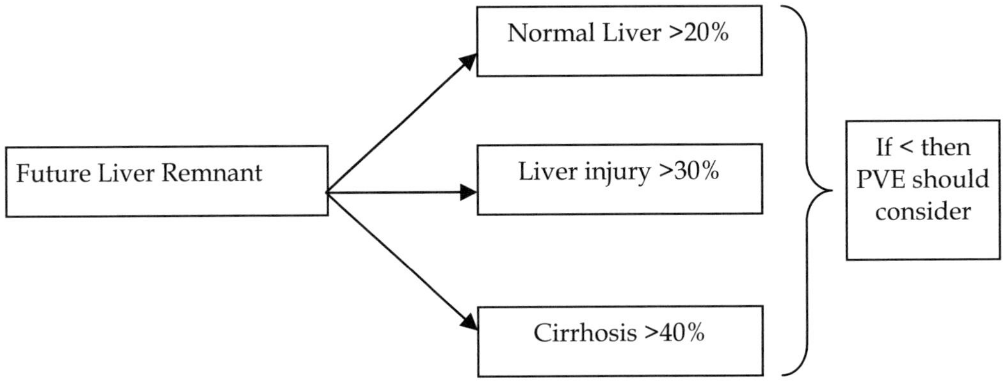

Fig. 2. Minimum FLR volume needed for safe liver resection in patients with normal, intermediate disease or cirrhotic liver (Zorzi et al. 2007).

When the future liver remnant (FLR) is insufficient PVE should be considered. PVE also constitutes a dynamic pre-operative test on the capacity of the liver to respond to the surgical aggression. If a hypertrophy greater than 5% is achieved after PVE, there is a low risk of a terrible post-operative liver insufficiency (Ribero et al. 2007). Chemotherapy does not seem to affect the hypertrophy induced by PVE. A few studies using bevazucimab recommend a 6 week waiting period between the last dose and the hepatectomy, although its influence on the hypertrophy is unclear.

PVE is well tolerated with minimum side effects such as fever, nausea, and transient abnormality of liver function test. The complication rate is below 5% (Abdallah et al. 2001). Azoulay et al. reported that PVE increased the feasibility of liver resection by 19% and that the actuarial survival rate was 40% at 5 years, similar to that of patients resected without PVE (Azoulay et al. 2000).

5.3 Two-stage hepatectomy

Two-stage hepatectomy is one of the methods to increase the resectability of liver tumours. Its objective is to eliminate the entire tumour burden. The first stage can also be performed together with laparoscopic colorectal resection. It consists of combining two sequential and planned liver resections when it is impossible to resect all liver metastases in a single procedure, while preserving at least 30% of functional liver volume to avoid post-operative liver failure. Frequently, it is associated with peri-operative systemic chemotherapy and PVE, although it is not a rule (Jaeck et al. 2004) (Figure 3).

The first hepatectomy attempts to resect the majority of liver tumours and to get hypertrophy of the remnant liver with or without PVE. The second hepatectomy is performed at least 4 weeks later to allow time for growth and hypertrophy of the FLR. The design of the technique must be meticulous well in advance of the first resection as an important strategy to achieve complete removal, admitting that around 30% of patients will not be rescued on the second hepatectomy.

Usually, on the first hepatectomy the future remnant liver is cleared out of tumours with non-anatomic resections and/or radiofrequency ablation or at most a single segment resection. As mentioned, it can be associated to the removal of the primary colorectal tumour, preferably through a laparoscopic approach or using a "J" incision if it is located on the right colon. After 2 to 4 weeks after the clearance of the FRL, percutaneous PVE is performed. Alternatively, PVE can be done during the first hepatectomy through the ligation and alcoholization of the right portal vein, which is the side more often embolized. The second hepatectomy can be done on the fourth of fifth week after PVE, when an adequate hypertrophy of the non-embolized hemi-liver is achieved.

Some authors recommend pre-operative chemotherapy during the entire process. This should be determined by the criteria of the multidisciplinary team according to each individual case (Adam et al. 2000). We carry out this procedure by performing PVE in the first hepatectomy with or without the removal of the primary tumour. After a 4 week waiting period and a CT confirming an adequate FRL, a second hepatectomy is performed. If during the second stage hepatectomy new liver metastases or extrahepatic lesions are discovered, such as localized peritoneum implants, the procedure can still be performed if a R0 resection can be achieved. A recent series reports a 5 year overall survival rate of 32% for patients on whom the procedure had been completed (Narita et al. 2011).

Two factors affect the success of two-stage hepatectomy: patient selection and optimal chemotherapy regimen. This procedure may be the only therapy able to provide long-term survival and a possible cure for patients with initially unresectable multiple and bilobar CRC liver metastases.

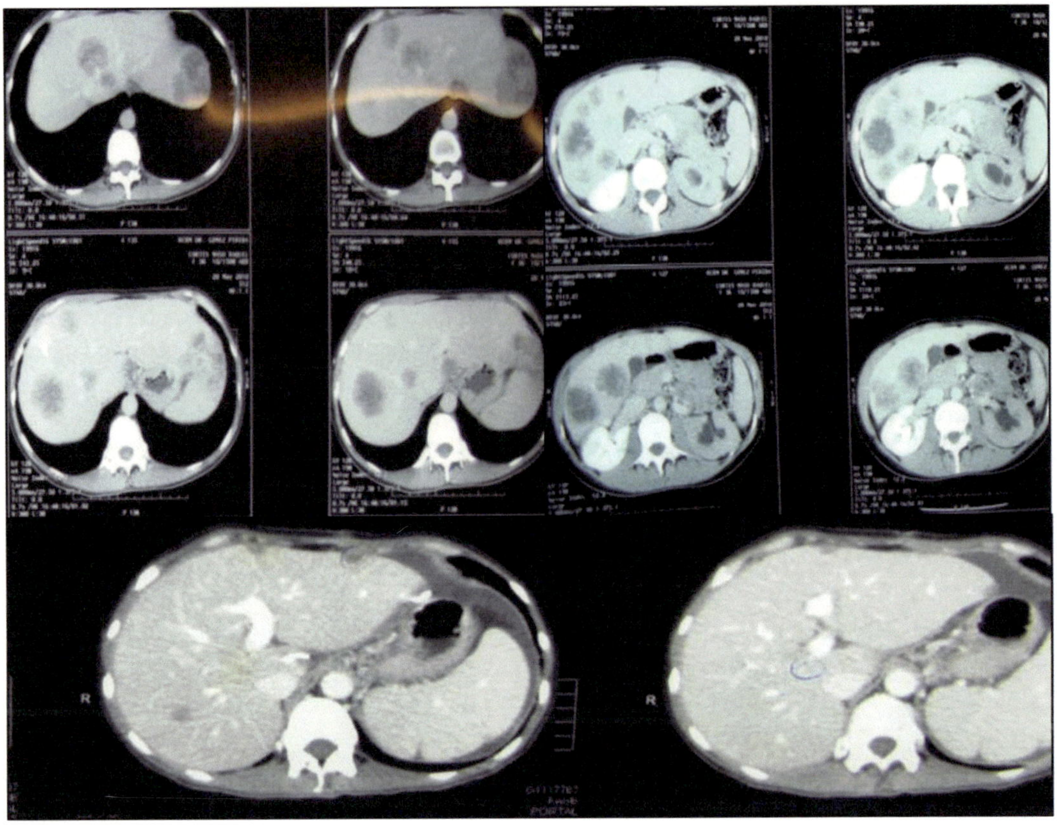

Fig. 3. Multiple and bilobar metastases, right hydronephrosis and rectum cancer involving the right ovarium in a 37 year old woman. After chemotherapy treatment, first stage surgery consisted of tumour clearance of the left liver, anterior colorectal resection, right oophorectomy and right PVE (lower pictures). Five weeks later an extended right hepatectomy was performed.

5.4 Synchronicity: Colorectal tumour and liver metastases

On the international registry of liver metastasis from CRC, LiverMet Survey, a 51.7% of synchronicity has been recorded in January 2011 (table 1). This frequent sort of presentation, together with the expansion of the criteria of resectability and the laparoscopic approach for the colorectal and liver surgery, have created a new insight within the multidisciplinary teams.

Sinc/Metac	Number of patients	1 year	3 year	5 year	10 year
Sincronic	6112	90%	58%	39%	22%
Metacronic	5724	90%	60%	43%	26%

Table 1. LiverMet Survey, January 2011. Survival rates in 11836 patients after hepatectomy (with permission).

As mentioned, colon resection can be done on the first stage, or a liver approach can be done first after a downstaging of the liver tumour/tumours. What should be done first depends on the primary tumour (mainly in cases of rectal cancer that require an ultralow resection or are T3 or T4) and on the volume of liver parenchyma that needs to be removed. If the patient has been downstaged to resectability, the liver should be approached first (if possible) and the colorectal tumour should be operated 4 to 6 weeks later (Figure 4).

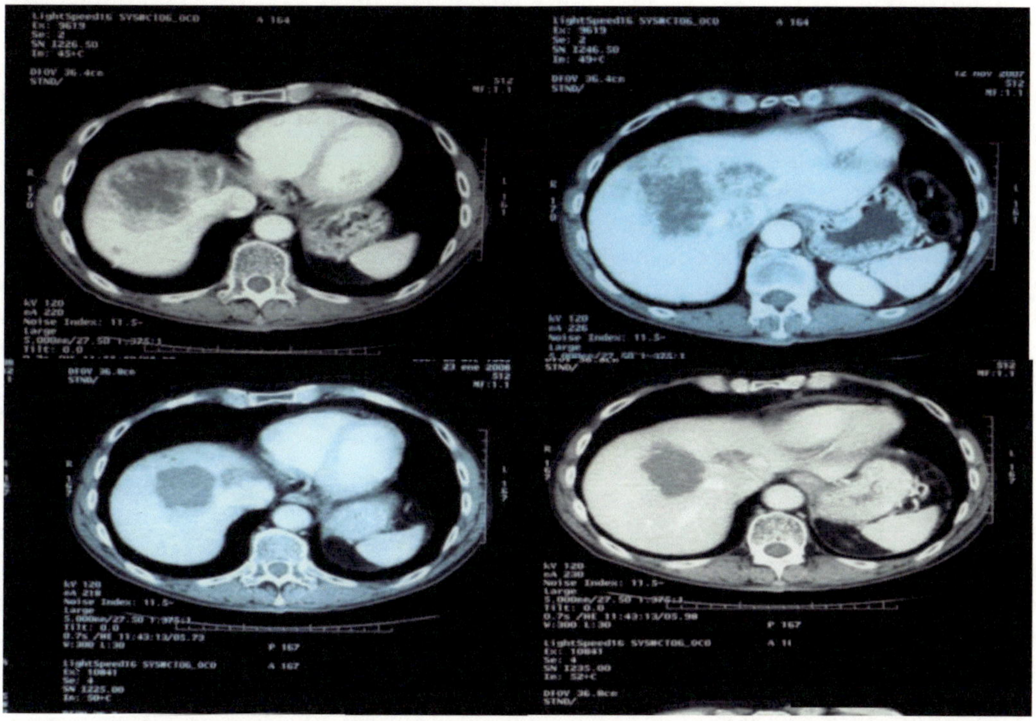

Fig. 4. Large liver metastasis involving the three hepatic veins (upper pictures) in a 61 year old patient with rectal cancer. After 3 months of chemotherapy (lower pictures) the patient underwent left hepatectomy, segment (Sg) 1 and Sg 8 segmentectomies and right hepatic vein reconstruction. Six weeks later the rectal cancer was resected.

5.5 Ante-situ, in-situ and ex-situ procedures: Extreme liver surgery

Liver transplantation has brought with it advances in techniques that can be applied to nontransplant hepatic surgery. The lessons learned from reducing adult-sized livers for implantation in children, living related donor liver transplantation and split liver transplantation can all be applied in the nontransplant setting. Tumours that were considered unresectable with standard techniques can now be considered for resection using in-situ, ante-situ and ex vivo or bench liver surgery. In the last technique, the liver is completely removed from the patient and perfused with preservation solution. A bloodless transection of hepatic parenchyma can then be performed allowing complex reconstruction of hepatic veins or portal structures after which the liver is reimplanted in the patient. The ex vivo technique was first performed by Pichlmayr and colleagues in 1988 and has been applied sparingly in selected patients since then (Hemming et al. 2000).

The common basis for in-situ, ante-situ and ex-situ resection is the total vascular exclusion (TVE) of the liver, and the perfusion of the organ by preservation hypothermic solution.

The principles are the same for the three techniques, which differ only in the extent to which liver is mobilized from its vascular connections, hylum and caval vein. Generally, a veno-venous bypass is used to avoid venous congestion during prolonged caval and portal crossclamping and a hypothermic preservation solution is instilled through the portal vein (Fortner et al. 1978). In a study population about liver resection under TVE, Azoulay et al. concluded that standard TVE of any duration with hypothermic perfusion of the liver, in this issue in-situ procedure, was associated with a better tolerance to ischemia. Furthermore, compared with TVE ≥ 60 minutes, it was associated with better post-operative liver and renal functions and lower morbidity (Azoulay et al. 2005). The main indications of the three techniques are tumours that involve vascular structures of the hylum, venous confluence or inferior vena cava (IVC), or are in close proximity to them. The technique can be used for benign, primary or metastatic tumours. The decision about what technique to use depends on the tumour location and its relationship with the three hepatic veins and caval vein. It is important to notice that the ex-situ technique is losing support due to its high morbidity and mortality. The location of the lesion or lesions in or near the suprahepatic IVC represents a true challenge due to the impossibility of using conventional resection techniques. Furthermore, optimal peri-operative anaesthetic management is crucial in this setting, and the anaesthesia team should be familiar with the hepatic transplant procedure.

The involvement of the inferior vena cava does not necessarily preclude resection (Figure 5). Liver resection with reconstruction of the IVC can be performed in selected cases. The resected IVC may then be replaced with an autogenous vein graft or a prosthetic material. The mortality rate of resection IVC is 4.5-25% and morbidity up to 40% (Azoulay et al. 2005). The increased risk associated with the procedure appears to be balanced by the possible benefits, particularly when the lack of alternative approaches is considered (Hemming et al. 2004).

In conclusion, liver resections, due to the adoption of several advanced techniques, such as vascular exclusion, veno-venous bypass, hypothermic perfusion of the liver (in-situ, ante-situ or ex-situ), have become more common and, when IVC is involved, resection of the vein is no longer considered a contraindication.

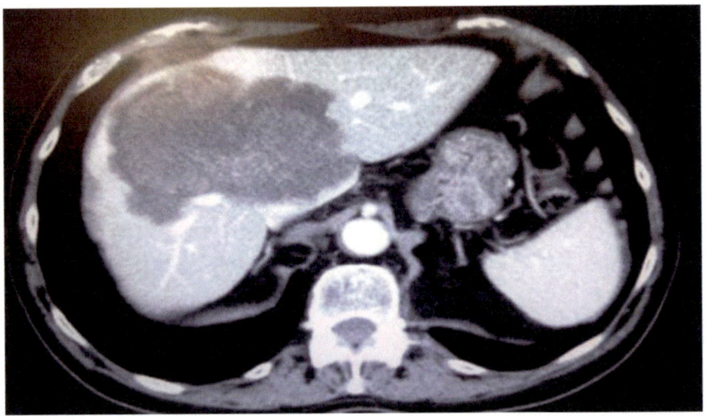

Fig. 5. Huge liver metastasis in a 64 year old patient with colon cancer. First surgery was an extended right hepatectomy plus Sg 1 segmentectomy, after PVE of right and Sg 4 portal veins. A left hemicolectomy was performed 7 weeks later.

6. Repeat resections

The first large series of liver resections for secondary tumours was reported in 1978 (Foster 1978). By improvement in surgical techniques, peri-operative patient's care and management of complications, the morbidity and mortality associated with liver resection were reduced. This has been a very important factor to increase the aggressiveness of the surgical approach.

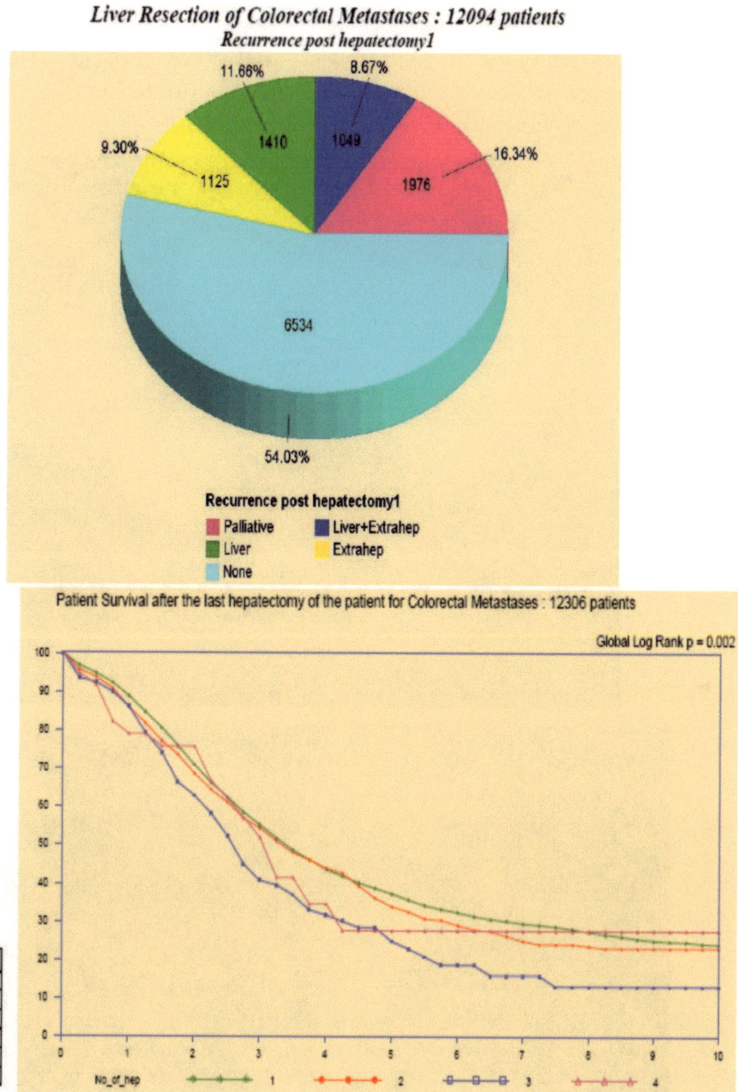

Details : Log rank p

		proba
1	2	0.086
1	3	0.0004
1	4	0.65
2	3	0.012
2	4	0.8
3	4	0.35

Survival %

No_of_hep	1 yr	2 yrs	3 yrs	4 yrs	5 yrs	6 yrs	7 yrs	8 yrs	9 yrs	10 yrs
1	89%	71%	55%	44%	37%	32%	30%	27%	25%	24%
2	86%	69%	54%	44%	34%	29%	25%	24%	23%	23%
3	86%	63%	41%	32%	25%	19%	16%	13%	13%	13%
4	79%	76%	52%	35%	28%	28%	28%	28%	28%	28%

Fig. 6. LiverMet database, with permission.

Liver recurrence of CRC is common (Figure 6) but only 5-27% of the patients are candidates for potentially curative repeated hepatectomy. About 70% of recurrences will be observed within the first 12 months after resection and 92% will be apparent within 24 months (Langenhoff et al. 2009). In medically fit patients, repeat hepatectomy has emerged as a safe and effective procedure under the same criteria of selection of the first hepatectomy. Although the prognostic variables provide rough indicators of prognosis, they should not be used as absolute contraindications to surgery. The multidisciplinary team should plan the strategy individually. Each new re-hepatectomy needs a particular and specific evaluation: disease-free interval, number of metastases, quality of life, general health condition, resectable extrahepatic disease, assessment of residual liver volume, etc. by the multidisciplinary team (Figure 7).

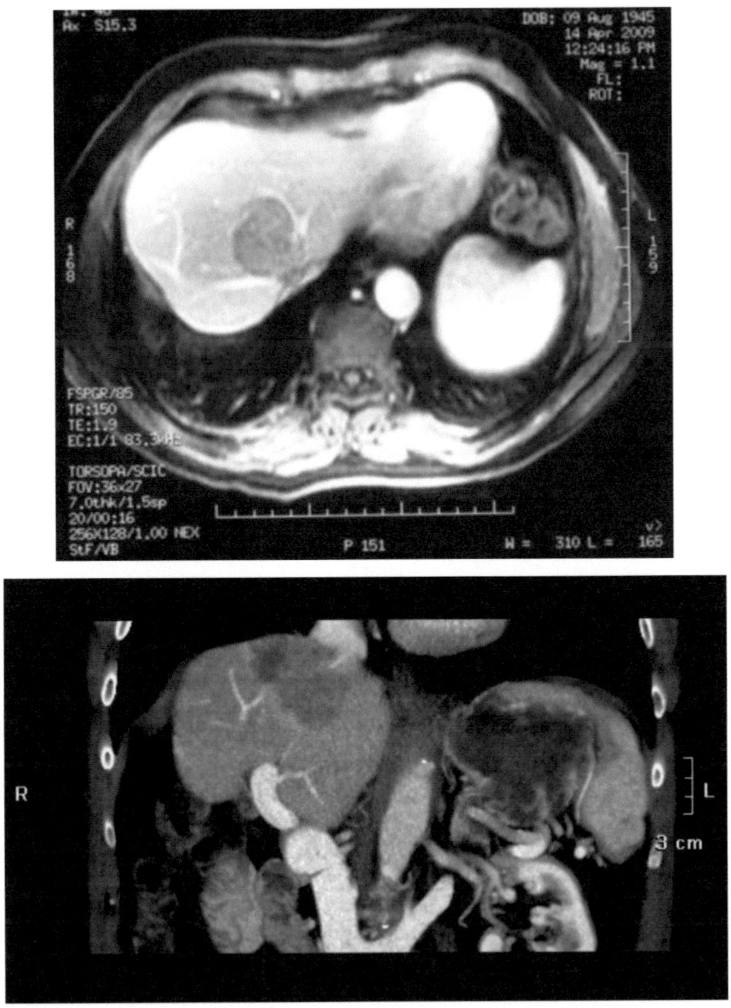

Fig. 7. A 63 year old patient with right hepatectomy plus Sg 4a resection; 24 months later a recurrence involving the only hepatic vein (left hepatic vein) appeared. Tumour was removed and the left hepatic vein was reimplanted in the caval vein using graft prosthesis (less than 60 minutes of total vascular exclusion).

The LiverMet Survey includes 12448 liver resections of which 14.5% are repeated hepatectomies (Figure 8, Table 2). Patients likely to benefit of this approach represent a small and highly selected group. Maybe, an accurate genetic, immunohistochemical and histological profile of the patient's tumour will be able to conclude who will benefit from this aggressive treatment.

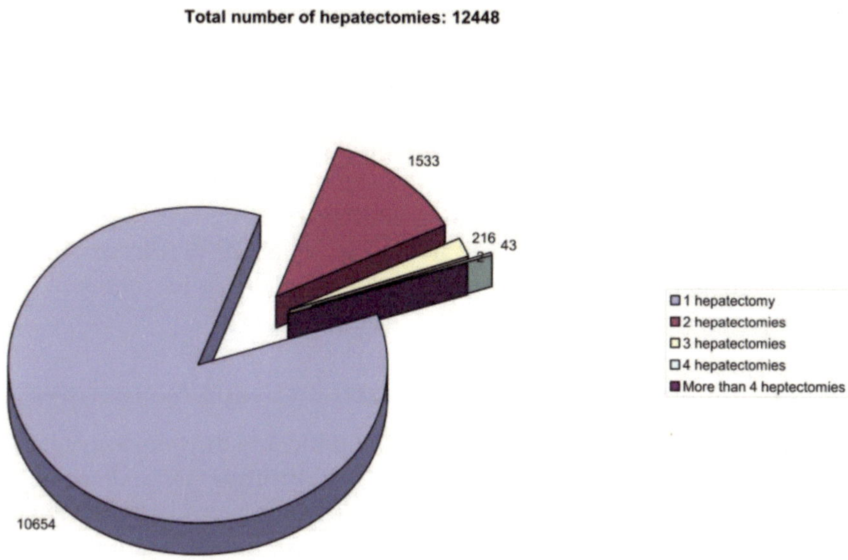

Fig. 8. LiverMet Survey: number of hepatectomies.

Repeat hepatectomies	Patients	% over initial resection	3-years SV	5-years SV
LiverMetsurvey (2011)	1794	15	58	37
Adam et al. (2003)	199	32	54	35
Fernandez - Trigo et al. (1995)	170	No reported		28
Petrowsky et al. (2002)	126	8	51	34
Nordlinger et al. (1994)	116	6	33	
Ishiguro et al. (2006)	111	No reported	74	41
Thelen et al. (2007)	94	12	55	38
Yamamoto et al. (1999)	75	21	48	31
Shaw et al. (2006)	66	9	68	44
Adam et al. (1997)	64	26	60	41
Yan, et al. (2007)	55	14		49
Nishio et al. (2007)	54	10	53	46

Table 2. Repeat hepatectomies series and survival rates.

Recurrence after repeat hepatectomy has been reported in 60–80% of patients (Smith & McCall 2009). A few have resectable disease limited to the liver and may be candidates for a third or even fourth hepatic resection. In our group there are two patients with five hepatectomies. Reports of large repeated hepatectomy series show that 9-30% of patients who underwent a second hepatectomy for colorectal liver metastases had a third resection (Fong et al 1999; Söreide et al. 2008; Yamamoto et al. 1999; Petrowsky et al. 2002) and 4% of them had a fourth resection (Adam et al. 2003; Yamamoto et al. 1999). The safety of multiple repeated hepatic resections has been demonstrated in recent reports, and long-term survivors have been documented (Adam et al. 2003; Nordlinger et al, 1994; Yamamoto et al. 1999; Petroswsky et al. 2002). LiverMet Survey published the largest series (n = 251) of third hepatectomies for recurrent CRC liver metastases with a survival benefit of 29% at 5 years. Adam et al. published a large series of patients who underwent a third liver resection with zero mortality and a morbidity rate of 5%, not significantly different from those who have had only one or two liver resections. In addition, patients with a third liver resection had a survival benefit of 32–38% at 5 years (Adam et al. 2003; Yamamoto et al. 1999). Major hepatectomy is possible in a minority of these patients, who represent a small and highly selected group (Petrowsky et al. 2002).

7. Inmunohistochemical markers based on tissue microarrays

The ideal marker predictor of outcome should include the following characteristics: of low cost and easy measure, reproducibility across institutions, and measurable both before and after treatment. Most importantly, this factor would predict major differences in outcome that significantly impact treatment. A clinical example is K-ras status as a predictor of response to therapy with cetuximab, a monoclonal antibody against the EGFR. In a prospective randomized controlled trial, patients with advanced CRC were randomized to receive treatment with or without cetuximab. When stratified for K-ras status, patients with wild type K-ras tumours demonstrated a significant survival advantage compared to those with mutated K-ras tumours, who derived no benefit from the agent. Therefore, patients with mutated K-ras do not receive cetuximab therapy and are spared the toxicity associated with a treatment with no proven benefit. To date, there is no specific clinical risk score or biomarker that specifically prognosticates or guides therapy for patients with resectable CRC liver metastases to this degree. This marker may combine the immunohistochemical markers of cell proliferation and cell cycle control, p53 and Ki67.

Surface antigen CD133 is a cell membrane glycoprotein that is considered as a cell surface marker expressed in stem cells of hematopoietic immature cells, but not in mature blood cells. CD133 has also been shown to be a marker of immature neuronal stem cells (Karoui et al. 2006). Two antibodies, CD133/1 or AC133 and CD133/2 (AC141), recognize it. CD133+ cells in colon cancer are helpful markers for detection of tumour initiating cells (Karoui et al. 2006) (Figure 9).

CD44 is considered as a cell membrane marker or epithelial cell adhesion molecule (*EpCAM*). Its phenotype $EpCAM^{high}$-$CD44^{+}$ is becoming established as a good marker for immature stem cells of human colon mucosa in certain series (Ieta et al. 2008) (Figure 10).

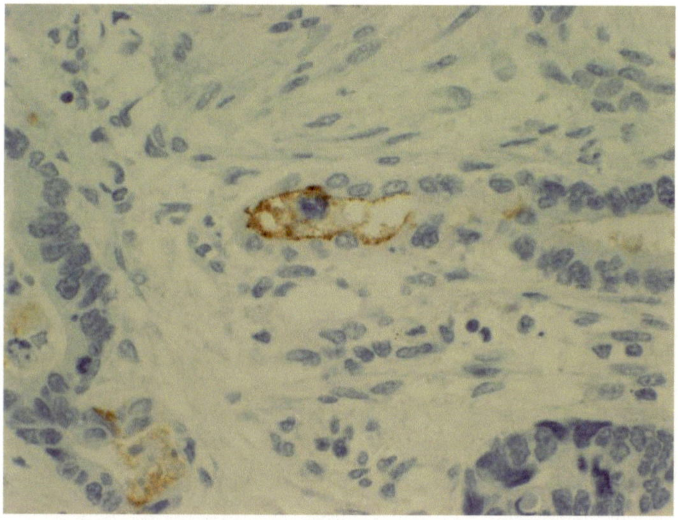

Fig. 9. Immunohistochemical pathological study. Positive membrane staining for stem cell markers CD133, CS-130127, CD133 (32AT1672) in most cells of metastatic adenocarcinoma. Santa Cruz Biotechnology®, Inc (x100).

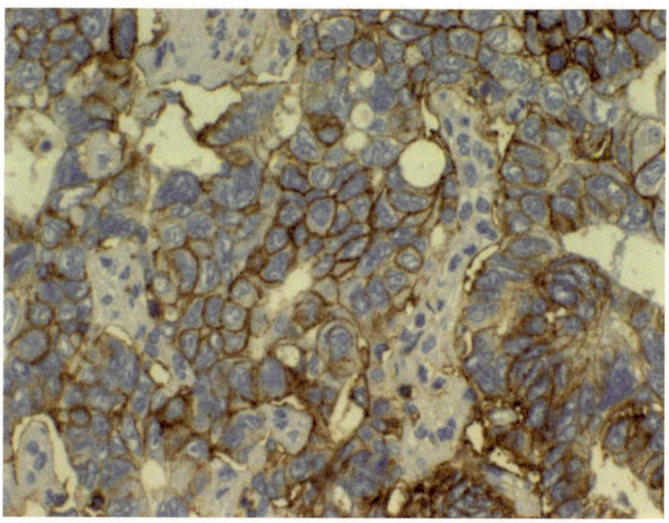

Fig. 10. Immunohistochemical pathological study. Positive membrane staining for stem cell markers CD44, *EpCAM*^{high}-CD44^{+} in most cells of metastatic adenocarcinoma. Santa Cruz Biotechnology®, Inc (x400).

CD166 is considered as a marker for both cell membrane or epithelial cell adhesion molecule (*EpCAM)* and cytoplasm (Figure 11). It is a marker of mesenchymal stem cells whose role in carcinogenesis is not fully clear (Ieta et al. 2008). Its phenotype *EpCAM*^{high}-CD166^{+} added to *EpCAM*^{high}-CD44^{+} is starting to be considered as an additional marker of immature stem cells in human colon mucosa (Dalerba et al. 2007).

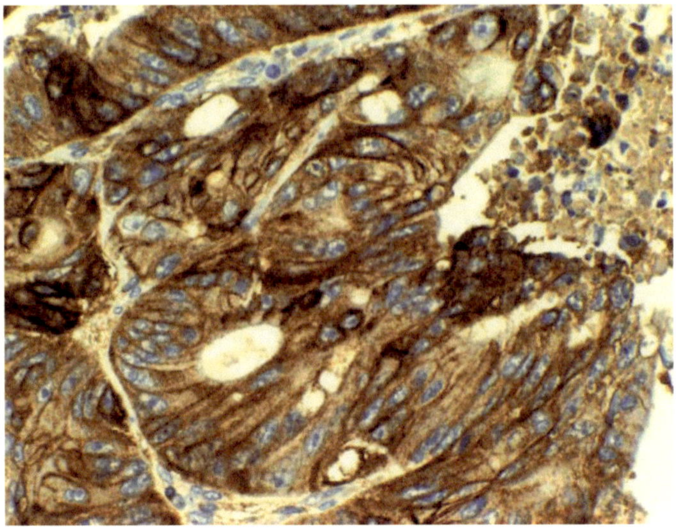

Fig. 11. Immunohistochemical pathological study. Positive membrane staining for stem cell markers CD166, 35264, CD166 LYO 1 mL *EpCAM*^{high}-CD166^{+} in most cells of metastatic adenocarcinoma. Menarini Diagnostics® (x40).

Borrego et al. (2010) analyzed, as did Kokudo et al. (2002), p53 expression. The immunohistochemical markers tested in their study (p53, Ki-67) were not poor prognostic factors, in agreement with Saw et al. (2002). By contrast, authors such as Tanaka et al. 2004 reported that p53 or Ki-67 expression had a negative impact on survival. It should be noticed, however, that in Borrego-Estella et al.'s study survival was longer than 5 years in patients with high Ki-67 levels and in those with a high mitotic index (>10 mitosis/mm^2), which is also another expression of the tumour proliferation index. However, no significant relationship was found between cell proliferation, as measured by Ki-67 and p53, whose changes express a loss of cell cycle control, and survival.

For O'Brien et al. (2007), most CD133+ stem cells had a 200-fold greater oncogenic potential than CD133- cells for development of CRC. In addition, this subpopulation is able to maintain itself and to differentiate and become established again as a tumour when transplanted in certain solid organs of experimental animals. For Borrego-Estella et al. significant trends were found in their series with regard to membrane CD133 and CD166 markers. According to O'Brien et al. and Ricci-Vitiani et al. 2007, in several CRC, CD44 was more determinant than CD133, because CD44 was expressed in tumour lines not expressing CD133.

To compare the results of Borrego et al. with other groups is difficult since many authors (Fong et al. 1999; Pawlik et al. 2005) did not performed immunohistochemical studies. However, regarding immunohistochemical markers, more significant results were not achieved probably because the only technique performed was immunohistochemistry array, but not flow cytometry or other molecular biology techniques.

Another interesting marker, microsatellite instability, is a measure of the inability of the DNA mismatch repair system to correct errors that occur during DNA replication. It is the alternative pathway to chromosomal instability with loss of heterozygosity in colorectal carcinogenesis. Microsatellite instability has been suggested to be prognostic for survival and predictive for response to therapy in patients with colorectal cancer.

In conclusion, many studies have analyzed pre-operative prognostic factors in patients undergoing liver resection for hepatic metastases from CRC in order to select patients for surgery. However, intraoperative and post-operative factors have been poorly analyzed. Future studies should establish post-operative prognostic factors through histological and immunohistochemical tests based on the tissue microarray technique.

8. References

Abdalla EK., Adam R., Bilchik AJ., Jaeck D., Vauthey JN., Mahvi R. (2006). Improving Resectability of Hepatic Colorectal Metastases: Expert Consensus Statement. *Annals of Surgical Oncology*, 13(10): 1271-1280

Abdallah EK., Hicks ME., Vauthey JN. (2001) Portal vein embolization: rationale, technique and future prospects. *Br J Surg* 88: 165-175

Adam R., Laurent A., Azoulay D., Castaing D., Bismuth H. (2000). Two-stage hepatectomy: a planned strategy to treat unresectable liver tumour. *Ann Surg* 232: 777-785

Adam R., Bismuth H., Castaing D., Waechter F., Navarro F., Abascal A., Majno P., Engerran L. (1997) Repeat hepatectomy for colorectal liver metastases. *Ann Surg* 225: 51 -60

Adam R., Pascal G., Azoulay D., Tanaka K., Castaing D., Bismuth H. (2003) Liver resection for colorectal metastases: the third hepatectomy. Ann Surg 238: 871 - 83

Adam R., de Haas RJ., Wicherts DA., Aloia TA., Delvart V., Azoulay D., Bismuth H., Castaing D. (2008) Is hepatic resection justified after chemotherapy in patients with colorectal liver metastases and lymph node involvement? *J Clin Oncol* 26(22): 3672-80

Adam R., Delvart V., Pascal G., Castaing D., Azoulay D., Giacchetti S., Paule B., Kunstlinger F., Ghémard O., Levi F., Bismuth H. (2004) Rescue surgery for unresectable colorectal liver metastases downstaged by chemotherapy: a model to predict long-term survival. *Ann Surg* 240:644-657

Adam R., Pascal G., Castaing D., Azoulay D., Delvart V., Paule B., Levi F., Bismuth H. (2004) Tumour progression while on chemotherapy: a contraindication to liver resection for multiple colorectal metastases? *Ann Surg* 240:1052-1061.

Adam R., Lucidi V., Bismuth H. (2004) Hepatic colorectal metastases: methods of improving resectability. *Surg Clin N Am* 84 659–671

Al-Hajj M., Wicha MS., Benito-Hernandez A., Morrison SJ., Clarke MF. (2003) Prospective identification of tumourigenic breast cancer cells. *Proc Natl Acad Sci USA*; 100:3983-3988

Altendorf-Hofmann A., Scheele J. (2003) A critical review of the major indicators of prognosis after resection of hepatic metastases from colorectal carcinoma. *Surg Oncol Clin N Am* 12: 165–192

Artigas V., Marín Hargreaves G., Marcuello E., Pey A., González JA., Rodríguez M., Moral A., Monill JM., Sancho J., Pericay C., Trías M. (2007) Surgical resection of liver metastases from colorectal carcinoma. Experience in Sant Pau Hospital. *Cir Esp* 81: 339-44

Azoulay D., Castaing D., Smail A., Adam R., Cailliez V., Laurent A., Lemoine A., Bismuth H. (2000). Resection of non-resectable liver metastases from colorectal cancer after percutaneous portal vein embolization. *Ann Surg* 4: 480-486

Azoulay D., Eshkenazy R., Andreani P. Castaing D., Adam R., Ichai P., Naili S., Vinet E., Saliba F., Lemoine A., Gillon MC., Bismuth H. (2005). In situ hypothermic perfusion of the liver versus standard total vascular exclusion of complex liver resection. *Ann Surg* 241: 277-285

Battifora H. (1986) The multitumour (sausage) tissue block: novel method for immunochemical antibody testing. *Lab Invest* 55:244-8

Belli G., D'Agostino A., Ciciliano F., Fantini C., Russolillo N., Belli A . (2002) Liver resection for hepatic metastases: 15 years of experience. *J Hepatobiliary Pancreat Surg* 9 (5): 607 - 613

Benoist S., Brouquet A., Penna C., Julié C., El Hajjam M., Chagnon S., Mitry E., Rougier P., Nordlinger B. (2006) Complete response of colorectal liver metastases after chemotherapy: does it mean cure? J Clin Oncol 20;24(24):3939-45

Bipat S., van Leeuwen MS., Comans EF., Pijl ME., Bossuyt PM., Zwinderman AH., Stoker J. (2005). Colorectal liver metastases: CT, MR imaging, and PET for diagnosis-meta-analysis. *Radiology* 237: 123-31

Bipat S., van Leeuwen MS., IJzermans JNM., Comans EFI., Planting AST., Bossuyt PMM., Greve J-W., Stoker J. (2007) Evidence-based guideline on management of colorectal liver metastases in the Netherlands. *Ned J Med* 63(1): 1-14

Bismuth, H. (1982) Surgical anatomy and anatomical surgery of the liver. *World J Surg* 6: 3-9, ISSN 0364-2313

Bluemke DA., Paulson EK., Choti MA., DeSena S., Clavien PA. (2000) Detection of Hepatic Lesions in Candidates for Surgery: Comparison of Ferumoxides-Enhanced MR Imaging and Dual-Phase Helical CT. *AJR* 175: 1653–1658

Bonnet D., Dick J. (1997) Human acute myeloid leukemia is organized as a hierarchy that originates from a primitive hematopoietic cell. *Nature Medicine* 3:730-737

Borrego V., Serrablo A., Hörndler C. (2010). Study of liver metastases of colorectal cancer with surgical rescue. Identification of prognostic biological markers. University of Salamanca Editions. Collection VITOR. 1st Ed. pp. 243-248. ISBN: 978-84-7800-205-4.

Casanova D., Figueras J., Pardo F. (2004) Metástasis hepáticas. In: Guía Clínica de la Asociación Española de Cirugía: Cirugía hepática. Arán, Madrid; pp 164-76.

Cellini C., Hunt SR., Fleshman JW., Birnbaum EH., Bierhals AJ., Mutch MG. (2010) Stage IV rectal cancer with liver metastases: is there a benefit to resection of the primary tumour? *World J Surg* 34(5): 110

Chami L., Lassau N., Malka D., Ducreux M., Bidault S., Roche A., Elias D. (2008). Benefits of Contrast-Enhanced Sonography for the Detection of Liver Lesions: Comparison with Histologic Findings. *AJR* 190: 683–690

Charnsangavej C, Clary B, Fong Y., Grothey A., Pawlik TM., Choti MA. (2006). Selection of patients for resection of hepatic colorectal metastases: expert consensus statement. *Ann Surg Oncol* 13 (10): 1261-1268.

Choti M., Sitzmann J., Tiburi ME., Sumetchotimetha W., Rangsin R., Schulick RD., Lillemoe KD., Yeo CJ., Cameron JL. (2002). Trends in long term survival following liver resection for hepatic colorectal metastases. *Ann Surg* 235: 759-66.

Coenegrachts K., De Geeter F., ter Beek L., Walgraeve N., Bipat S., Stoker J., Rigauts H. (2009). Comparison of MRI (including SS SE-EPI and SPIO-enhanced MRI) and FDG-PET/CT for the detection of colorectal liver metastases. *Eur Radiol* 19(2): 370-379

Couinaud C (1957). Le Foie, Études Anatomiques et Chirurgicales. Masson

Dalerba P., Cho RW., Clarke MF. (2007) Cancer stem cells and tumour metastasis: first steps into uncharted territory. *Ann Rev Med* 58:267-284.

de Haas R J., Wicherts DA., Andreani P., Pascal G., Saliba F., Ichai P., Adam R., Castaing D., Azoulay D. (2011) Impact of Expanding Criteria for Resectability of Colorectal Metastases on Short- and Long-Term Outcomes After Hepatic Resection. *Ann Surg* 253(6): 1069–1079

Doan P L., Vauthey JN., Palavecino M., Morse MA. (2010) Colorectal Liver Metastases. In: *Malignant Liver Tumours. Current and Emerging Therapies.* Clavien PA, Breitenstein S (Ed), pp. 342-6, Wiley-Blackwell

Donadon M., Ribero D., Morris-Stiff G., Abdalla EK., Vauthey JN. (2007) New Paradigm in the Management of Liver-Only Metastases From Colorectal Cancer. *Gastrointest Cancer Res* 1(1): 20-27

El Khodary M., Milot L., Reinhold C. (2011) Imaging of Hepatic Metastases. In: *Liver Metastasis: Biology and Clinical Management.* Brodt P (Ed), pp. 307-353, Springer Science+Business Media B.V., ISBN 978-94-007-0291-2, New York

Elias D., Liberale G., Vernerey D., Pocard M., Ducreux M., Boige V., Malka D., Pignon JP., Lasser P. (2005) Hepatic and extrahepatic colorectal metastases: when resectable, their localization does not matter, but their total number has a prognostic effect. *Ann Surg Oncol* 12: 900-909.

Elias D., Ouellet JF., Bellon N. (2003) Extrahepatic disease does not contraindicate hepatectomy for colorectal liver metastases. *Br J Surg* 90: 567-574.

Fernandez-Trigo V., Shamsa F., Sugarbaker PH.. (1995) Repeat liver resections from colorectal metastasis. Repeat Hepatic Metastases Registry. *Surgery* 117: 296–304

Fernandez FG., Drebin JA., Linehan DC., Dehdashti F., Siegel BA., Strasberg SM. (2004) Five-year survival after resection of hepatic metastases from colorectal cancer in patients screened by positron emission tomography with F-18 fluorodeoxyglucose (FDG-PET). *Ann Surg* 240(3): 438-50

Figueras J., Burdio F., Ramos E., Torras J., Llado L., Lopez-Ben S., Codina-Barreras A., Mojal S. (2007). Effect of subcentimeter nonpositive resection margin on hepatic recurrence in patients undergoing hepatectomy for colorectal liver metastases. Evidences from 663 liver resections. *Annals of Oncology* 18: 1190–1195

Fioole B., de Haas RJ., Wicherts DA., Elias SG., Scheffers JM., van Hillegersberg R., van Leeuwen MS., Borel Rinkes IH. (2008) Additional value of contrast enhanced intraoperative ultrasound for colorectal liver metastases.. *Eur J Radiol* 67(1): 169-7

Fong Y., Fortner J., Sun RL., Brennan MF., Blumgart LH. (1999) Clinical score for predicting recurrence after hepatic resection metastatic colorectal cancer: analysis of 1001 consecutive cases. *Ann Surg* 230:309-18.

Fortner JG., Kim DK., MacLean BJ., Barrett MK., Iwatsuki S., Turnbull AD., Howland WS., Beattie EJ Jr. (1978). Major hepatic resection for neoplasia: personal experience in 108 patients. *Ann Surg* 188: 363-371

Foster JH. (1978) Survival after liver resection for secondary tumours. *Am J Surg* 135: 389-394

Fusai G., Dadvison BR. (2003) Strategies to increase the resectability of liver metastases from colorectal cancer. *Cancer* 20: 431-496.

Galli R., Binda E., Orfanelli U., Cipelletti B., Gritti A., De Vitis S., Fiocco R., Foroni C., Dimeco F., Vescovi A. (2004) Isolation and characterization of tumourigenic, stem like neural precursors from human glioblastoma. *Cancer Res* 64:7011-7021.

Garden OJ., Rees M., Poston GJ., Mirza D., Saunders M., Ledermann J., Primrose JN., Parks RW. (2006). Guidelines for resection of colorectal cancer liver metastases. *Gut* 55 (Suppl 3): iii1–iii8

Guglielmi A., Pachera S., Ruzzenente A. Surgical Therapy of Hepatic Metastases. In: Delaini GG. Rectal Cancer: New Frontiers in Diagnosis, Treatment and Rehabilitation. © Springer-Verlag Milan 2005

Harmantas A., Rotstein LE., Langer B. (1996) Regional versus systemic chemotherapy in the treatment of colorectal carcinoma metastatic to the liver. Is there a survival difference? Metanalysis of the published literature. *Cancer* 78: 1639-45. PMID: 8859174.

Hemming AW., Chari RS., Cattral MS. (2000). Ex vivo resection. *Can J Surg* 43(3): 222-224

Hemming AW., Reed AI., Langham MR Jr., Fujita S., Howard RJ. (2004) Combined Resection of the Liver and Inferior Vena Cava for Hepatic Malignancy. *Ann Surg* 239: 712–721

Hill RP. (2006) Identifying cancer stem cells in solid tumours: case not proven. *Cancer Res* 66: 1891-1895.

Hoti E., Salloum C., Azoulay D. (2011) Hepatic resection with in situ hypothermic perfusion is superior to other resection techniques. *Dig Sur*; 28(2): 94-9

Ieta K., Tanaka F., Haraguchi N., Kita Y., Sakashita H., Mimori K. (2008) Biological and genetic characteristics of tumour initiating cells in colon cancer. *Ann Sur Oncol* 15: 638-648.

Ishiguro S., Akasu T., Fujimoto Y., Yamamoto J., Sakamoto Y., Sano T., Shimada K., Kosuge T., Yamamoto S., Fujita S., Moriya Y. (2006) Second hepatectomy for recurrent colorectal liver metastasis: analysis of preoperative prognostic factors. *Ann Surg Oncol* 13: 1579 – 87

Jaeck D. (2003) The significance of hepatic pedicle lymph nodes metastases in surgical management of colorectal liver metastases and of other liver malignancies. *Ann Surg Oncol* 10: 1007–1011

Jaeck D., Oussoultzoglou E., Rosso E., Greget M., Weber JC., Bachellier P. (2004) Two-stage hepatectomy procedure combined with portal vein embolization to achieve curative resection for initially unresectable multiple and bilobar colorectal liver metastases. *Ann Surg* 240: 1037-1049.

Jordan CT., Guzman ML., Noble M. (2006) Cancer stem cells. *N Engl J Med* 355: 1253-1261.

Karoui M., Penna C., Amin-Hashem M., Mitry E., Benoist S., Franc B., Rougier P., Nordlinger B. (2006) Influence of preoperative chemotherapy on the risk of major hepatectomy for colorectal liver metastases. *Ann Surg* 243: 1-7.

Kinkel K., Lu Y., Both M., Warren RS., Thoeni RF. (2002) Detection of hepatic metastases from cancers of the gastrointestinal tract by using noninvasive imaging methods (US, CT, MR Imaging, PET): a meta-analysis. *Radiology* 224: 748-756

Koh DM., Scurr E., Collins DJ., Pirgon A., Kanber B., Karanjia N., Brown G., Leach MO., Husband JE. (2006) Colorectal hepatic metastases: quantitative measurements using single-shot echo-planar diffusion-weighted MR imaging. *Eur Radiol* 16: 1898–1905

Koike N., Cho A., Nasu K., Seto K., Nagaya S., Ohshima Y., Ohkohchi N. (2009) Role of diffusion-weighted magnetic resonance imaging in the differential diagnosis of focal hepatic lesions. *World J Gastroenterol* 14; 15(46): 5805-5812

Kokudo N., Miki Y., Sugai S., Yanagisawa A., Kato Y., Sakamoto Y., Yamamoto J., Yamaguchi T., Muto T., Makuuchi M. (2002). Genetic and histological assessment of surgical margins in resected liver metastases from colorectal carcinoma: minimum surgical margins for successful resection. *Arch Surg* 137: 833-40

Kong G., Jackson C., Koh D., Lewington V., Sharma B., Brown G., Cunningham D., Cook G. (2008) The use of 18F-FDG PET/CT in colorectal liver metastases-comparison with CT and liver MRI. *Eur J Nucl Med Mol Imaging* 35(7): 1323-1329

Kononen J., Bubendorf L., Kallioniemi A., Bärlund M., Schraml P., Leighton S., Torhorst J., Mihatsch MJ., Sauter G., Kallioniemi OP. (1998) Tissue microarrays for high-throughput molecular profiling of tumour specimens. *Nat Med* 4: 844-7.

Kopez S., Vauthey JN. (2008) Perioperative chemotherapy for resectable liver metastases. *Lancet* 22: 371(9617): 1007-16

Kronawitter U., Kemeny N., Heelan R., Fata F., Fong Y. (1999) Evaluation of chest computed tomography in the staging of patients with potentially resectable liver metastases from colorectal cancer. *Cancer* 86: 229-35

Laghi A., Sansoni I., Celestre M., Paolantonio P., Passariello R. (2005) Computed Tomography. In: Focal Liver Lesions Detection, Characterization, Ablation. Lencioni R, Cioni D, Bartolozzi C (Ed). Springer-Verlag Berlin Heidelberg

Langenhoff BS., Krabbe PF., Ruers TJ. (2009) Efficacy of follow-up after surgical treatment of colorectal liver metastases. *Eur J Surg Oncol* 35: 180-186

Larsen LPS. (2010) Role of contrast enhanced ultrasonography in the assessment of hepatic metastases: A review. *World J Hepatol* 27; 2(1): 8-15

Laurent C., Sa Cunha A., Couderc P., Rullier E., Saric J. (2003) Influence of postoperative morbidity on long-term survival following liver resection for colorectal metastases. *Br J Surg* 90(9): 1131-6

Leen E., Ceccotti P., Moug SJ., Glen P., MacQuarrie J., Angerson WJ., Albrecht T., Hohmann J., Oldenburg A., Ritz JP., Horgan PG. (2006) Potential value of contrast-enhanced intraoperative ultrasonography during partial hepatectomy for metastases: an essential investigation before resection? *Ann Surg* 243: 236-240

Li C., Heidt DG., Dalerba P., Burant CF., Zhang L., Adsay V., Wicha M., Clarke MF., Simeone DM. (2007) Identification of pancreatic cancer stem cells. *Cancer Res* 67: 1030-1037.

Lordan JT., Karanjia ND. (2007) Size of surgical margin does not influence recurrence rates after curative liver resection for colorectal cancer liver metastases. *Br J Surg* 94: 1133-1138

Lucey BC., Varghese J., Soto JA. (2006) Hepatic Disorders: Colorectal Cancer Metastases, Cirrhosis, and Hepatocellular Carcinoma. In: Evidence-Based Imaging. Medina LS, Blackmore CC. Springer Science+Business Media, Inc. New York

Marín C., Robles R., Pérez D., López A., Parrilla P. (2009) Prognostic factors after resection of colorectal cancer liver metastases. *Cir Esp* 85: 32-39

Mehrabi A., Fonouni H., Golriz M., Hofer S., Hafezi M., Rahbari NN., Weitz J., Büchler MW., Schmidt J. (2011) Hypothermic ante situm resection in tumours of the hepatocaval confluence. *Dig Surg* 28(2): 100-8

Milanes-Yearsley M., Hammond ME., Pajak TF., Cooper JS., Chang C., Griffin T., Nelson D., Laramore G., Pilepich M. (2002) Tissue microarray: a cost and time-effective method for correlative studies by regional and national cancer study groups. *Mod Pathol* 15: 1366-1373

Nakano H., Ishida Y., Hatakeyama T., Sakuraba K., Hayashi M., Sakurai O., Hataya K. (2008) Contrast-enhanced intraoperative ultrasonography equipped with late

Kupffer-phase image obtained by sonazoid in patients with colorectal liver metastases. *World J Gastroenterol* 28; 14(20): 3207-3211

Narita M., Oussoultzoglou E., Jaeck D., Fuchschuber P., Rosso E., Pessaux P., Marzano E., Bachellier P. (2011) Two-stage hepatectomy for multiple bilobar colorectal liver metastases. *Br J Surg* 98(10): 1463-75

Niekel MC., Bipat Sh., Stoker J. (2010) Diagnostic Imaging of Colorectal Liver Metastases with CT, MR Imaging, FDG PET, and/or FDG PET/CT: A Meta-Analysis of Prospective Studies Including Patients Who Have Not Previously Undergone Treatment. *Radiology* 257(3): 674-684

Nishio H., Hamady ZZ., Malik HZ., Fenwick S., Rajendra Prasad K., Toogood GJ., Lodge JP. (2007) Outcome following repeat liver resection for colorectal liver metastases. *Eur J Surg Oncol* 33: 729–34

Nomura K., Kadoya M., Ueda K., Fujinaga Y., Miwa S., Miyagawa S. (2007) Detection of Hepatic Metastases From Colorectal Carcinoma: Comparison of Histopathologic Features of Anatomically Resected Liver With Results of Pre-operative Imaging. *J Clin Gastroenterol* 41(8)789-95

Nordlinger B., Vaillant JC., Guiguet M., Balladur P., Paris F., Bachellier P., Jaeck D. (1994) Survival benefit of repeat liver resections for recurrent colorectal metastases: 143 cases. Association Francaise de Chirurgie. *J Clin Oncol* 12 :1491-6

Nordlinger B., Guiguet M., Vaillant JC., Balladur P., Boudjema K., Bachellier P. (1996) Surgical resection of colorectal carcinoma metastases to the liver. A prognostic scoring system to improve case selection, based on 1568 patients. *Cancer* 77: 1254-62

Nondlinger B., Sorbye H., Glimelius B., Poston GJ., Schlag PM., Rougier P., Bechstein WO., Primrose JN., Walpole ET., Finch-Jones M., Jaeck D., Mirza D., Parks RW., Collette L., Praet M., Bethe U., Van Cutsem E., Scheithauer W., Gruenberger T. (2008) Perioperative chemotherapy with FOLFOX4 and surgery versus surgery alone for resectable liver metastases from colorectal cancer (EORTC Intergroup trial 40983): a randomised controlled trial. *Lancet* 371: 1007-16

O'Brien CA., Pollett A., Gallinger S., Dick JE. (2007) Chemotherapy and cancer stem cells. *Nature* 445: 106-10

Ohlsson B., Stenram U., Tranberg KG. (1998) Resection of colorectal liver metastases: 25 year experience. *World J Surg* 22: 268-76

Oldenburg A., Albrecht T. (2008) Baseline and contrast-enhanced ultrasound of the liver in tumour patients. *Ultraschall Med* 29(5): 488-98. Abstract

Oldhafer KJ., Lang H., Malago M., Testa G., Broelsch CE. (2001) Ex-situ resection and resection of the in-situ perfused liver: are there still indications? *Chirurg* 72(2): 131-7. Abstract

Patel S., McCall M., Ohinmaa A., Bigam D., Dryden DM. (2011) Positron emission tomography/computed tomographic scans compared to computed tomographic scans for detecting colorectal liver metastases: a systematic review. *Ann Surg* 253(4): 666-71

Pawlik T., Assumpcao L., Vossen J., Buijs M., Gleisner A., Schulick R., Choti M. (2009) Trends in nontherapeutic laparotomy rates in patients undergoing surgical therapy for hepatic colorectal metastases. *Ann Surg Oncol* 16(2): 371-378

Pawlik TM., Schulik RD., Choti MA. (2008) Expanding Criteria for Resectability of Colorectal Liver Metastases. *Oncologist* 13(1): 51-64

Petrowsky H., Gonen M., Jarnagin W., Lorenz M., DeMatteo R., Heinrich S., Encke A., Blumgart L., Fong Y. (2002) Second liver resections are safe and effective treatment for recurrent hepatic metastases from colorectal cancer: a bi - institutional analysis. *Ann Surg* 235: 863–71

Power DG., Kemeny NE. (2010) Role of adjuvant therapy after resection of colorectal cancer liver metastases. *J Clin Oncol* 28(13): 2300-9

Prince ME., Sivanandan R., Kaczorowski A., Wolf GT., Kaplan MJ., Dalerba P., Weissman IL., Clarke MF., Ailles LE. (2007) Identification of a subpopulation of cells with cancer stem cell properties in head and neck squamous cell carcinoma. *Proc Natl Acad Sci USA* 104: 973-8

Reya T., Morrison SJ., Clarke MF., Weissman IL. (2001) Applying the principles of stem cell biology to cancer. *Nature* 414: 105-11

Ribero D., Abdallah EK., Madoff DC., Donadon M., Loyer EM., Vauthey JN. (2007) Portal vein embolization before major hepatectomy and its effects on regeneration, resectability and outcome. *Br J Surg* 94: 1386-96

Ricci-Vitiani L., Lombardi DG., Pilozzi E., Biffoni M., Todaro M., Peschle C., De Maria R. (2007) Phenotypic characterization of human colorectal cancer stem cells. *Nature* 445: 111-5

Saw RP., Koorey D., Painter D., Gallagher PJ. (2002) p53, DCC and thymidylate synthase as predictors of survival after resection of hepatic metastases from colorectal cancer. *Br J Surg* 89: 1409-15

Schwartz L., Brody L., Brown K., Covey A., Tuorto S., Mazumdar M., Riedel E., Jarnagin W., Getrajdman G., Fong Y. (2006) Prospective, blinded comparison of helical CT and CT arterial portography in the assessment of hepatic metastasis from colorectal carcinoma. *World J Surg* 30(10): 1892 -901

Selzner M., Hany TF., Wildbrett P., McCormack L., Kadry Z., Clavien PA. (2004) Does the novel PET/CT imaging modality impact on the treatment of patients with metastatic colorectal cancer of the liver? *Ann Surg* 240: 1027-34

Shaw IM., Rees M., Welsh FK., Bygrave S., John TG. (2006). Repeat hepatic resection for recurrent colorectal liver metastases is associated with favourable long - term survival. *Br J Surg* 93: 457-64

Singh SK., Hawkins C., Clarke ID., Squire JA., Bayani J., Hide T., Henkelman RM., Cusimano MD., Dirks PB. (2004) Identification of a subpopulation of cells with cancer stem cell properties in head and neck squamous cell carcinoma. *Nature* 432: 396-401

Shimada H., Tanaka K., Endou I., Ichikawa Y. (2009). Treatment of colorectal liver metastases: a review. *Langenbecks Arch Surg* 394 (6): 973-83

Smith MD., McCall JL. (2009) Systematic review of tumour number and outcome after radical treatment of colorectal liver metastases. *Br J Surg* 96(10): 1101-13

Söreide JA., Eiriksson K., Sandvik O., Viste A., Horn A., Johnsen G., Grønbech JE. (2008) Surgical treatment of liver metastases from colorectal cancer. *Br J Surg* 128: 50-3.

Sørensen M., Mortensen FV., Høyer M., Vilstrup H., Keiding S. and The Liver Tumour Board at Aarhus University Hospital. (2007). FDG-PET improves management of patients with colorectal liver metastases allocated for local treatment: a consecutive prospective study. *Scand J Surg* 96: 209–13

Tanaka K., Shimada H., Miura M.., Fujii Y., Yamaguchi S., Endo I., Sekido H., Togo S., Ike H. (2004) Metastatic tumour doubling time: most important prehepatectomy predictor of survival and nonrecurrence of hepatic colorectal cancer metastasis. *World J Surg* 28: 263-70

Thelen A., Jonas S., Benckert C., Schumacher G., Lopez-Hänninen E., Rudolph B., Neumann U., Neuhaus P. (2007) Repeat liver resection for recurrent liver metastases from colorectal cancer. *Eur J Surg Oncol* 33: 324-8

Torzilli G., Del Fabbro D., Palmisano A., Donadon M., Bianchi P., Roncalli M., Balzarini L., Montorsi M. (2005) Contrast-enhanced intraoperative ultrasonography during hepatectomies for colorectal cancer liver metastases. *J Gastrointest Surg* 9: 1148-53

Udayasankar U., Chamsuddin A., Mittal P., Small WC. (2008) Diagnostic Imaging and Image-Guided Interventions of Hepatobiliary Malignancies. In: Imaging in Oncology. Blake MA, Kalra MK. Springer Science+Business Media, LLC. New York

Valls C., Andia E., Sanchez A., Guma A., Figueras J., Torras J, Serrano T. (2001) Hepatic Metastases from Colorectal Cancer: Preoperative Detection and Assessment of Resectability with Helical CT. *Radiology* 218: 55-60

Valls C., Martinez L., Ruiz S., Alba E. (2009). Radiological Imaging of Liver Metastases. In: *Liver Metastases*. Vauthey JN, Hoff PMG, Audisio RA, Poston GJ (Eds), pp. 1-13 Springer-Verlag London, ISBN 978-1-84628-946-0

van Erkel AR., Pijl MEJ., van den Berg-Huysmans AA., Wasser MNJM., van de Velde CJH., Bloem JL. (2002). Hepatic Metastases in Patients with Colorectal Cancer: Relationship between Size of Metastases, Standard of Reference, and Detection Rates. *Radiology* 224: 404–9

Vauthey JN. (2007) Colorectal Liver Metastases: Treat Effectively Up Front and Consider the Borderline Resectable. *J Clin Oncol* 25(29): 4524-5

Vauthey JN. The AHPBA 2006 Consensus Conference: Focus on Improving Resectability in Patients With Hepatic Colorectal Metastases. Medscape Oncology. Posted: 03/31/2006. Available from: http://www.medscape.org/viewarticle/524135

Vidiri A., Carpanese L., D'Annibale M., Caterino M., Cosimelli M., Zeuli M., David V., Crecco M. (2004) Evaluation of Hepatic Metastases from Colorectal Carcinoma with MR-Superparamagnetic Iron Oxide. *J Exp Clin Cancer Res* 23(1): 53-60

Wagman LD., Byun TE. (2009) Managing colorectal cancer liver metastases. *Oncology* 23 (12): 1063-71

Wiering B., Krabbe PFM., Jager GJ., Oyen WJG., Ruers TJF. (2005) The Impact of Fluor-18-Deoxyglucose-Positron Emission Tomography in the Management of Colorectal Liver Metastases: A Systematic Review and Metaanalysis. *Cancer* 104 (12): 2658-70

Woodington GF., Waugh JM (1963). Results of resection of metastastic tumours of the liver. *Am J Surg* 105:24

Yamamoto J., Kosuge T., Shimada K., Yamasaki S., Moriya Y., Sugihara K. (1999) Repeat liver resection for recurrent colorectal liver metastases. *Am J Surg* 178: 275-81

Yan T., Sim J., Black D., Niu R., Morris DL. (2007) Systematic review on safety and efficacy of repeat hepatectomy for recurrent liver metastases from colorectal carcinoma. *Ann Surg Oncol* 14: 2069-77

Yang S., Ho S., Hanna SS., Gallinger S., Wei AC., Kiss A., Law C. (2010) Utility of preoperative imaging in evaluating colorectal liver metastases declines over time. *HPB* 12(9): 605-9

Zorzi D., Laurent A., Pawlik TM., Lauwers GY., Vauthey JN., Abdalla EK. (2007) Chemotherapy-associated hepatotoxicity and surgery for colorectal liver metastases. *Br J Surg* 94(3): 274-86

10

Expanding Local Control Rate in Liver Cancer Surgery – The Value of Radiofrequency Ablation

Alexander Julianov
Department of Surgery, Thracian University Hospital, Stara Zagora, Bulgaria

1. Introduction

Hepatic resection still remains the golden standard treatment for patients with primary and metastatic liver cancer and offers the best chance for cure and survival (Agrawal & Belghiti, 2011). However the vast majority of the patients with malignant liver tumors are not suitable for hepatectomy due to number or distribution of the hepatic lesions relative to future liver remnant volume. Aiming to overcome these limitations various local tumor ablation techniques were developed. Among them radiofrequency ablation (RFA) gained popularity in the past decade and became the most used local ablation technique worldwide. The principles of RFA are well described and discussed elsewhere (Rhim et al, 2001; Ahmed & Goldberg, 2004; Chen et al, 2004). In brief - needle electrode/-s and high frequency electric current generator are used during RFA, in order to heat and coagulate neoplastic tissue (Figure 1).

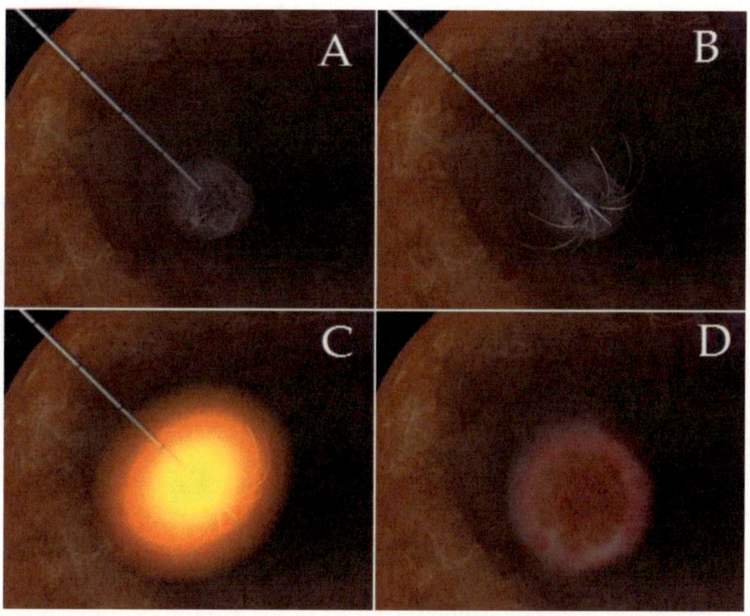

Fig. 1. Schematic view of the RFA process with the LeVeen needle electrode.

A sufficient rim of healthy liver parenchyma should also be destroyed as a safety margin. The size and geometry of created ablation zone depends mainly on the ablation protocol, electrodes used, tissue impedance and proximity of large vessels. Various RFA devices and electrodes are present on the market (Pereira et al, 2004), and they should be carefully evaluated before starting a clinical RFA program. Whenever possible the RFA devices should be tested in animal laboratory in order to become more familiar with the chosen technique before its clinical application. Clinical RFA of liver tumors currently is being performed percutaneously or during operation. Intraoperative RFA can be performed either as a sole procedure or (more frequently) as an adjunct to hepatic resection in order to control the functionally unresectable disease in the remnant liver (Figure 2). This chapter will discuss the rationale and technical aspects of intraoperative RFA in the treatment of patients with liver tumors.

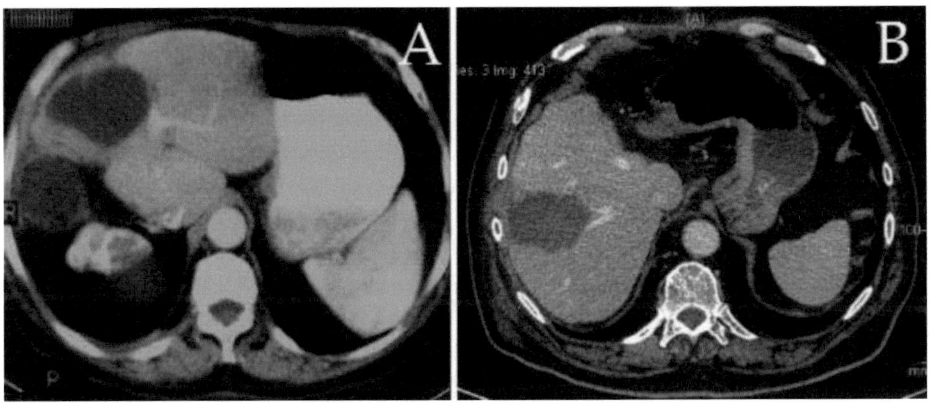

Fig. 2. Follow-up computed tomografy of patients after combined RFA and right hepatectomy (A) or left hepatectomy (B) for colorectal liver metastases.

2. Indications for RFA

Before considering RFA as a treatment option it should be remembered that hepatic resection still remains the standard treatment for patients with malignant liver tumors and offers the best chance for cure and survival. The volume of the liver remnant after resection is the most important factor when hepatic surgery is considered in a patient with liver cancer. Currently any hepatic involvement by a cancer is considered resectable if during surgery sufficient amount of tumor-free liver parenchyma can be spared, with preserved or reconstructed inflow, outflow and bile drainage. Otherwise RFA alone or in combination with resection can be performed to control the malignant disease in the liver.

2.1 Hepatocellular carcinoma

HCC in patients with viral hepatitis and/or cirrhosis is the most common indication for RFA. The limited hepatic functional reserve of a cirrhotic patient frequently is a cause of functional unresectability. In these patients RFA was proven as an effective treatment modality as well as a useful bridge to transplantation in transplant-candidates. Compared to various other local treatment modalities in both randomized and non-randomized studies RFA is more effective in terms of less recurrence of HCC or improved safety. However compared to liver resection RFA demonstrates significantly more recurrences and shorter time to recurrence (Sutherland et al, 2006). Important local factors, which influence the effectiveness of RFA of HCC, are the size and growth pattern of the tumor. For medium and large HCC, an infiltrating growth pattern (portal invasion, irregular margins, extranodal growth) is associated with higher risk of local recurrence than a noninfiltrating growth pattern (well-circumscribed margins or surrounded by a capsule). However some authors reported safe and effective, mainly intraoperative RFA of large HCC up to 8cm (Poon et al, 2004). For small HCC the presence or absence of a capsule did not influence the risk of local recurrence. There is an evidence from multivariate meta-analysis that RFA approach (percutaneous or intraoperative) influences significantly the effectiveness of ablation for both primary and metastatic liver malignancies regardless of the size of the tumor (Table 1, Mulier et al, 2005).

	Percutaneous RFA	RFA by laparotomy/laparoscopy
< 3 cm (small)	16.0	3.6
3-5 cm (medium)	25.9	21.7
> 5 cm (large)	60.0	50.0

Table 1. Local recurrence rates (in %) after RFA according to the approach.

The possibilities for more precise placement of the electrodes and for obtaining both inflow and outflow vascular control are among the most important factors contributing to the superiority of surgical RFA (Julianov et al, 2008, Julianov, 2009) (Figure 3).

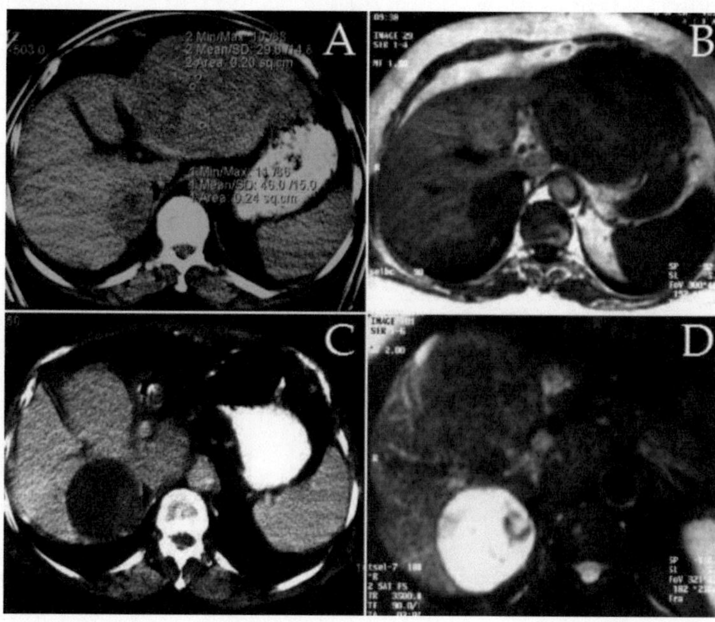

Fig. 3. Preoperative CT (A) and MRI (B) images of a patient with bilobar HCC. Follow-up CT (C) and MRI (D) five years after combined operation - RFA of a right-sided lesion which was adjacent to vena cava and resection of the dominant left-sided tumor, demonstrates control of the disease.

The route of application also influences the safety of the RFA. Although the morbidity is insignificantly higher in more invasive surgical approaches (by laparotomy/laparoscopy), the possibility to control complications during treatment, results in virtually no mortality from intraoperative RFA for both primary and metastatic liver cancer (Table 2, Mulier et al, 2002).

	percutaneous RFA	RFA by laparotomy	RFA by laparoscopy
Morbidity	7.2	9.5	9.9
Mortality	0.5	0	0

Table 2. Morbidity and mortality rates (in %) after RFA according to the approach.

Short- and intermediate-term survival rates after RFA for small HCC are as high as 100% and 98% for 1- and 2-years, with corresponding local recurrence-free rates of 98% and 96% respectively (Lencioni et al, 2003). However with time progression and for medium- and large-sized HCC the results worsened sharply. Except from the lower complete ablation rates obtained in larger lesions, this situation is explained by the frequent presence of microscopic satellite tumor nodules in HCC. In small HCC microscopic tumor extends more than 1 cm beyond visible tumor borders in 60% of patients. In larger lesions this microscopic extension is more than 2 cm in 67% (Lai et al, 1993). It is important to note also that even in early HCC < 2 cm microscopic portal vein invasion is present in 25% of lesions (Kojiro, 2002). According to the above data it is reasonable to recommend RFA with at least 1.5 cm security ablation margin for small HCC and with ≥2.5 cm margin for larger lesions, with concomitant inflow- and/or outflow control during ablation. In cases with bilobar/multiple tumors RFA can be recommended as an adjunct to surgical resection or as an alternative treatment option if the disease is deemed inoperable at laparotomy/laparoscopy. RFA can be a valuable treatment option for patients with unresectable HCC up to 8 cm. Surgical approach offers significantly better local control rates compared with percutaneous RFA independent of tumor size. Thus percutaneous RFA should be reserved for patients who refuse or cannot tolerate surgery.

2.2 Liver metastases

The liver is a common site for metastases from almost all solid malignancies. Hepatic resection is the standard treatment for liver metastases from various primary sites. However curative resection is frequently precluded by insufficient volume of the planned future liver remnant. Hepatectomy is not useful also in patients in poor general condition or in those who refuse liver resection. In these circumstances RFA was intensely explored as a treatment option for metastatic liver disease in unresectable cases. Currently RFA is used for treatment of unresectable liver metastases from different primaries including colorectal, neuroendocrine, sarcoma, breast etc. (Livraghi et al, 2003; Pawlik et al, 2006; Sutherland et al, 2006). Almost all of the published clinical data show that RFA can improve survival in patients with metastatic liver cancer compared with chemotherapy alone. In our study in 130 patients, RFA as an adjunct to surgical resection significantly improves both the local control and survival rate in primary and metastatic liver cancer (Julianov, 2009). However there is no a randomized controlled trial comparing RFA with liver resection for metastatic liver disease. For many reasons such a trial does not seem ethical to be conducted in a near future (Julianov & Karashmalakov, 2011). It is clear that RFA still cannot replace hepatic resection in the treatment of the liver metastases. For example - incomplete necrosis rates after percutaneous RFA for colorectal liver metastases reach 40% even in the treatment of small lesions <3 cm by most experienced hands (Livraghi et al., 2003). Moreover, the MD Anderson Cancer Center group reports stressing and still poorly explained data: no 5-year disease-free survivors in the RFA-treated group of 30 patients with solitary colorectal liver metastasis, even among patients with lesions < 3 cm. The comparison with the results of the liver resection in the same report clearly demonstrates that resection determines the outcome—5-year overall- and disease-free survival 27% and 0% for RFA versus 71% and 50% for resection, respectively (Aloia et al, 2006). Regarding the route of application of RFA (percutaneous or surgical) there is evidence that short-term benefits of lower invasiveness of percutaneous RFA for liver tumors do not outweigh the longer-term higher risk of local recurrence. As mentioned above - surgical RFA results in superior local control, independent of tumor size, and percutaneous RFA should be reserved for patients who cannot tolerate laparoscopy or laparotomy (Mulier et al, 2005).

3. Technique of intraoperative RFA

3.1 General considerations

Irrespective whether RFA is planned or not, any operation for liver tumor begins with through exploration of abdominal cavity for presence of previously unrecognized extrahepatic disease. Exploration of the liver with intraoperative ultrasound (IOUS) is a key step of the operation. All of the current imaging studies, including PET-CT, have well known limits to detect small hepatic and extrahepatic lesions compared with intraoperative staging, which includes IOUS. The latter fact ultimately adds unpredictable bias in estimating "new" lesions in any study of percutaneous RFA of liver metastases (Elias et al, 2005). In our study, as in many others IOUS demonstrates significantly higher sensitivity compared with other diagnostic methods for detection of hepatic lesions (Table 3; Julianov, 2008). More than 90% of the missed lesions are < 1cm and frequently had subcapsular location.

Diagnostic method used	Sensitivity	p
Preoperatively		
US	64 %	0,001
CT	79 %	0,001
US + CT	82 %	0,001
Intraoperatively		
Inspection & palpation	78 %	0,01
IOUS	92 %	0,01

Table 3. Sensitivity of different diagnostic methods for detection of hepatic tumors.

Resectable extrahepatic disease is not longer considered as a contraindication for liver surgery. However in most cases the presence of unresectable extrahepatic disease is a contraindication for a liver-directed procedure. Currently the exception from this rule can be made for some patients with peritoneal carcinomatosis, if cytoreductive surgery plus intraperitoneal chemotherapy can be performed simultaneously with the liver-directed surgical treatment. In every case any attempt should be made initially for R0 resection even as a staged procedure. Survival rates following two-step hepatectomy for liver metastases still are better than those of combined RFA+liver resection procedures. RFA is recommended in some cases before portal vein embolisation to control small centrally placed lesion in the planned future liver remnant. When R0 hepatectomy deemed impossible RFA+resection can be considered. The aim of the procedure is to resect as much as possible of the lesions, treating smaller and centrally placed ones with RFA in order to preserve sufficient amount of residual healthy liver. However in patients with unresectable recurrence after liver resection, in high-risk patients with severe comorbidities or in those refusing hepatic resection RFA is a treatment option as a sole procedure (Figure 4).

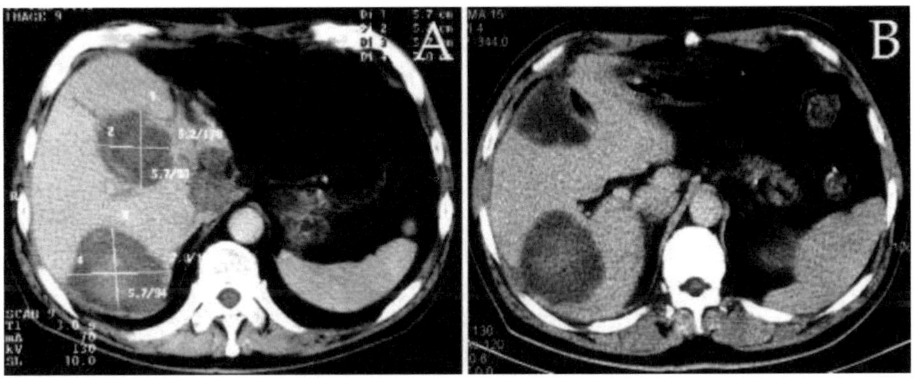

Fig. 4. Follow-up CT after intraoperative RFA of recurrent colorectal liver metastases after previous resection (A), and of colorectal metastases in a high-risk patient (B) .

In selected patients with synchronous bilobar metastases and resectable extrahepatic disease simultaneous RFA plus liver and extrahepatic resection can be safely performed (Julianov et al, 2004, 2006). A substantial survival advantage can be expected in patients in whom local control is achieved with RFA/RFA+resection, compared with those patients treated with chemotherapy only. In our study of patients with liver metastases there were no 2-year survivors between patients deemed unresectable at operation and further treated with chemotherapy only. For comparison - the 3-year survival rate for patients treated with liver resection alone was 71% vs. 34% for those treated with combined RFA+resection or RFA alone. However the mean number of liver metastases was 2.5 in the resection group vs. 5 in the combined treatment group (Julianov, 2009).

3.2 Technique of intraoperative RFA in different situations

When performing intraoperative RFA some principal rules should be followed. IOUS guidance is mandatory for proper positioning of the RFA probe. A free-hand puncture technique usually allows more freedom to manipulate when compared to the puncture through guide, attached to the US-transducer. Mobilization of the liver is not mandatory but is sometimes necessary in order to achieve more comfortable positioning of the RFA electrode, to isolate the liver from adjacent organs/structures in order to protect them from thermal injury, or for the purposes of outflow vascular control. The most deep and closest to the major vessel part of the lesion is treated first, to eliminate further cooling effect ("heat sink") of the blood flow on ablation process. During RFA we always apply Pringle-maneuver, starting at 5 minutes after beginning of each ablation cycle till its end. Finally the probe is cauterized before removing it from the liver, in order to minimize the risk of needle-tract seeding of viable tumor cells.

RFA near major blood vessels. Proximity of a major vessel was identified as an independent limiting factor for successful hepatic RFA (Mulier et al, 2005). In animal experiments with RFA a rim of viable tissue has been always observed around the large vessels >5mm (Lu et al, 2002). Thus vascular control becomes important adjunct to RFA procedure, when tumors near major vessels are treated in both normal and cirrhotic livers (Rossi et al, 2000; De Baere et al, 2002; Washburn et al, 2003). Pringle-maneuver is sufficient vascular control technique for lesions located near inflow vessels. However inflow occlusion does not eliminate the "heat sink" when the tumor located near major hepatic vein is treated. In this situation the backflow cooling from the hepatic vein can be simply controlled by finding with IOUS the respective vein confluence to the inferior vena cava, and compressing the vein with the transducer until its lumen disappears on IOUS-screen (Julianov, 2008, 2009). Even the lesions adjacent to the vena cava can be successfully treated if proper vascular control techniques are used during RFA (Julianov et al, 2008; Figure 3).

RFA near hilar bile ducts. RFA for a lesion near the hepatic hilum is considered dangerous because of the high risk from thermal injury and subsequent stricture of hilar bile ducts. However successful and safe RFA of a hepatic tumor near the hepatic hilum can be performed (Figure 5).

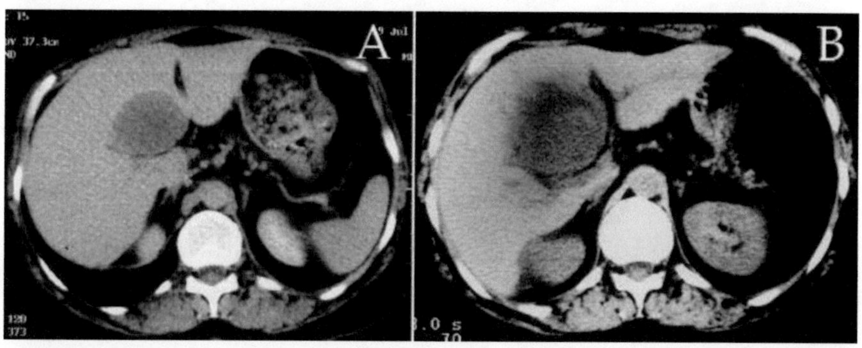

Fig. 5. Computed tomography of a patient with liver metastasis from gastrointestinal stromal tumor (A). RFA with cooling of bile ducts was performed (B).

For this purpose the left and right main duct should be protected. One option is to place the stents in both ducts through ERCP. Another option proven in both experimental and clinical setting is to cool the bile ducts during ablation. Our preferred option is to cool the biliary tree by perfusion of cold 5% isotonic glucose solution in the bile ducts using catheters inserted through small incision of the common bile duct, as proposed by D. Elias (Elias et al, 2001).

Large-volume RFA. For large lesions, more than a single positioning of the RFA probe is frequently necessary to control the tumor with appropriate safety margin. In such cases it is important to plan the whole RFA procedure with all positions of the electrode before starting the ablation. RFA causes changes in the coagulated liver parenchyma, which will affect further proper positioning of the probe under US-guidance (Figure 6). The geometry of overlapping ablations can vary widely, and they should be planned with respect of the size of the target lesion. A well-designed protocol for RFA of larger lesions should be used in order to ensure high success rate of complete ablation (Chen et al, 2004).

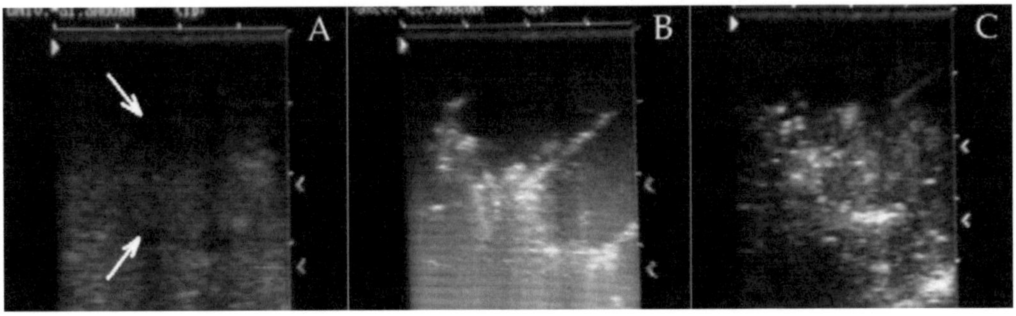

Fig. 6. IOUS images. Isoechoic liver metastasis with hypoechoic rim before treatment (A). The lesion is punctured with the LeVeen needle electrode and ablation started (B). The RFA cycle is finished (C).

To date the physiologic response of large-volume RFA (Figure 7), has not reported to be different from the more limited "usual" ablation volumes in clinical practice. However the safety limit of clinical RFA of the liver remains unknown.

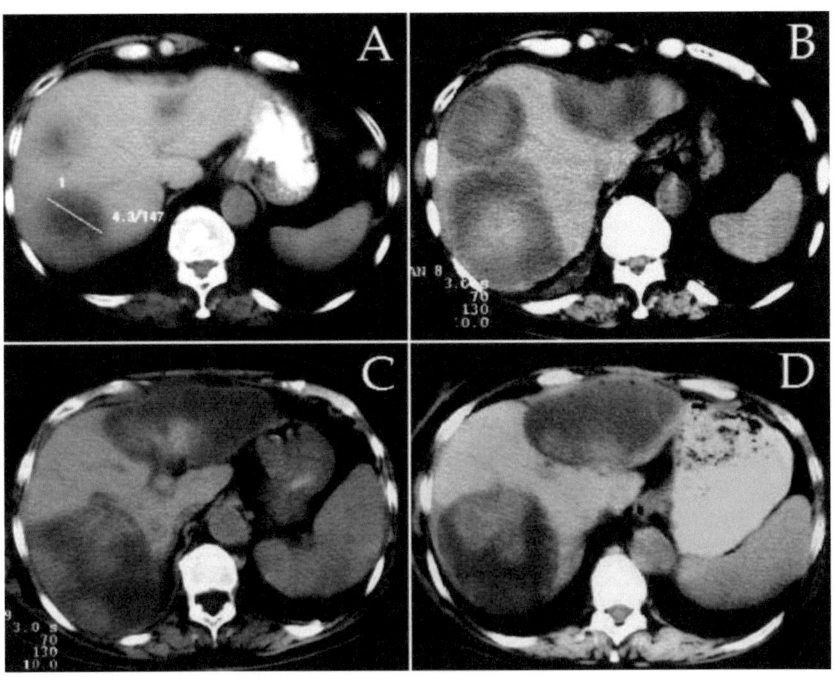

Fig. 7. Computed tomography of a patient with colorectal liver metastases before (A) and one week after large-volume RFA (B). Posttreatment follow-up CT of a patient two weeks (C) and 6 months (D) after large volume RFA.

In animal model of RFA a 40% of the liver volume is ablated without mortality in healthy livers whereas in cirrhotic liver up to 20% can be ablated safely, without significant systemic inflammatory response (Ng et al, 2006). It is not clear whether these data are applicable in clinical setting. In our experience, the posttreatment course of patients with even very large volumes of hepatic RFA does not show any specific difference from more "usual" cases.

3.3 Complications after RFA

The postoperative care after RFA does not require specific treatment, irrespective whether RFA is performed as a sole procedure or simultaneously with various hepatic and/or extrahepatic resections. However the possibility of a potential life-threatening complication after RFA should always be kept in mind (Figure 8).

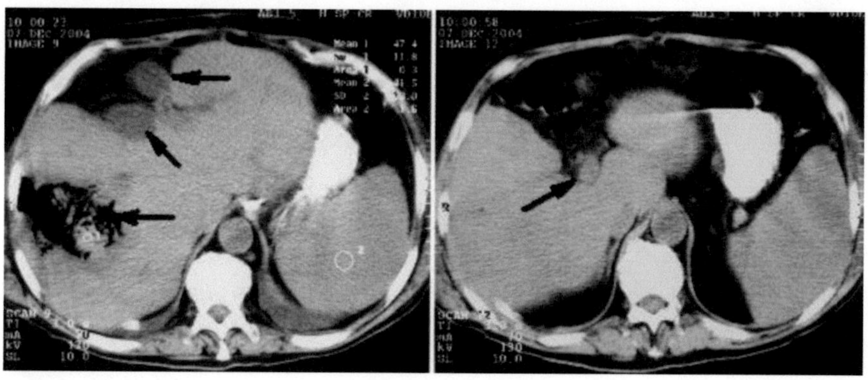

Fig. 8. Computed tomography of a patient after simultaneously performed bowel and liver resection plus RFA. Hepatic abscesses occurred at resection- and RFA sites (arrows).

Although RFA of the liver is a well-tolerated and safe procedure, complications and rarely death may occur after RFA-treatment. The most common complications after RFA of the liver are bleeding, abscessus and biloma formation and they sometimes may be fatal (Enne et al, 2003). The life-threatening complications from the thermal injury of organs adjacent to the liver were reported mainly for percutaneous RFA. Surgical approaches permit protection and isolation of endangered organs from inadvertent burn injury during hepatic RFA. In patients with cirrhosis, delayed portal vein thrombosis can occur after RFA near the main portal vein branches. Rare complication as a gas gangrene after RFA was also reported (Kvitting et al, 2006). Any complication after hepatic RFA require immediate treatment and when necessary interventions (surgical or image-guided) should be regarded as life saving and performed without delay. This approach permits avoiding mortality even in most critical situations (Julianov, 2008)

4. Conclusions

The two crucial questions must be always addressed when considering RFA as a treatment option in a patient with primary or metastatic liver cancer: 1. Whether RFA is equal in curability to surgical resection for resectable malignant liver tumor, and 2. What additional survival benefit does RFA has over modern systemic therapies in the treatment of unresectable disease? The long-term results from clinical studies to date showed significantly better survival obtained from surgical resection for all types of resectable malignant liver tumors. Thus RFA cannot be regarded as an equally effective alternative of liver resection. On the other hand, if compared with systemic treatment alone there is enough clinical data to demonstrate that when local control is achieved by RFA it offers survival advantage (and even cure) for patients with unresectable disease. Unfortunately these facts are frequently misinterpreted and lead to misuse or abuse with RFA. In a survey from Germany 25.9% of patients undergoing RFA had a resectable tumor (Birth et al, 2004). This is partly because of the public pressure on physicians to refer their patients for minimally invasive treatment, rather than for major surgery, becomes heavier today. As a consequence many radiologists and gastroenterologists start to treat with percutaneous RFA patients with resectable tumors. On the other hand, surgeons that have no experience with hepatic surgery start to perform RFA as an alternative to resection in resectable cases, rather than referring these patients to the experienced liver surgeon. As the philosopher Abraham Maslow once said, "If the only tool you have is a hammer, then you tend to see every problem as a nail." However, when RFA is properly used in patients with primary and metastatic liver cancer its clinical benefits in terms of prolonged survival and even cure are indisputed. Today the RFA-device clearly is a necessary tool in the armamentarium of a liver surgeon.

5. References

Agrawal, S. & Belghiti, J. (2011). Oncologic Resection for Malignant Tumors of the Liver. *Ann Surg*, Vol.253, pp. 656–665, ISSN 0003-4932

Ahmed, M. & Goldberg, S. (2004). Radiofrequency tissue ablation: principles and techniques. In: *Radiofrequency ablation for cancer: current indications, techniques and outcomes*, L. Ellis, S. Curley & K. Tanabe, (Eds.), Springer-Verlag, ISBN 978-1-4419-3058-3, New York, USA

Aloia, T.; Vauthey, J.; Loyer, E. et al. (2006). Solitary colorectal liver metastasis: resection determines outcome. *Arch Surg*, Vol.141, pp. 460–466, ISSN 0004-0010

Birth, M.; Hildebrand, P.; Dahmen, G. et al. (2004). Present state of radio frequency ablation of liver tumors in Germany. *Chirurg*, Vol.75, pp. 417–423, ISSN 0009-4722

De Baere, T.; Bessoud, B.; Dromain, C. et al. (2002). Percutaneous Radiofrequency Ablation of Hepatic Tumors During Temporary Venous Occlusion. *AJR*, Vol.178, pp. 53–59, ISSN 0361-803X

Chen, M.; Yang, W.; Yan, K. et al. (2004). Large Liver Tumors: Protocol for Radiofrequency Ablation and Its Clinical Application in 110 Patients—Mathematic Model, Overlapping Mode, and Electrode Placement Process. *Radiology*, Vol.232, pp. 260–271, ISSN 0033-8419

Elias, D.; Azzedine, E.; Alain, G. et al. (2001). Intraductal cooling of the main bile ducts during intraoperative radiofrequency ablation. *J Surg Oncol*, Vol.76, pp.297-300, ISSN 1096-9098

Elias, D.; Sideris, L.; Pocard, M. et al. (2005). Incidence of unsuspected and treatable metastatic disease associated with operable colorectal liver metastases discovered only at laparotomy (and not treated when performing percutaneous radiofrequency ablation). *Ann Surg Oncol*, Vol.12, pp. 298–302, ISSN 1068-9265

Enne, M.; Pacheco-Moreira, L.; Cerqueira, A.; Balbi, E. et al. (2003). Fatal hemobilia after radiofrequency thermal ablation for hepatocellular carcinoma. *Surgery*, Vol.135, pp. 460-461, ISSN 0148-7043

Julianov, A.; Karachmalakov, A.; Rachkov, I. & Hristov, H. (2004) Treatment of Colorectal Cancer with Synchronous Bilobar Liver Metastases with Simultaneous Bowel and Liver Resection plus Radiofrequency Ablation. *Hepatogastroenterology*, Vol.51, pp. 643-645, ISSN 0172-6390

Julianov, A. & Karachmalakov, A. (2006) Simultaneous pulmonary metastasectomy and hepatic radiofrequency ablation to treat recurrent metastases from rectal cancer. *Eur J Cancer Care*, Vol.15, pp. 369-370, ISSN 1365-2354

Julianov, A. (2008). *Possibilities for the treatment of liver tumors with resection and intraoperative radiofrequency ablation*. Dissertation, Thracian University, Stara Zagora, Bulgaria

Julianov, A.; Rachkov, I. & Karashmalakov, A. (2008). A five-year disease-free survival after combined hepatectomy and radiofrequency ablation of large hepatocellular carcinoma adjacent to vena cava. *Cent Eur J Med*, Vol.3, pp. 370-373, ISSN 1895-1058

Julianov A. (2009). *Radiofrequency ablation for liver cancer*. DugaPlus, ISBN 978-954-9387-47-6, Stara Zagora, Bulgaria

Julianov A. & Karashmalakov A. (2011). Percutaneous Radiofrequency Ablation as First-Line Treatment in Patients With Early Colorectal Liver Metastases Amenable to Surgery: Is It Justified? *Ann Surg*, Vol.254, pp. 178, ISSN 0003-4932

Kojiro, M. (2002). The evolution of pathologic features of hepatocellular carcinoma. In: *Viruses and Liver Cancer*, E. Tabor, (Ed.), Elsevier, ISBN 0-444-50580-6, Amsterdam, Netherlands

Kvitting, J.; Sandstrom, P.; Thorelius, L. et al. (2006). Radiofrequency ablation of a liver metastasis complicated by extensive liver necrosis and sepsis caused by gas gangrene. *Surgery*, Vol.139, pp. 123-125, ISSN 0148-7043

Lai, E.; You, K.; Ng, I. et al. (1993). The pathological basis of resection margin for hepatocellular carcinoma. *World J Surg*, Vol.17, pp. 786–791, ISSN 0364-2313

Lencioni, R.; Allgaier, H.; Cioni, D. et al. (2003). Small hepatocellular carcinoma in cirrhosis: randomized comparison of radio-frequency thermal ablation versus percutaneous ethanol injection. *Radiology*, Vol.228, pp. 235-240, ISSN 0033-8419

Livraghi, T.; Solbiati, L.; Meloni, F. et al. (2003) Percutaneous radiofrequency ablation of liver metastases in potential candidates for resection: the "test-oftime approach". *Cancer*, Vol.97, pp. 3027–3035, ISSN 1097-0142

Lu, D.; Raman, S.; Vodopich, D. et al. (2002). Effect of Vessel Size on Creation of Hepatic Radiofrequency Lesions in Pigs: Assessment of the "Heat Sink" Effect. *AJR*, Vol.178, pp. 47–51, ISSN 0361-803X

Mulier, S.; Ni, Y.; Jamart, J. et al. (2005). Local recurrence after hepatic radiofrequency coagulation: multivariate meta-analysis and review of contributing factors. *Ann Surg*, Vol.242, pp. 158–171, ISSN 0003-4932

Mulier, S.; Mulier, P.; Ni, Y. et al. (2002). Complications of radiofrequency coagulation of liver tumours. *Br J Surg*, Vol.89, pp. 1206-1222, ISSN 0007-1323

Ng, K.; Lam, C.; Poon, R. et al. (2006). Safety Limit of Large-Volume Hepatic Radiofrequency Ablation in a Rat Model. *Arch Surg*, Vol.141, pp. 252-258, ISSN 0004-0010

Pawlik, T.; Vauthey, J.; Abdalla, E. et al.. (2006). Results of a Single-Center Experience With Resection and Ablation for Sarcoma Metastatic to the Liver. *Arch Surg*, Vol.141, pp. 537-544, ISSN 0004-0010

Pereira, P.; Trubenbach, J.; Schenk, M. et al. (2004). Radiofrequency Ablation: In Vivo Comparison of Four Commercially Available Devices in Pig Livers. *Radiology*, Vol.232, pp. 482–490, ISSN 0033-8419

Poon, RT.; Ng, KC.; Lam, C. et al. (2004). Effectiveness of Radiofrequency Ablation for Hepatocellular Carcinomas Larger Than 3 cm in Diameter. *Arch Surg*, Vol.139, pp. 281-287, ISSN 0004-0010

Rhim, H.; Goldberg, S.; Dodd, G. et al. (2001). Essential Techniques for Successful Radiofrequency Thermal Ablation of Malignant Hepatic Tumors. *RadioGraphics*, Vol.21, pp. S17–S39, ISSN 0271-5333

Rossi, S.; Garbagnati, F.; Lencioni, R. et al. (2000). Percutaneous Radio-frequency Thermal Ablation of Nonresectable Hepatocellular Carcinoma after Occlusion of Tumor Blood Supply. *Radiology*, Vol.217, pp. 119–126, ISSN 0033-8419

Sutherland, L.; Williams, J.; Padbury, R. et al. (2006). Radiofrequency Ablation of Liver Tumors: A Systematic Review. *Arch Surg*, Vol.141, pp. 181-190, ISSN 0004-0010

Washburn, W.; Dodd, G.; Kohlmeier, E. et al. (2003). Radiofrequency Tissue Ablation: Effect of Hepatic Blood Flow Occlusion on Thermal Injuries Produced in Cirrhotic Livers. *Ann Surg Oncol*, Vol.10, pp. 773-777, ISSN 1068-9265

11

Improving the Tumor-Specific Delivery of Doxorubicin in Primary Liver Cancer

Junfeng Zhang, Zhen Huang and Lei Dong
Nanjing University
China

1. Introduction

Primary liver cancer is the fifth most common cancer worldwide and the third most common cause of cancer mortality. More than 500 000 new cases are currently diagnosed yearly, with an age-adjusted worldwide incidence of 5.5–14.9 per 100 000 population (Jemal et al., 2011). Doxorubicin remains the first line of treatment for liver cancer ever since its discovery in 1971 (Yoshikawa & Kitaoka, 1971). Unfortunately, clinical effectiveness of this class of drugs is limited by cumulative cardiotoxicity which occurs in significant percentage of patients at cumulative dose in the range 450-600 mg/m^2 (Ganz et al., 1993). Therefore, various strategies have been developed to reduce cardiotoxicity of doxorubicin and its analogues (Haley & Frenkel, 2008). Commercialized doxorubicin has high cytotoxicity, good solubility and high affinity to nuclear (Viale & Yamamoto, 2008). There is no need to improve its ability to penetrate cell membrane and accumulation into cell nuclear. The aim of delivery techniques is to alter its in vivo distribution, enhance its deposition in the liver tumor sites and reduce its cardiotoxicity. Formulations of doxorubicin should have the ability to specifically release the drug in response to the tumor micro-environment.

Doxorubicin can insert in the double strand of DNA and preferentially bind to double-stranded 5′-GC-3′ or 5′-CG-3′ to form tightly coupled complex without chemical bond links (Vicent, 2007). Once the DNA was digested, the doxorubicin can be released. Cationic polymers are often used as carriers for the DNA drugs' delivery because they can combine DNA to form nanoscale particles by the interaction between their positive charge and the negative charge on the DNA chain (Bodley et al., 1989). Upon these two aspects, we developed a nanoscale formulation of doxorubicin. Doxorubicin was complexed into polyGC double-strand DNA fragments to form the DOX-polyGC intercalation. After that, the DOX-polyGC intercalation was combined by a bio-degradable cationic polymer, cationic gelatin, to form nanoscale particles. Cationic gelatin can be effectively digested by gelatinase (GA) that is a mixture of two kinds of matrix metalloproteinase (MMP) highly expressed by the tumor tissue (Eliyahu, 2005). This makes the complex composed by cationic gelatin, DNA and doxorubicin (CPX1) can be specifically digested and release the doxorubicin in tumor sites (Figure 1). To avoid the accumulation into the liver which also produces gelatinase in a relatively high level (Emonard & Grimaud, 1990), a pH-sensitive material, histamine-modified alginate (His-alginate) was used to cover CPX1 to form CPX2. His-alginate has a pKa of about 6.9 which shows a cationic state when $pH < 6.9$ and an anionic state when pH > 6.9. His-alginate combined CPX1 at physiological pH (7.2) via its anion interact with the cation on the surface of CPX1. In tumor micro-environment, the pH varied from 6.2-6.7 according to different physical states. At such a pH, His-alginate turned it anionic state to a cationic one and dissociated from CPX2. To enhance the ability of CPX2 to escape from the reticuloendothelial system, PEG 2000 was conjugated to His-alginate to form PEG-His-alginate (PHA). The construct scheme was shown in Figure 1.

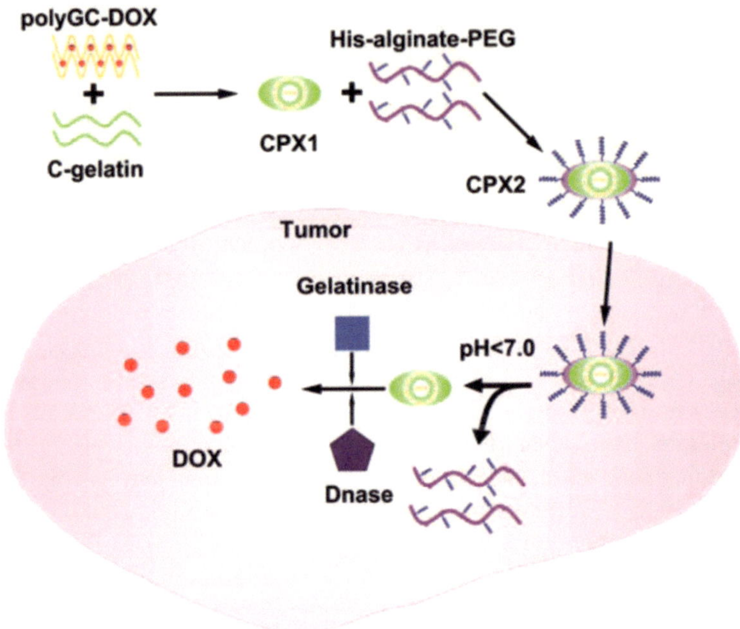

Fig. 1. Fabrication scheme of CXP1 and CPX2.

2. Materials and methods

2.1 Materials synthesis

Poly-GC and Poly-AT were synthesized by Invitrogen (Shanghai, China) with a length of 20 bases. Cationic gelatin was synthesized by using Ethylenediamine-modification according to the reported methods (Matsumoto et al., 2006). The conversion rate of carboxyl groups to amino groups was measured by the TNBS method to characterize the product (Eklund, 1976). PEG-His-modified alginate was synthesized according the following methods: A total of 500 mg of alginate (Sigma) was dissolved in 20 ml of 10 mM N,N,N',N'-tetramethylethylenediamine (TEMED) / HCl buffer solution (pH 4.7). A total of 1.0 g of EDC was added to this solution and stirred at 40 ◦C for 24 h. Then, different1.5 g histidine were added and stirred for another 24 h at 40 ◦C. The resulting His-alginate were dialyzed for 4 days against Milli Q water and lyophilized. The resulted His-alginate was examined for its pKa value. The following Pegylation was achieved by conjugating a 2000 Da mPEG-NH2 to the His-alginate using a Pegylation kit (YARE Chem, Shanghai, China). Rhodamine-labled

PEG-His-alginate and FITC-labled cationic gelatine was synthesized by using fluorescence-label kits (DAZHI Biotech, Nanjing, China) injected into liver tumor bearing mice.

2.2 Cells and animals

Hepa 1-6 is a mouse hepatoma cell line derived from the BW7756 mouse hepatoma which arose in C57/L mouse (ATCC). Hepa 1-6 cells were cultured in DMEM supplemented with 10% FCS. Female ICR mice (18-20g) of the same background were purchased from the experimental animal center of Nanjing Medical University. All animals received human care according to Chinese legal requirements. To generate the allograft model of liver cancer, Hepa 1-6 cells (1×10^7 cells/ml, 10 μl) were injected into the hepatic lobe of anesthetized mice using a microinjector (Cheng et al., 2011).

2.3 Preparation of CPX1 and CPX2

PolyGC-DOX intercalation was obtained by mixing 2 mg/ml DOX with DNA solutions with different concentrations to find the DOX/DNA ratio at which free DOX can insert into DNA chain completely. The fluorescence (exciting: 480 nm; emission: 590nm) of DOX quenched when inserting in the DNA. By detecting the fluorescence of DOX, the formation of the intercalation could be determined. CPX1 was formed by mixing PolyGC-DOX intercalation with cationic gelatin solution at different DNA/Gelatin weight ratio. CPX2 was obtained by mixing CPX1 solution with the some volume of 2mg/ml PEG-His-alginate solution by gently agitation for 1 hour. The physical stability of each complex was studied by agarose gel electrophoresis (0.8% agarose in TAE buffer). The diameters and zeta potential of the complex were analyzed by photon correlation spectroscopy by using 90 Plus Particle Sizer (Brookhaven Instruments, Holtsville, NY). The DOX fluorescence of CPX1 was also examined to investigate whether the combination between the intercalation and cationic gelatin release the DOX from DNA chain.

2.4 Dox release from the complexes

CPX1 and CPX2 were digested by gelatinase and Dnase I in PBS buffers with different PH values, and the resulted solution was examined by DOX fluorescence quantification.

The digestion abilities of mouse plasma, the supernatant of the tumor homogenate (THS) and liver homogenate (LHS) on CPX1 and CPX2 were also examined. CPX1 and CPX2 solutions were mixed with mouse plasma or the tissue homogenate supernatants for 2 hours. After that, the mixtures were examined by quantification of the DOX fluorescence.

To further confirm the tumor-specific drug-release ability of CPX2, in vivo experiments was performed. Rhodamine labeled PEG-His-alginate (PHA) and FITC-labeled cationic gelatin was used to form CPX2. Hoechst 33258 was used to substitute for DOX because Hoechst 33258 also possess high DNA-affinity like DOX and it show blue fluorescence which could be discriminated from the red fluorescence of PHA and green fluorescence of C-gelatin. PolyAT was used to substitute for polyGC because Hoechst 33258 specifically binds AT in DNA (Jong et al., 1991). This PHA-C-gelatin-polyAT-Hoechst complex was injected into the tumor and liver separately. One hour later, sections of the liver and tumor was examined under microscope.

2.5 Bio-distribution of doxorubicin

CPX1 and CPX2 solutions and free DOX solution were separately injected into liver tumor bearing mice via tail vain at a dose of 20 mg/kg body weight. Different organs were harvested from the experimental mice bearing implanted tumors. Doxorubicin in the organ was extracted according a reported method and quantified by the examination of its fluorescence intensity at 590 nm (Bigotte, 1985).

2.6 Toxicology investigation

Healthy mice were given CPX1, CPX2 or free DOX to examine their toxicity. CPX1, CPX2 and DOX were intravenously injected into animals at the doses of 20 mg DOX/kg body weight and 30 mg DOX/kg body weight. The changes of their body weights were examined every day for one week. The mortality of the animals was also calculated. For histological examination, different tissues were harvested at the 4th day after the drugs were given and sectioned and analyzed by hematoxylin and eosin staining. Animal plasma activity of alanine transaminase (ALT) and creatine kinase (CK) were determined for the evaluation of the functions of livers and hearts.

2.7 Anti-cancer activity

Animals bearing implanted liver tumors were intravenously given CPX1, CPX2 and free DOX at a dose of 10 mg DOX/kg body weight every two days from day 5 after the allograft model establishment. All tumors were separated, weighed and sectioned for pathological analyze on day 21. For the calculation of survives, testing animals bearing tumors were divided into 4 group, 10 animals each. CPX1 and CPX2 at a dose of 10 mg DOX/kg body weight were given intravenously every two days with free doxorubicin and saline as controls.

2.8 Statistical analysis

Results are expressed as the mean ± standard error of the mean (S.E.M). The differences between groups were analyzed by Mann-Whitney U test and, if appropriate, by Kruskal-Wallis ANOVA test. Survival curves were analyzed by the Kaplan-Meyer log-rank test. Changes in body weight were compared by use of the Wilcoxon matched-pair signed-rank test. A value of $P < 0.05$ was considered significant.

3. Results

3.1 Preparation of CPX1 and CPX2

The anthracycline class of drugs, including doxorubicin, has fluorescence properties that become quenched after intercalation into DNA. Fluorescence spectroscopy was used to examine the binding of doxorubicin to DNA and the drug encapsulation efficiency of CPX1 and CPX2. A series of weight ratio of DOX/polyGC was tested. DOX could be completely combined by polyGC at the weight ratio of 2:1. Cationic gelatin could combine with DOX-polyGC intercalation at a weight ratio of polyGC/C-gelatin = 1:2. In CPX1, weight ratio of DOX/polyGC/C-gelatin = 2:1:2. Its zeta potential was +18 mV. PEG-His-alginate was added to the solution of CPX1 at the C-gelatin/PEG-His-alginate ratio of 1:1

to form CPX2. The zeta potential of CPX2 was -1.2 mV. Figure 2A show the fluorescence intensity of doxorubicin, DOX-polyGC, CPX1 and CPX2. Figure 2B show the particle sizes of CPX2.

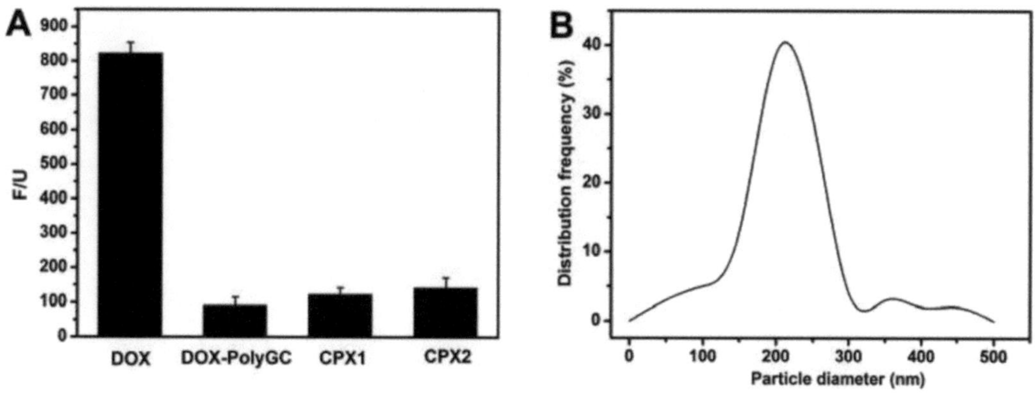

Fig. 2. Preparation of CPX1 and CPX2. A) Fluorescent intensity of free DOX, DOX-polyGC intercalation (weight ratio : DOX:polyGC = 2:1), CPX1 (weight ratio: C-gelatin : polyGC : DOX = 2:1:2) and CPX2 (weight ratio: PEG-His-alginate : C-gelatin : polyGC : DOX = 2:2:1:2) at 590nm; B) Size distribution of CPX2 in saline.

3.2 DOX release from the complexes

The most important property of the complex is to response to PH and gelatinase. PHA-C-gelatin-polyAT-Hoechst complex was used in vivo instead of CPX2 to test the drug release property of CPX2 in response to tumor acidic microenvironments. Results shown in Figure 3A demonstrated that the three kinds of fluorescence were completely overlapped in liver sections. In liver tumor sections, blue "drug" could be seen in a separated area from the green and red fluorescence.

The ability of gelatinase and Dnase I (DA1) to free DOX from CPX1 and CPX2 in PBS buffers with different pH values was tested. The results in Figure 3B demonstrated that DOX in CPX1 could be released under both PH values of 7.2 and 6.5 while CPX2 could only be digested when PH was 6.5. CPX1 and CPX2 were incubated with tumor tissue homogenate supernatant (THS) and then were examined for the released DOX. Serum and normal liver tissue homogenate supernatant (LHS) was used as the control. The results were shown in Figure 3C and Figure 3D. DOX in CPX1 or CPX2 was not released in serum while THS could efficiently release free DOX from CPX1 and CPX2. LHS could only release free DOX from CPX1. CPX2 remained stable in LHS. Figure 3E demonstrated that more than 60% DOX was released from both CPX1 and CPX2 within 2 hours when incubated with THS. When incubated with LHS, CPX1 was also destructed and released DOX very quickly while CPX2 remained stable and kept the DOX from release for more than 20 hours.

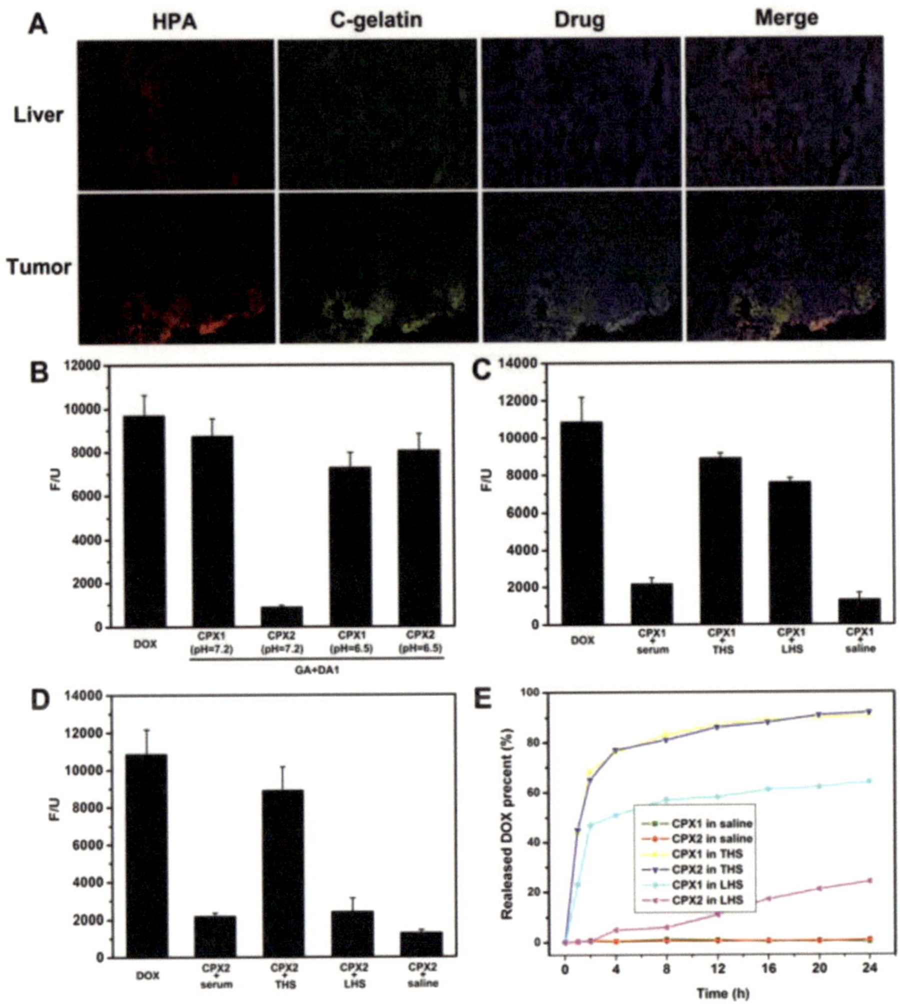

Fig. 3. Release of DOX from CPX1 and CPX2. A) Tumor-specific drug release of CPX2. 0.2 mg Hoechst 33258 contained in multi-fluorescence-labeled CPX2 (polyGC was substituted by polyAT) was injected into the tumor or animal liver after the animals were anesthetized 1 hour before the tissues were separated, sectioned and analyzed by microscope. B) Fluorescent intensity of CPX1 and CPX2 digested by 5 U/ml gelatinase (GA) and 0.5 U/ml Dnase I (DA1) in PBS buffer with PH value of 7.2 or 6.5 for 2 hours at 37 ˚C at 590nm; C) Fluorescent intensity of CPX1 digested by plasma, THS or LHS for 2 hours at 37 ˚C at 590nm; D) Fluorescent intensity of CPX2 by plasma, THS or LHS for 2 hours at 37 ˚C at 590nm; E) DOX release rates from the complexes in THS or LHS. In all experiments, the concentration of DOX contained in CPX1 and CPX2 in the solution is 0.2mg/ml.

3.3 Bio-distribution of doxorubicin

Free DOX, CPX1 and CPX2 were administrated into mice via tail vein at a dose of 20 mg DOX per kg body weight. Different tissues and organs were harvested 48 hours later. The concentration of DOX in these tissues was measured. Data in Figure 4A indicated that CPX2 efficiently enhanced the accumulation of DOX in tumor tissue and reduced the deposition of the drug in heart and the other organs. As a control, CPX1 not only enhanced the drug concentration in tumor but also in liver. The concentration of DOX delivered by CPX1 was 2 times higher than free DOX. Figure 4B and Figure 4C described the variation of DOX concentrations in tumor and liver after CPX1, CPX2 or free DOX was administrated. CPX2 dramatically increased the deposition of DOX in tumor and decreased the liver concentration of the drug. CPX1 could increase the concentration of DOX in both tumor and liver.

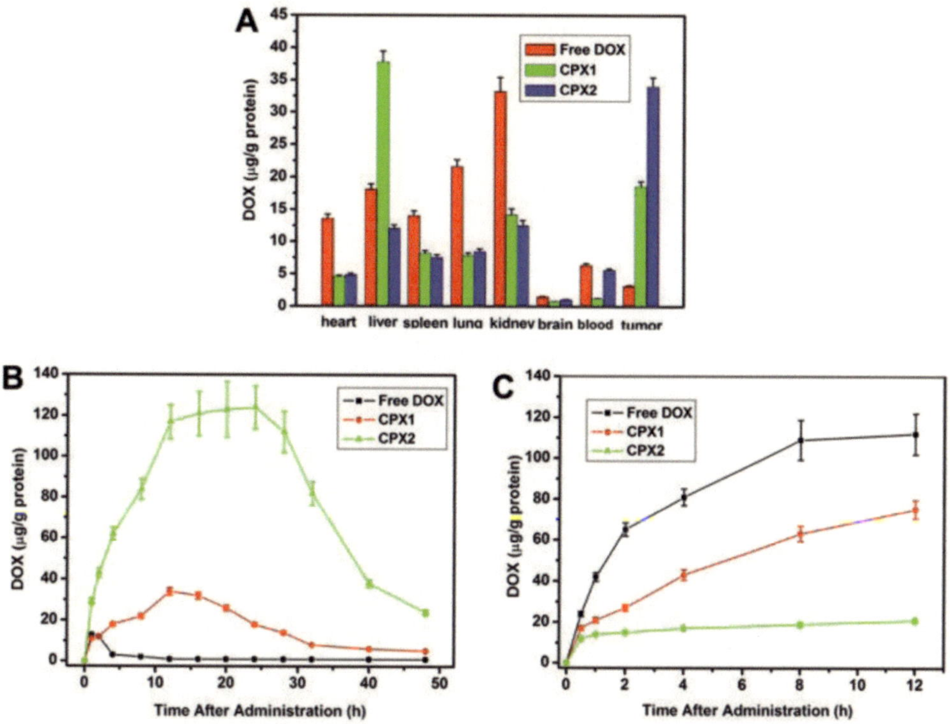

Fig. 4. A) Bio-distribution of free DOX or delivered by CPX1 and CPX2 given i.v. at a dose of 20 mg/kg body weight; B) DOX concentrations in tumor after free DOX, CPX1 or CPX2 were injected i.v. at the dose of 20 mg/kg body weight; C) DOX concentrations in liver after free DOX, CPX1 or CPX2 were injected i.v. at the dose of 20 mg/kg body weight.

3.4 Toxicology investigation

Daily injection of doxorubicin exhibited serious toxicity which resulted in loss of weight, cardiac toxicity and death. CPX1 and CPX2 remarkably reduced the toxicity of doxorubicin, which caused less weight loss than free DOX (Figure 5A). 30 and 20 mg/kg body weight of DOX caused 100% and 60% death in 5 days. The same dose of DOX in the form of CPX1 caused 50% and 20% death in up to 8 days while 20 mg/kg body weight DOX in the form of CPX2 cause no death and the extreme high dose of 30 mg/kg body weight only caused 10% death (Figure 5B).

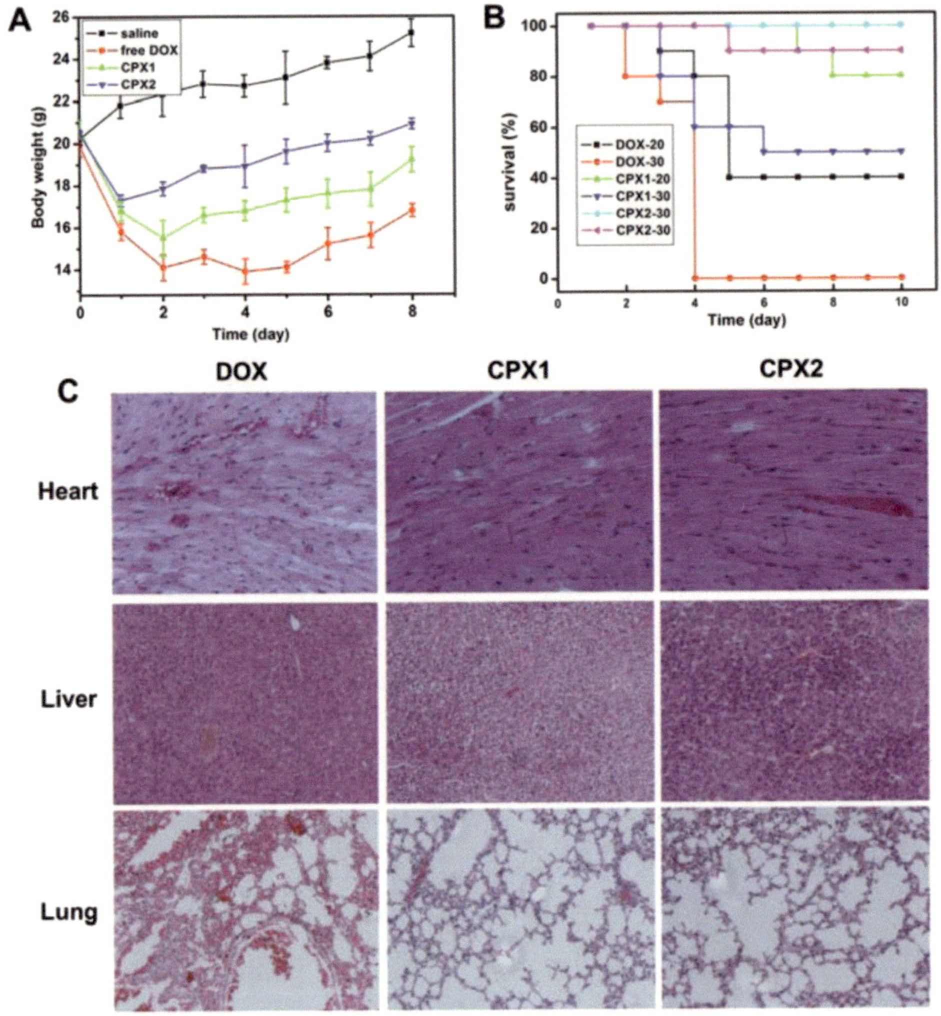

Fig. 5. Toxicology analysis. A) Body weight changes of animals received i.v. injections of saline, free DOX, CPX1 or CPX2 at a dose of 20 mg/kg body weight; B) Mortality caused by free DOX, CPX1 or CPX2 at different doses; C) H & E stained heart, liver and lung tissue sections of animal treated by 20 mg/kg body weight free DOX or delivered by CPX1 and CPX2.

Treatment with free doxorubicin caused massive myocardial degeneration (Figure 5C), which resulted in the increase of the plasma level of CK and LDH (Table 1) and heart failure which induced significant pulmonary congestion (Figure 5C). This toxicity was greatly reduced when DOX was delivered by CPX1 and CPX2 (Figure 5C and Table 1). CPX1 showed more hepatotoxicity than free doxorubicin at the same dose, which resulted in the necrosis of hepatocytes (Figure 5C) and increase in plasma levels of ALT (Table 1) while CPX2 did not cause this toxicity. CPX2 also reduced the nephrotoxicity of doxorubicin which was demonstrated by the decrease of BUN level (Table 1).

	ALT (IU)	AST (IU)	CK (U/ml)	LDH (U/l)	BUN (U/l)
Healthy mice	26.9	32.1	0.23	489.2	10.3
Mice given DOX	29.5	29.7	1.28	562.9	12.7
Mice given CPX1	42.3	34.1	0.26	461.3	10.9
Mice given CPX2	28.3	30.5	0.24	462.7	10.2

Table 1. Serological analysis of mice treated with free DOX, CPX1 and CPX2.

3.5 Anti-cancer activity of CPX1 and CPX2

The anti-tumor activity was evaluated in a mouse orthotopic allograft liver cancer model using a hepatoma cell line, Hepa 1-6. Figure 6A shows the photograph of tumors separated from animals 16 days after they received free DOX, CPX1, CPX2 and saline in vein. From the results of histological analyze of tumor sections (Figure 6B), massive cancer cell remissions could be observed from the sections of tumors treated with CPX1 and CPX2. CPX2 exhibited the most efficiency on prevention of cancer cell's expansion.

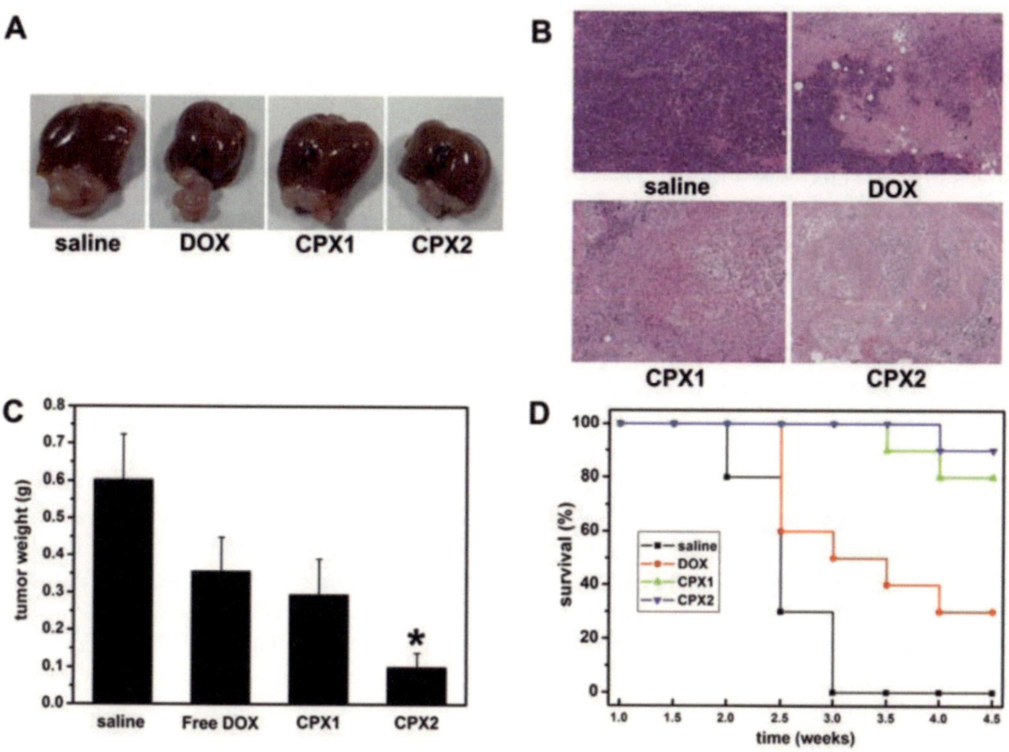

Fig. 6. Anti-tumor activity. A) Representative Tumors separated from animals received intravenous injections of saline, free DOX, CPX1 or CPX2. B) Sections of tumor tissues taken from animal received intravenous injections of saline, free DOX, CPX1 or CPX2. C) Mean weights of tumors separated from animals received of saline, free DOX, CPX1 or CPX2 intravenously. D) Survive rates of animals implanted tumors received treatments with saline, free DOX, CPX1 or CPX2 in more than 4 weeks. *$p < 0.05$ compared with saline treated group.

The mean weight of the tumors isolated from the liver was shown in figure 6C. CPX2 exhibited more than 1 times higher anti-tumor activity than free DOX. Results of the examination of animal survive shown in Figure 6D. Animals bearing tumors and received saline as control died within 4 weeks. Free doxorubicin kept 30% animals from death within 5 weeks while CPX2 rescued 90% of them in more than 4 weeks.

4. Discussion

Doxorubicin, as a chemotherapy drug, has been commonly used in the treatment of hepatocellular carcinoma, but is thwarted by a key obstacle-cumulative cardiotoxicity. To improve its anti-cancer activity and reduce its toxicity, a number of doxorubicin formations such as pegylated liposomal doxorubicin, doxorubicin-eluting-bead has been performed in liver cancer clinical trials recently. Among them, anthracycline-DNA complexes as therapeutic reagents have been used for the treatment of liver cancer for a long history, due its easy-fabrication, no change in the structure of the drug molecules and its anti-cancer activity (Trouet, 1979a). Clinical trials were also carried out to evaluate their enhancement in the performances in effectiveness and toxicology compared to free anthracycline (Trouet, 1979b). However, except a few of *in vitro* reports about successfully reducing the toxicity of the anthracycline by using the complexes, there is no convincing results demonstrating the advantages of using the complexes instead of free anthracycline (Dorr et al., 1991). One of the most important reasons underlies the ineffectiveness of the intercalation between DNA and anthracycline is that there is abundant Dnase in circulation and body fluids which digests un-protected DNA molecular with extremely high efficiency (Paik & Kim, 1970). The anthracycline-DNA complexes were destroyed soon after their injection into the body. The anthracycline in complexes was released very quickly and did not change their pharmaceutical properties any more.

Protection of DNA from destroying by Dnase is necessary for gene delivery technology (Tranchant et al., 2004). Non-viral gene delivery practices take the advantage of using cationic polymers to combine DNA, which prevents the exposure of DNA molecules to Dnases (Wagner, 2004). DNA complexed with cationic polymers could totally resist the degradation of Dnase I or serum Dnases in reported *in vivo* and *in vitro* tests (Paleos et al., 2009). These researches instruct us cationic polymers could be used to combine the intercalation of anthracycline-DNA to form an anthracycline-DNA-cationic polymer ternary complex. Such a complex can avoid the unexpected early release of anthracycline into serum by protecting DNA from the digestion of Dnases. In our experimets, cationic gelatin was used to combine DNA-DOX intercalation. This simple process generated regular nanocomplexes that could be observed. It is difficult to release DOX in short time using Dnase I alone to digest the complex, which suggested that DNA is well protected by cationic gelatin. Additionally, in the present study, synthesized GC oligonucleotide was used to substitute the natural DNA fragments, which increased the drug-loading capacity of DNA. Moreover, the combination between DOX and polyGC is more stable than DOX-natural DNA intercalation fragments which may release DOX when combined by some kind of cationic polymer. No DOX release was observed in the study when DOX-polyGC was combined by cationic gelatin.

A lot of cationic polymers are used as gene carriers, such as polyether imide (PEI), polylysine (PLL), cationic polysaccharides and other polycation materials (Bodley et al.,

1989). To ensure the sufficient release of anthracycline in tumor sites, the cationic polymer used to form the anthracycline-DNA-cationic polymer ternary complex must be biodegradable, especially in tumor. Cationic gelatin is a derivate of gelatin by conjugating ethylenediamine, spermine or other compounds with multiple amino groups to the gelatin molecules. Cationic gelatin is a proved effective DNA carrier for gene delivery *in vitro* and *in vivo*. It can protect DNA and even RNA from the degradation of Dnases (Kushibiki et al., 2003). More importantly, cationic gelatin can be easily digested by gelatinase (Ganea et al, 2007). Gelatinase belong to the matrix metallopeptidase (MMP) family. It is composed of MMP-2 and MMP-9 (Eliyahu, 2005). Recent investigations suggest that gelatinase is involved in the genesis, development and metastasis of most kinds of tumors, which is highly expressed in solid tumors (Deryugina & Quigley, 2006). That means cationic gelatin could be effectively digested in tumor. To address this, tumor homogenate supernatant was tested for its ability to digest cationic gelatin in CPX1 and release DOX. Compared to plasma, THS exhibited much higher efficiency of releasing the DOX from CPX1. This implies CPX1 can be destroyed and DOX can be released specifically in tumor sites.

However, only gelatinase-response is not sufficient to enable the tumor-specific drug release ability of the delivery system because gelatinase is relatively high-expressed in liver (Emonard & Grimaud, 1990). In our experiments, CPX1 notablely enhanced the liver accumulation of DOX and caused serious hepatotoxicity which weakened the efficacy of the drug. To avoid this, a pegylated PH-responsive alginate was introduced in the system. After the surface of CPX1 was covered with this polymer (Formed CPX2), it could resist the digestion of gelatinase under physiological conditions. The environment intra tumor is acid which could trigger a change of the charge on the polymer from negative to a positive one, which resulted in the dissociation of the polymer form CPX1 and the digestion of CPX1 by gelatinase in the tumor. Because of the pegylation, CPX2 acquired stronger enhanced permeability and retention (EPR) effect that increased the distribution of the drug in tumor than CPX1 and greatly reduced the liver accumulation.

Cardiotoxicity is the main drawback of anthracycline, which restraints more effective application of this drug to liver cancer patients (Ferreira et al., 2008). Myocardial degeneration is the most commonly encountered side-effects of anthracycline (Combs & Acosta, 1990). It can cause serious heart failure and even death (Ferrans, 1978). In our study, CPX2 efficiently reduced the accumulation of DOX in heart, which greatly alleviated the cardiotoxicity of DOX. It completely rescued animals from death caused by high doses of DOX. Additionally, controlled-release and tumor site specifically release of DOX also eased the acute toxicity-induced loss of body weight.

5. Conclusion

In our present study, a PH-/enzyme responsive complex composed by self-assemble of doxorubicin, CpG DNA fragments, cationic gelatin and a PH-sensitive alginate was developed. This complex increased the accumulation of doxorubicin in tumor, reduced its deposition in heart and could specifically release doxorubicin in tumor sites, which resulted in the enhanced anti-cancer activity and decreased cardiotoxicity of doxorubicin. When tested in animal model of implanted tumor, the complex exhibited high effective in preventing the growth of the tumors and dramatically alleviated toxicity compared to free doxorubicin. All results suggest that this easy- manufactured, cost-effective nanoscale formulation of doxorubicin hold great promise to be used to clinical practices.

6. Acknowledgements

This work was supported by National Natural Science Foundation of China (50673041, 30771036 and BK2007144), National Basic Research Foundation of China (973 Program 2006CB503909, 2004CB518603), Key Program for Science and Technology Research from Chinese Ministry of Education (01005), Young Investigator Grant (NCET-04-0466), the Chinese National Programs for High Technology Research and Development (863 Program 2006AA02Z177), China Postdoctoral Science Fundation 200801364 and 20080431077.

7. References

Bigotte, L. (1985). Doxorubicin as a fluorescent nuclear marker in tumors of the human nervous system: a simple and reliable staining technique. *Clinical Neuropathology.* Vol. 4, No.5, (September 1985), pp. 220-6, ISSN 0722-5091

Bodley, A.; Liu, LF. & Israel, M. (1989). DNA topoisomerase II-mediated interaction of doxorubicin and daunorubicin congeners with DNA. *Cancer Research.* Vol. 49, No.21, (October 1989), pp. 5969-78, ISSN 0008-5472

Cheng, X.; Gao, F. & Xiang, J. (2011). Galactosylated alpha,beta-poly[(2-hydroxyethyl)-L-aspartamide]-bound doxorubicin: improved antitumor activity against hepatocellular carcinoma with reduced hepatotoxicity. *Anticancer Drugs.* Vol. 22, No.2, (February 2011), pp. 136-47, ISSN 0959-4973

Combs, AB. & Acosta, D. (1990). Toxic mechanisms of the heart: a review. *Toxicologic Pathology.* Vol. 18, No.4, (January 1990), pp. 583-96, ISSN 0192-6233

Deryugina, EI. & Quigley, JP. (2006). Matrix metalloproteinases and tumor metastasis. *Cancer and Metastasis Reviews.* Vol. 25, No.1, (March 2006), pp. 9-34, ISSN 0167-7659

Dorr, RT.; Shipp, NG. & Lee, KM. (1991). Comparison of cytotoxicity in heart cells and tumor cells exposed to DNA intercalating agents in vitro. *Anticancer Drugs.* Vol. 2, No.1, (February 1991), pp. 27-33, ISSN 0959-4973

Eklund, A. (1976). On the determination of available lysine in casein and rapeseed protein concentrates using 2,4,6-trinitrobenzenesulphonic acid (TNBS) as a reagent for free epsilon amino group of lysine. *Analytical Biochemistry.* Vol. 70, No.2, (February 1976), pp. 434-9, ISSN 0003-2697

Eliyahu, H.; Barenholz, Y. & Domb, AJ. (2005). Polymers for DNA delivery. *Molecules.* Vol. 10, No. 1, (November 2005), pp. 36-64, ISSN 1420-3049

Emonard, H. & Grimaud, JA. (1990). Matrix metalloproteinases. A review. *Cellular and Molecular Biology.* Vol. 36, No. 2, (January 1990), pp. 131-53, ISSN 0415-5680

Ferrans, VJ. (1978). Overview of cardiac pathology in relation to anthracycline cardiotoxicity. *Cancer treatment reports.* Vol. 62, No. 6, (June 1978), pp. 955-61, ISSN 0361-5960

Ferreira, AL.; Matsubara, LS. & Matsubara, BB. (2008). Anthracycline-induced cardiotoxicity. *Cardiovascular and Hematological Agents in Medicinal Chemistry.* Vol. 36, No. 2, (January 2008), pp. 131-53, ISSN 0415-5680

Ganea, E.; Trifan, M. & Laslo, AC. (2007). Matrix metalloproteinases: useful and deleterious. *Biochemical Society Transactions*. Vol. 35, No. Pt4 , (August 2007), pp. 689-91, ISSN 0300-5127

Ganz, WI.; Sridhar, KS. & Forness, TJ. (1993). Detection of early anthracycline cardiotoxicity by monitoring the peak filling rate. *American Journal of Clinical Oncology*. Vol. 16, No.2, (April 1993), pp. 109-12, ISSN 0277-3732

Haley, B. & Frenkel, E. (2008). Nanoparticles for drug delivery in cancer treatment. *Urologic Oncology: Seminars and Original Investigations*. Vol. 26, No.1, (January 2008), pp. 57-64, ISSN 1078-1439

Jemal, A.; Bray, F. & Center MM. (2011). Global cancer statistics. *CA: A Cancer Journal for Clinicians*. Vol.61, No.2, (March 2011), pp. 69-90, ISSN 1542-4863

Jong, J.; Guérand, WS. & Schoofs, PR. Simple and sensitive quantification of anthracyclines in mouse atrial tissue using high-performance liquid chromatography and fluorescence detection. *Journal of Chromatography*. Vol. 570, No.1, (September 1991), pp. 209-16, ISSN 0021-9673

Kushibiki, T.; Tomoshige, R. & Fukunaka, Y. (2003). In vivo release and gene expression of plasmid DNA by hydrogels of gelatin with different cationization extents. *Journal of Controlled Release*. Vol. 90, No.2, (June 2003), pp. 207-16, ISSN 0168-3659

Matsumoto, G.; Kushibiki, T. & Kinoshita, Y. (2006). Cationized gelatin delivery of a plasmid DNA expressing small interference RNA for VEGF inhibits murine squamous cell carcinoma. *Cancer Science*. Vol.97, No.4, (April 2006), pp. 313-21, ISSN 1347-9032

Paik, WK. & Kim, S. (1970). Comparison of the acetylation of proteins and nucleic acids. *Biochemical Journal*. Vol.116, No.4, (February 1970), pp. 611-5, ISSN 0264-6021

Paleos, CM.; Tziveleka, LA. & Sideratou, Z. (2009). Gene delivery using functional dendritic polymers. *Expert Opinion on Drug Delivery*. Vol. 6, No.1, (January 2009), pp. 27-38, ISSN 1742-5247

Tranchant, I.; Thompson, B. & Nicolazzi M. (2004). Physicochemical optimisation of plasmid delivery by cationic lipids. *The Journal of Gene Medicine*. Vol. 6, No.1, (February 2004), pp. S24-35, ISSN 1099-498X

Trouet, A. & Campeneere, DD. (1979a). Daunorubicin-DNA and doxorubicin-DNA. A review of experimental and clinical data. *Cancer Chemotherapy and Pharmacology*. Vol.2, No.1, (January 1979), pp. 77-9, ISSN 0344-5704

Trouet ,A & Sokal, G. (1979b). Clinical studies with daunorubicin-DNA and adriamycin-DNA complexes: a review. *Cancer treatment reports*. Vol.63, No.5, (May 1979), pp. 895-8, ISSN 0361-5960

Viale, PH. & Yamamoto, DS. (2008). Cardiovascular toxicity associated with cancer treatment. *Clinical Journal of Oncology Nursing*. Vol.12, No.4, (August 2008), pp. 627-38, ISSN 1092-1095

Vicent, MJ. (2007). Polymer-drug conjugates as modulators of cellular apoptosis. *The AAPS Journal*. Vol.9, No.2, (October 2007), pp. E200-7, ISSN 1550-7416

Wagner E. (2004). Strategies to improve DNA polyplexes for in vivo gene transfer: will "artificial viruses" be the answer? *Pharmaceutical Research*. Vol.21, No.1, (January 2004), pp. 8-14, ISSN 0724-8741

Yoshikawa, K. & Kitaoka, H. (1971). Prolonged intra-aortic infusion therapy with anti-tumor agents for advanced cancer of the stomach, colon and rectum. *The Japanese Journal of Surgery*. Vol. 1, No.4, (December 1971), pp. 256-62, ISSN 0047-1909